Barry G. Silverman, Ashlesha Jain, Ajita Ichalkaranje, Lakhmi C. Jain (Eds.)

Intelligent Paradigms for Healthcare Enterprises

Studies in Fuzziness and Soft Computing, Volume 184

Editor-in-chief
Prof. Janusz Kacprzyk
Systems Research Institute
Polish Academy of Sciences
ul. Newelska 6
01-447 Warsaw
Poland
E-mail: kacprzyk@ibspan.waw.pl

Further volumes of this series
can be found on our homepage:
springeronline.com

Vol. 169. C.R. Bector, Suresh Chandra
Fuzzy Mathematical Programming and Fuzzy Matrix Games, 2005
ISBN 3-540-23729-1

Vol. 170. Martin Pelikan
Hierarchical Bayesian Optimization Algorithm, 2005
ISBN 3-540-23774-7

Vol. 171. James J. Buckley
Simulating Fuzzy Systems, 2005
ISBN 3-540-24116-7

Vol. 172. Patricia Melin, Oscar Castillo
Hybrid Intelligent Systems for Pattern Recognition Using Soft Computing, 2005
ISBN 3-540-24121-3

Vol. 173. Bogdan Gabrys, Kauko Leiviskä, Jens Strackeljan (Eds.)
Do Smart Adaptive Systems Exist?, 2005
ISBN 3-540-24077-2

Vol. 174. Mircea Negoita, Daniel Neagu, Vasile Palade
Computational Intelligence: Engineering of Hybrid Systems, 2005
ISBN 3-540-23219-2

Vol. 175. Anna Maria Gil-Lafuente
Fuzzy Logic in Financial Analysis, 2005
ISBN 3-540-23213-3

Vol. 176. Udo Seiffert, Lakhmi C. Jain, Patric Schweizer (Eds.)
Bioinformatics Using Computational Intelligence Paradigms, 2005
ISBN 3-540-22901-9

Vol. 177. Lipo Wang (Ed.)
Support Vector Machines: Theory and Applications, 2005
ISBN 3-540-24388-7

Vol. 178. Claude Ghaoui, Mitu Jain, Vivek Bannore, Lakhmi C. Jain (Eds.)
Knowledge-Based Virtual Education, 2005
ISBN 3-540-25045-X

Vol. 179. Mircea Negoita, Bernd Reusch (Eds.)
Real World Applications of Computational Intelligence, 2005
ISBN 3-540-25006-9

Vol. 180. Wesley Chu, Tsau Young Lin (Eds.)
Foundations and Advances in Data Mining, 2005
ISBN 3-540-25057-3

Vol. 181. Nadia Nedjah, Luiza de Macedo Mourelle
Fuzzy Systems Engineering, 2005
ISBN 3-540-25322-X

Vol. 182. John N. Mordeson, Kiran R. Bhutani, Azriel Rosenfeld
Fuzzy Group Theory, 2005
ISBN 3-540-25072-7

Vol. 183. Larry Bull, Tim Kovacs (Eds.)
Foundations of Learning Classifier Systems, 2005
ISBN 3-540-25073-5

Vol. 184. Barry G. Silverman, Ashlesha Jain, Ajita Ichalkaranje, Lakhmi C. Jain (Eds.)
Intelligent Paradigms for Healthcare Enterprises, 2005
ISBN 3-540-22903-5

Barry G. Silverman
Ashlesha Jain
Ajita Ichalkaranje
Lakhmi C. Jain
(Eds.)

Intelligent Paradigms for Healthcare Enterprises

Systems Thinking

Springer

Dr. Barry G. Silverman
Professor of Engineering/ESE & CIS
Wharton/OPIM, and Medicine
Towne Bldg, Rm 251
University of Pennsylvania
Philadelphia, PA 19104-6315
United States of America
E-mail: barryg@seas.upenn.edu

Dr. Ajita Ichalkaranje
Independant Living Centre
Adelaide, South Australia
SA 5086
Australia

Dr. Ashlesha Jain
Queen Elizabeth Hospital
Adelaide, South Australia
SA 5011
Australia

Professor Lakhmi C. Jain
Professor of Knowledge-Based Engineering
University of South Australia
Adelaide, South Australia
SA 5095
Australia
E-mail: lakhmi.jain@unisa.edu.au

ISBN 978-3-642-06175-2 e-ISBN 978-3-540-32362-4

ISSN print edition: 1434-9922
ISSN electronic edition: 1860-0808

Springer is a part of Springer Science+Business Media
springeronline.com

Softcover reprint of the hardcover 1st edition 2005

Foreword

The practice of medicine is information intensive, yet systemic thinking is confined to how the body works rather than how the healthcare system works. So it is refreshing to have the perspectives this book assembles in one place. That is, information systems in medical practices historically have tended to focus on automating individual functions (e.g., billing, procedure or room scheduling, and record keeping). Like other large industries that learned to contain runaway costs, healthcare is now automating more and more of these functions across larger expanses of the enterprise. As this happens, the debate is shifting beyond specific functions and basic transaction processing to ways to interoperate in order to improve performance and reduce errors. As with other more automated sectors, the focus is now turning to how to better engineer the knowledge and information management cycles that exist throughout the healthcare field, and ways to adapt and develop the healthcare enterprise itself. This is where stepping back and taking a systems view becomes important.

What makes the systems approach so challenging is that one must simultaneously shift the institutional focus to patient-centric; use that focus and improve interactions with patient communities; and also seek to improve the internal workflow and knowledge management for doctors, nurses, and other employees. These three perspectives (institution, consumers, and providers) are exactly what this book helps the reader to focus on.

In the International Journal of Medical Informatics that I co-edit, we recently published a vision piece by a group on "Healthcare in the information society. A prognosis for the year 2013," *Int J Med Inf* , 2002 Nov;66(1-3):3-21 (Haux R, Ammenwerth E, Herzog W, Knaup P.). That group identified a number of the topics also found in this book as important goals for the further development of information processing in healthcare.

In that regard the current book is timely. It spans the topics from 'what are virtual online patient communities chatting and thinking about?' to 'what are the ways to improve the knowledge management that providers use when thinking about patient problems?' Likewise it straddles technologic topics from DNA processing and automating medical second opinions in the lab, to telemedicine and chat spaces for rural patient outreach, among many others. In terms of management concerns, this book also explores systems approaches such as automated clinical guidelines, institutional workflow management, and best practices and lessons learned with actual applications.

This compendium under the editorship of B.G. Silverman, A. Jain, A. Ichalkaranje, and L.C. Jain brings together leading researchers in the field, addressing the plethora of issues involved in advanced intelligent paradigms. Barry Silverman is an expert in artificial intelligence, a professor in the School of Engineering, School of Medicine, and Wharton at University of Pennsylvania, and is Director of the Ackoff Center for the Advancement of the Systems Approach. Lakhmi Jain is a Professor of Knowledge-Based Engineering at the University of South Australia.

This work comes at a critical moment of development, as the world goes online and communication between all people is fostered at an ever-increasing rate. Hopefully, healthcare managers and informaticians worldwide will utilize the ideas and practices addressed in this book to help advance the systems approach being used in their own organizations.

Charles Safran, MD, MS
Associate Clinical Professor of Medicine, Harvard Medical School
Chairman, American Medical Informatics Association

Preface

Healthcare organizations need to consider their existence from a systems perspective and transform themselves accordingly. In the systems perspective, three viewpoints are important. Organizations exist as purposeful systems with their own goals and ideals (the control problem). But they contain as parts, individual employees who also are purposeful and have their own needs (the humanization problem). Finally, organizations exist as parts of a larger system and have responsibilities to the interests of those stakeholders as well (the environmentalization problem). It is incumbent upon managers to think through the needs and balance the interests of all three levels, not for some academic goal, but to survive and adapt in a changing world. The managers who can continually anticipate and balance the needs of all three perspectives will find they have organizations that adapt and develop, that survive and flourish, regardless of the turns in the road.

Healthcare is a challenging field with potential for runaway costs and its limiting focus on sickness care only. While there are economic, legal, and social issues yet to be resolved (and outside the scope of this volume), the intelligent paradigms explored in this book raise the prospects of future healthcare enterprises repositioned to effectively tackle each of the three systems levels: (1) Chapters One and Three explore control issues and how enterprise-wide knowledge and workflow management help managers to resolve them; (2) Chapters Two, Six, and Seven turn to the humanization issues, particularly as concerns the 'knowledge worker' and how to more deeply understand their thought processes and support system needs in order to free them and help them work more effectively; and (3) Chapters Four, Five, and Eight focus our attention on environmentalization issues and a sea change in shifting from institution-centric to consumer-centric approaches including removal of limits of time, distance, and computer interface, respectively.

For the healthcare manager, this book can be read as an overview of strategic investments that might payoff for the enterprise. For the informatician, this book can be read at a more detailed level. The chapters are filled with meat about how to implement each of these paradigm shifts and lessons learned in actual efforts to date. Specifically, the reader will get ideas for efficiency enhancements (by lowering costs, effort, duplication, etc.); for improving effectiveness and quality of care (via best practice guidelines, latest evidence-based ideas, and more patient-centric service); and for increasing patient safety (reduce errors, improve treatment, tighten workflows). Many of the chapters touch on different aspects of these common concerns.

Over the past decade there has been much discussion about the "knowledge economy," knowledge workers, knowing organizations, and the knowledge transformation cycle. Certainly, this discussion is germane to the field of healthcare where knowledge is highly specialized, hundreds of specialties exist, and the half-life of knowledge in any specialty is relatively short. In the best evidence-based traditions, clinical trials continually push new knowledge out to the practitioners, and keeping up with the latest evidence is a daily challenge for these practitioners. One of the best proposals to assisting practitioners with knowledge management issues is via the adoption of clinical practice guidelines. As Gersende Georg in Chapter One points out, well-maintained guidelines offer a way to help practitioners keep up to date with the latest knowledge and evidence based approaches. They also provide a way for medical enterprises to assure all practitioners are applying a consistent standard of care. Lastly, they can provide dramatic cost savings by shifting patient care from strictly a reactive sickness-orientation, to a more preventive as well as chronic disease management approach. Healthcare, at the end of the day, should be about wellness care and not just sickness. This latter use of guidelines introduces a systems thinking approach into practice, and may be the best weapon health enterprises have to reducing errors and improving performance by keeping consumers out of the system to begin with. Georg goes on to point out that these many promising benefits come with an often overlooked cost – that of guideline knowledge management so they remain useful to and usable by the practitioners. Georg offers many useful approaches to those who would seek to implement clinical guideline practices in their organization.

Given that Practitioners are being asked to apply latest know-how and guidelines generated elsewhere, one is tempted to conclude that the science of medicine lies in the research and tertiary care centers. However, Pantzi, Arocha, and Moehr remind us in Chapter Two, that general practitioners are better thought of as applied scientists, conducting new studies on each patient who comes under their care. The authors are interested in how such individuals use their own reasoning when processing clinical knowledge and patient information. They examine 'case based reasoning' as the best fit intelligent paradigm for modeling the general practitioner. Case based reasoning is a well known paradigm in the intelligent systems field, and many argue that it mimics how humans actually reason by reusing and adapting solutions to past problems or cases that appear similar to the current one. As Pantzi, Arocha, and Moehr point out research on the case based reasoning paradigm holds many of the keys to improving diagnostic practice, patient care, and training of new practitioners. In their thoughtful chapter, they take the reader on a survey of what is known today and where are the challenges and further research needs in order to fully realize the potential practice and training benefits of better models of the practitioner's knowledge processing. This is, of course, part of the 'humanization problem'.

Good systems thinkers are never happy just with a better model of a part of the larger system, but always seek to improve their models and understanding of how the parts inter-relate and contribute to the operating of larger holisms. Davis and Blanco, in Chapter Three, challenge the reader to think about the bigger picture of workflow throughout the clinic and healthcare enterprise. For well over a decade, most successful enterprises in other industries have pursued workflow management as a best practice -- studying organizational performance, modeling workflows, and reengineering the enterprise to improve and automate workflow management. This is the very essence of how companies like Walmart and Dell have risen to the top of their respective industries. In healthcare, however, one can count on one's hands the number of organizations that appreciate the value of these system control practices and fewer still that actually have begun to implement better workflow paradigms and related intelligent technologies (IT) that help with implementation, and the attending performance boost, error reduction, and improvement in the bottom line. Davis and Blanco help the reader to understand why the healthcare industry is so far behind in adopting such a well understood best-practice, the challenges to moving forward, and state of the art methodologies and approaches that can help out. Although 'agent-oriented' modeling may sound exotic, Chapter Three offers a pragmatic look that helps the reader see concrete steps needed, the effort required, and real healthcare enterprise workflow cases with lessons learned.

Organizations are socio-technical entities that might best be thought of as organisms. Legally, they are treated as such, and we often talk about organizational growth, decay, and evolution, as if they are living entities. It is a truism that organizations must constantly evolve and develop if they are to stay healthy, to compete in a dynamic world, and to continually adapt to new complexities and realities. Many healthcare enterprises appreciate this and, in the US over the past decade, one can't help but observe the restructuring of the industry that occurred with isolated clinics becoming the anomaly and regional healthcare management enterprises purchasing these 'feeder' clinics and linking them with tertiary care centers. Part of that initiative was fueled by the attempt to reduce redundant assets (beds, imaging devices, surgical units, etc.), part of it was to achieve economies to scale, and part of it was to improve practice at the point of care across the region. This is but one of many possible forms that the healthcare enterprises might evolve to. In the age of the information superhighway, it is inevitable that healthcare enterprises will also experiment with bricks-and-clicks approaches much as other retail industries have done in the effort to improve their performance and their responsiveness to consumer needs. Chapters Four and Five examine some of the potential for this virtual organizational design space, the technologies that make it possible, and the social issues that variously are solved and/or arise and must be thought about.

Specifically, in Chapter Four, Demiris explores the many kinds of 'virtual communities' in healthcare – everything from virtual care-giver teams, to patient-provider collaborations, to self-help consumer groups. As healthcare enterprises rethink their delivery modes and begin to consider how to support virtual communities, a host of issues arise as reviewed by Demiris, not the least of which are security and privacy, identity and deception, provider and patient empowerment, self-reporting, sociability and usability, and ethical concerns, among others. As the chapter points out, virtual communities are increasing and the pressure is on healthcare enterprises to explore them in their quest to find new paradigms that improve performance and enhance responsiveness and care, without compromising patient safety. The paradigm shift from institution-centric to patient- and consumer-centric is a large jump, however, and Demiris cautions that significant ongoing research and monitoring of the "soft side" or human factors issues will be essential.

Chapter Five vividly illustrates how the quest to continually adapt the organization and provide care to new categories of consumers might run afoul of conventional wisdom for how best to operate the rest of the enterprise. That is, as in Chapter One, best practices advocate that organizations adopt clinical practice guidelines that help practitioners to follow the latest evidence based medicine and that ensure a consistent standard of care. Yet, telemedicine extends the reach of the healthcare enterprise to rural regions, less developed nations, and remote platforms (ships, spacecraft, oil rigs, etc.). In these domains, as Anogianakis, Klisarova, Papaliagkas, and Anogianakis point out; it may be sub-optimal to apply the same standards of care given constraints on the locally available drugs, treatments prospects, and care customs. This is an authoritative review for anyone interested in implementing telemedicine and a good example of how complex adaptive systems often need to decentralize decision making and permit what appear to be local optima in order to enhance overall system performance.

Chapter Six explores internal clinical decision support systems that might be harnessed in the effort to improve patient safety and care. Specifically, the clinical decision support systems reviewed in Chapter Six, focusing on the case of breast cancer and mammography, include the latest paradigms for how to manage computer-generated 'second opinions'. The origins of the field of artificial intelligence are intimately connected to medicine, and most of the early knowledge-based expert systems breakthrough of the 1970s and 1980s were initially made with medical diagnostic aids. However, clinical decision aids were not able to transition into useful practice, and an "intelligent system winter" resulted in the field of healthcare, even as these intelligent system paradigms paradoxically flourished and made great performance gains for other sectors of the economy. Tourassi in Chapter Six provides insights about this paradox -- the early intelligent aids in medicine were trying to solve the wrong problems with difficult-to-maintain knowledge and hard-to-use interfaces. That era should be past us now and healthcare needs to make the same gains with clinical decision support systems that other sectors have already realized. However, as Tourassi points out, old resistances can prove stubborn and this chapter provides a number of cautionary insights for those trying to alter the state of the practice with computer generated second opinions.

One of the largest recent breakthroughs of biomedical science was the successful mapping of the human genome. Yet this mapping is only the beginning of a new era. To harness the potential clinically, one needs to be able to diagnose disorders and recommend therapies at the level of DNA and gene expression. In Chapter Seven, Fukuoka, Inaoka, and Kohane review how DNA microarrays can be harnessed for this purpose in order to identify genes whose expression is highly differentiating with respect to disease conditions. After explaining some of the fundamentals, they survey applications of DNA microarrays to medical diagnosis and prognosis. To date, most of the success has come from studying certain types of cancer tumors. This is due to the ease of comparing a tumor cell to nearby healthy tissue. In other diseases, the diagnosis might involve multiple organs and tissues, and hence a simple comparative process is obviated. Headway is thus slower, though progress is occurring there as well. Major breakthroughs can be expected when and if automated datamining techniques mature for handling and interpreting microarray expressions. This is an important chapter for those interested in mapping their way to the future of healthcare informatics.

Every intelligent paradigm in this book holds the potential for a sea-change to arise in the healthcare enterprise. We have looked into ways to better manage knowledge (guidelines, case based reasoning) to organizational streamlining (workflow, virtual communities) to changing to a customer-centric model (virtual communities, telemedicine) to automating the clinical diagnosis and prognosis processes (mammography, DNA microarrays). It is fitting to end this book with a look at yet one more paradigm shift that healthcare could harness to improve the quality of care and to redesign itself yet again. Specifically, Glaris and Fotiadis in Chapter Eight focus on the paradigm shift connected with ubiquitous computing and wearable devices. While virtual communities, the Internet, decision support, and telemedicine are largely about immersing oneself into cyberspace, ubiquitous computing is the opposite. It is about making the computer invisible – how to get it to blend into the woodwork, the clothing we wear, and the everyday artifacts we use in our daily routines. Ubiquitous devices reviewed here can be broadly categorised according to their primary function into monitoring systems, rehabilitation assistance devices and long-term medical aids. Glaris and Fotiadis explore the thrust of such devices to further the consumer-centric shift and to help with preventive care and overall disease management. They close with a review of number of logistical, financial, and human factors that limit the adoption and spread of this approach and of what must happen to reduce those limits.

This book is a result of significant contributions made by the authors and the reviewers in this evolving area of research. We are grateful to Feng-Hsing Wang for his contribution during the evolution phase of this book.

Contents

1. Computerization of Clinical Guidelines: an Application of Medical Document Processing

Gersende Georg

SPIM ; Inserm ERM 202, 15 rue de l'École de Médecine, F-75006 Paris, France

1.1 Introduction: Clinical Guidelines as Normalized Documents

Clinical Guidelines are being developed as a tool to promote Best Practice in Medicine. They are usually defined as "systematically developed statements to assist practitioner and patient decisions about appropriate Healthcare for specific clinical circumstances" *(Institute of Medicine, 1990)*. The Institute's Committee on Practice Guidelines further clarified this definition by specifying *appropriate care* as: "the expected health benefit exceeds the expected negative consequences by a sufficient margin that the care is worth providing".

Clinical Guidelines bridge the gap between clinical science and practice. Their first concern is the growing awareness of large variations in clinical practice [1]. The second is the fact that Health professionals have difficulties in keeping up-to-date with the overwhelming volume of new scientific evidence for good clinical practice [2]. Another problem is the growing cost of Health services which prompts the need for Best Practice. A study conducted by the Juran Institute concluded that 30% of Health costs could be reduced and outcomes improved if quality issues were addressed [3]. As a result, Clinical Guidelines are touted as vehicles for improving the quality of Healthcare as well as decreasing costs.

Clinical Guidelines are also poised to play an important role in the diffusion and standardization of medical knowledge, as they rely on recent concepts of *Evidence-Based Medicine*. David Sackett defined *Evidence-Based Medicine* as "the conscientious, explicit and judicious use of current best evidence in making decisions about the care or individual patients. The practice of *Evidence-Based Medicine* means integrating individual clinical expertise with the best available clinical evidence from systematic research" [4]. However, we should emphasize that *Evidence-Based Medicine* is in no way downgrading medical standards to reduce costs. Indeed, in many cases, Clinical Guidelines incorporate the most current knowledge about Best Practice.

Recent studies have suggested that the diffusion of paper Guidelines only had a limited impact. Previous research on Clinical Guidelines concluded that their use was not widespread [5]. Many reasons have been put forward to account for this situation, among them the difficulty to use Clinical Guidelines (38% of respondents) [6]. Medin and Ross [7] hypothesize that this is due to the detailed processing required for written texts. However, another hypothesis invokes disagreements on the recommendations which may arise from the focus of the Guideline (*e.g.* the kind

G. Georg: *Computerization of Clinical Guidelines: an Application of Medical Document Processing*, StudFuzz **184**, 1–30 (2005)
www.springerlink.com

of patients for whom the Guideline is intended may differ from the actual patient under consideration [8]).

This is why, the same studies have demonstrated that the inclusion of Clinical Guidelines within Decision Support Systems (DSS) has a significant potential to improve compliance of Health professionals. Several studies have proposed to evaluate the impact of DSS. One of them systematically reviewed feedback directed to Healthcare providers or patients [9]. It concluded that reminders are more effective than feedback in modifying physician behavior. Patient-directed reminders can improve medication adherence as well. In a similar fashion, Lobach and Hammond [10] showed that DSS based on Clinical Guidelines are an effective tool for assisting clinicians in the management of diabetic patients. The effect of computer-generated advice on clinician behavior was measured through the rate of compliance with Guideline recommendations. Compliance for the group receiving recommendations was 32.0% versus 15.6% for the control group. As a result, the use of DSS based on Clinical Guidelines may improve the quality of medical care.

1.2 The Authoring of Clinical Guidelines

Computerization of Clinical Guidelines is a major challenge for their successful dissemination. Because of their textual nature and their relation to standardized medical knowledge, their computerization involves many different fields of Health Informatics, from document processing to knowledge-based systems. In this chapter, we discuss the computerization of Clinical Guidelines through the various aspects of their life cycle, from production to consultation and use (Figure 1).

1.2.1 Problems Encountered with Clinical Guidelines Authoring

Some studies have noticed the lack of a standard structure in the publication of text-based Clinical Guidelines. Indeed, Clinical Guidelines were being "produced and disseminated by a variety of government and professional organizations and because these Guidelines are largely in narrative-form, they are sometimes ambiguous and generally lack the structure and internal consistency that would allow execution by computer" [11]. This is why several studies are focusing on authoring and standardization of Clinical Guidelines through their computerization. Recently, Shiffman et al. [12] concluded that one major factor affecting the quality of Clinical Guidelines is the fact that Guideline development panels are commonly composed of people who are inexperienced in Guideline authoring. This important point explains some of the standardization problems encountered. On the other hand, Guideline production could be "intentionally ambiguous to satisfy a consensus process used to create it, or the Guideline may lack coverage (incomplete cases) or appear to be contradictory" [13].

Clinical Guidelines may be complex, and often composed of elaborate collections of procedures containing logical gaps or contradictions that can generate ambiguity. Many Clinical Guidelines also suffer from a complex structure, involving the nesting of procedures or complicated temporal or causal relations. An understanding of the semantics of Clinical Guidelines and of their potential interpretation by physicians may improve this, and ultimately the usability of Clinical Guidelines [8].

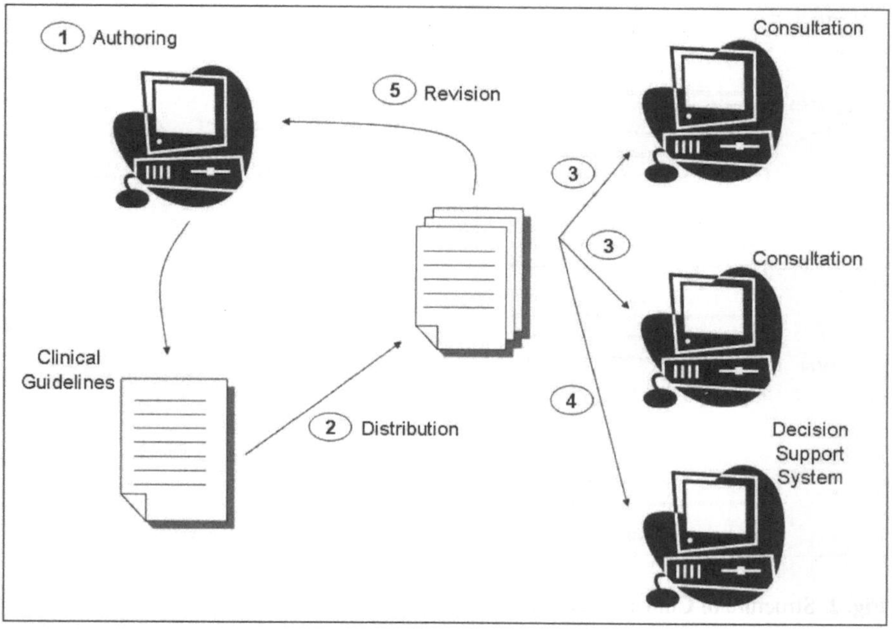

Fig. 1. The life cycle of Clinical Guidelines.

1.2.2 Clinical Guidelines' Structure

Clinical Guidelines focus on the management of specific diseases, such as diabetes or hypertension and are typically presented in textual and algorithmic forms. We can observe separate chapters for the different steps in disease management, for example diagnosis and therapeutic strategy (Figure 2).

Textual Guidelines consist of the description of a procedure, usually based on scientific evidence from clinical studies. To complement written Guidelines, algorithms (Figure 2) are often integrated into Clinical Guidelines that describe therapeutic or diagnostic procedures. Algorithmic representations organize all of the relevant information into a directly applicable form, and therefore may aid decision-making [14].

Clinical Guidelines can be characterized by their specific structure and their specific knowledge content. Their logical form has inspired much research in document processing, while their knowledge content has served as a starting point for experiments with knowledge-based systems. There is no standardized language in which to encode the elements of a Clinical Guideline in a consistent way which would support its computerization. Indeed, as traditional forms of Clinical Guidelines may not make it immediately clear how to apply the Guideline [11], research into their structure is a precondition to their computerization.

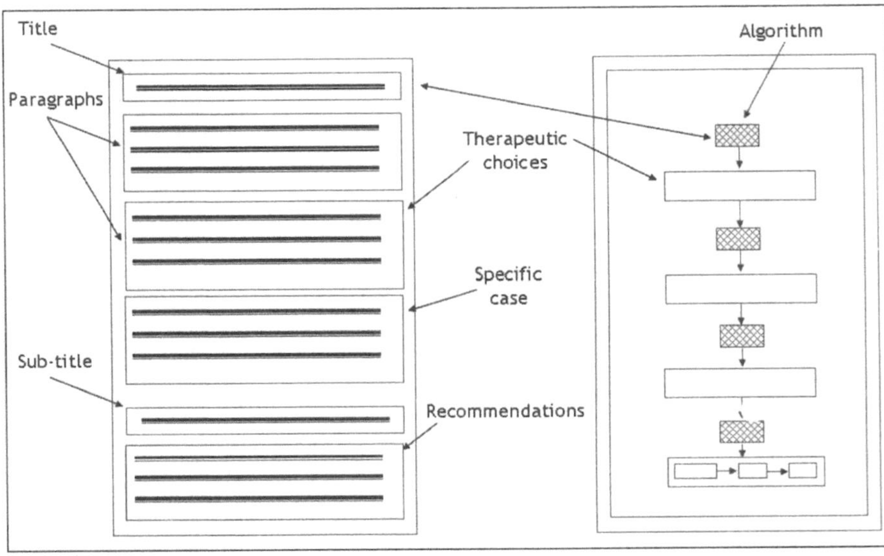

Fig. 2. Structure of Clinical Guidelines.

In this context, we present state-of-the-art research in document management techniques applied to Clinical Guidelines, and report recent results from our own work in the computerization of the Guideline production workflow.

The knowledge content of Clinical Guidelines can be characterized by two major dimensions. One consists in the representation of medical decision processes (for instance, the therapeutic strategy) and the other in the attempt at disseminating standardized clinical knowledge. Several authors have proposed knowledge representations for the decision process contained in Clinical Guidelines. For instance, the Guideline Interchange Format (GLIF) represents the decision processes as flowcharts [15], while the PRO*forma* model [16] enhances Guidelines' contents with task-based formalisms representing the decision processes as task models, while the GUIDE system [17] formalizes the decision process using Petri nets. Others researchers have proposed to relate the contents of Clinical Guidelines to Medical Logic Modules (MLM) embedding the standardized knowledge they convey [18].

1.3 Knowledge Representation of Clinical Guidelines

Several authors have proposed knowledge representations for the decision process contained in Clinical Guidelines. To highlight commonalities and differences between these approaches, we present them through a common example based on Chronic Cough management Guidelines, presented in a recent study [19]. This extract contains three recommendations:

(i) "Chronic cough is cough that lasts for at least 3 weeks."
(ii) "Chest radiographs should be ordered before any treatment is prescribed in nearly all patients with chronic cough (Grade II-2)."
(iii) "Chest radiographs do not have to be routinely obtained before beginning treatment, for presumed PNDS (post nasal drip syndrome) in young nonsmokers, in pregnant women, or before observing the result of discontinuation of an ACE-I (ACE Inhibitor) for 4 weeks for patients who developed cough shortly after beginning to take an ACE-I."

1.3.1 The Guideline Interchange Format (GLIF)

The GLIF formalism has been collaboratively developed by groups at Columbia, Stanford, and Harvard universities (working together as the InterMed Collaboratory). The main interest of GLIF derives from the importance of sharing Guidelines among different institutions and software systems. This model behaves as a meta-model for describing and representing the components of Clinical Guidelines.

1.3.1.1 Flowcharts' Customization and the Description of Decision Processes

The first version of GLIF [15] was published in 1998. GLIF supported Guideline modeling as a flowchart with a specific syntax. To tackle the complexity of Clinical Guidelines, the flowchart is extended to enable the specification of a Clinical Guideline as temporally ordered steps. The "Conditional Step" is the equivalent of the "if" part of the rule-based "if … then" structure. The "Action Step" is the equivalent of the "then" part of an "if … then" statement.

Concurrency was modeled using "Branch Steps" which specify multiple steps that can happen concurrently, and "Synchronization Steps" which synchronize the execution of the multiple branches.

1.3.1.2 Limitations of the GLIF Approach

Some GLIF studies [11] have found that the process of structuring Clinical Guidelines information into GLIF requires that users have extensive coding abilities (Figure 3). Without this, programmers often experience difficulties which result in substantial variability when encoding Clinical Guidelines into the GLIF format [11]. As a result, users require significant time to learn the GLIF language. Furthermore, studies have also found that by encoding a Clinical Guideline with GLIF, the original integrity of the text-based Guideline can sometimes be lost [20].

A non-exhaustive list of shortcomings may be raised: (i) GLIF does not specify how to structure important attributes of Clinical Guidelines steps; (ii) the integration with heterogeneous clinical systems is difficult; (iii) its semantics is a mixture of concurrency and decision making; and (iv) important concepts are lacking, for example those for describing iteration, patient-state, exception conditions, and events.

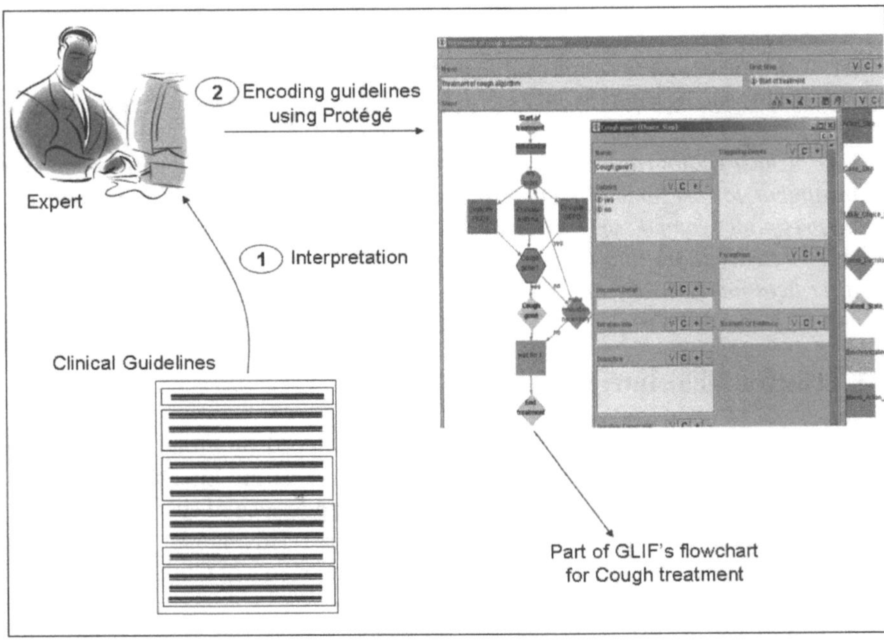

Fig. 3. Knowledge extraction from Clinical Guidelines using Protégé.

To tackle these problems, the latest release GLIF3 augments the GLIF2 specification to support versioning of GLIF-encoded Clinical Guidelines [21]. This is why three levels have been proposed to encode Clinical Guidelines with GLIF [22]: (1) The conceptual flowchart; (2) The computable specification (which is automatically checked for consistency); and (3) the implementable specification.

1.3.1.3 The Latest Release of GLIF: GLIF3

The Conceptual Flowchart

Flowcharts initially described in GLIF have been augmented using Unified Modeling Language (UML) class diagrams. This supports nesting mechanisms for representing complex Clinical Guidelines through iterative specification of Clinical Guidelines (for instance, through the nesting of Sub-Guidelines in action and decision steps). This provides a flexible decision model through a hierarchy of decision step classes (Figure 4).

For instance, using our standard example, Chronic Cough, which is shown in Figure 5 as an action step, can be expanded by zooming, through the nesting mechanism, to show its details in the form of yet another flowchart diagram. This decision hierarchy distinguishes between decision steps that can be automated (*case steps*) and those that have to be further specified by a physician (*choice steps*).

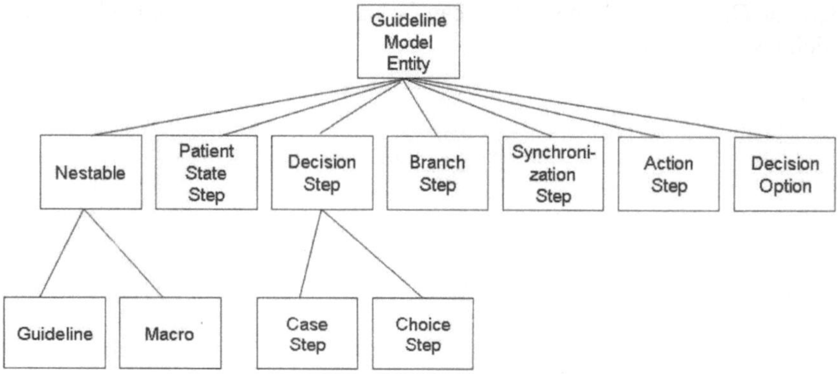

Fig. 4. Overview of the main classes in GLIF version 3.

The action specification model has been extended to include two types of actions: (1) Guideline-flow-relevant actions, such as invoking a Sub-Guideline, or computing values for clinical parameters; and (2) clinically relevant actions, such as issuing recommendations. Clinically relevant actions relate to the domain ontology such as prescriptions, laboratory tests, or referrals.

Finally, the branching and synchronization steps have been modified to remove redundancy in descriptions of parallel pathways in the Guideline flowchart.

Extending the Flowchart Representation

New representational features have been developed such as (i) describing *Iterations* and *Conditions* that control the iteration flow; (ii) describing *Events* and the triggering of actions by these events; (iii) describing *Exceptions* in Guidelines flow and associated exception-handling mechanisms; (iv) representing *Patient-State* as another Guideline step (a node in the flowchart). In this way, a *Patient-State Step* serves as an entry point into the Guideline.

The Computable Specification

The computable level stands between the abstract flowchart level (supported by GLIF2) and the implementation level (currently partially supported by GLIF3). The aim of the abstract flowchart level is to help authors and users visualize and understand the structure of Clinical Guidelines.

The Implementable Specification
A formal syntax for specifying expressions and criteria has been added to the model. It is based on a superset of the Arden Syntax logic grammar [22], and adds new operators such as "is a", "overlaps", "xor", "from now", "is unknown", and "at least *k* of …". This enables to describe a MLM (cf. section 'Arden Syntax') using a pattern of GLIF components which can be used to map GLIF encoded Clinical Guidelines into MLM.

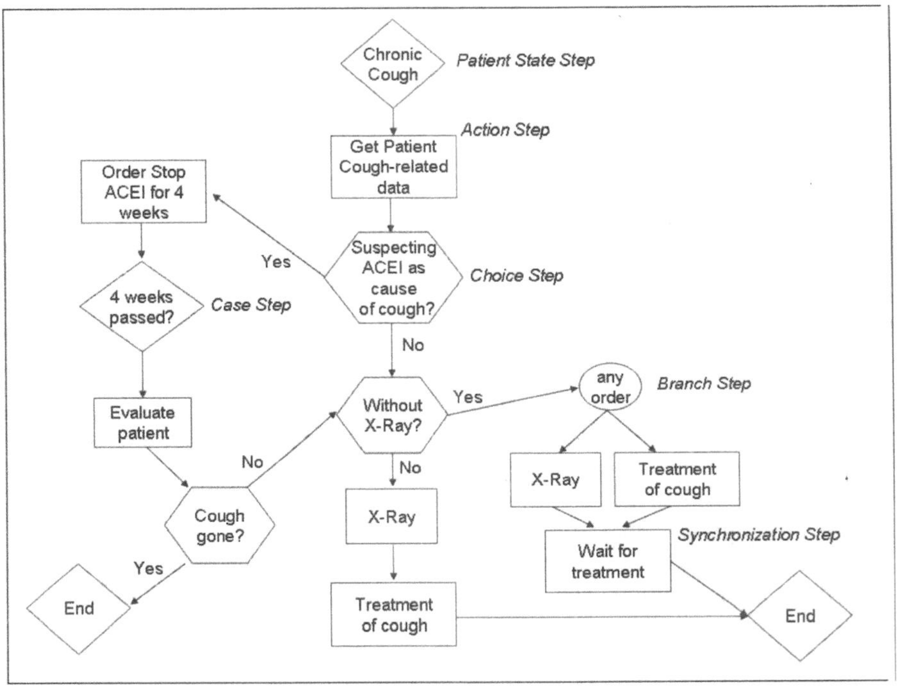

Fig. 5. Conceptual flowchart specification for part of the Chronic Cough Guideline.

GLIF3 is also based on a domain ontology that normalizes terms encoding. However, work on domain ontology in GLIF3 is still in progress. The proposed ontology is based on three layers. The *Core Layer* provides a standard interface to all medical data and concepts that may be represented and referenced by GLIF. The *Reference Information Model (RIM) Layer* provides a semantic hierarchy for medical concepts, and allows attribute specification for each class of medical data. The *Medical Knowledge Layer* contains a term dictionary (*e.g.*, UMLS) and can provide access to medical knowledge bases.

1.3.1.4 Current Research

Future versions of GLIF will explore structured representations for (1) specifying the various goals of each Guideline step, (2) incorporating probabilistic models for decision-making, and (3) incorporating patient preferences in each decision step.

Software tools are currently being developed for authoring, verifying, viewing, distributing, and executing Guidelines. The GLIF3's promoters are currently producing several examples Clinical Guidelines, described at these three levels, in order to evaluate GLIF3.

As a conclusion, this new version of GLIF combines the strengths of several knowledge representations, such as MLM, UML class diagram and ontologies. Standardization of Clinical Guidelines control-flow by HL7 also draws upon the GLIF model of linked Guideline steps. InterMed members are active participants of the HL7 Clinical Guidelines Special Interest Group and the Clinical Decision Support Technical Committee, thus contributing to the process of standardization of a shareable Guideline modeling language, which draws upon experiences from the GLIF project.

1.3.2 PRO*forma*

PRO*forma* is a formal knowledge representation language supported by acquisition and execution tools with the goal of supporting Guideline dissemination in the form of expert systems that assist patient care through active decision support and workflow management [16]. PRO*forma* was developed at the Advanced Computation Laboratory of Cancer Research, UK. The name PRO*forma* is a concatenation of the terms *proxy* ('authorized to act for another') and *formalize* ('give definite form to').

1.3.2.1 The Domino Autonomous Agent Model for Clinical Guidelines

PRO*forma* is an agent language which has developed out of research in logic-based decision making, workflow agents and process modeling [23]. The PRO*forma* model is based on the Domino autonomous agent model and includes several components such as: goals, situations (patient data), actions (clinical orders), candidate solutions, decisions (diagnosis, treatment), and plans (treatment and care plans).

PRO*forma* is based on predicate calculus augmented by non-standard logics. It has also a well-structured syntax, defined in a BNF-equivalent normal form for which applications can be developed using ordinary text editors and compilers. As a consequence, it combines logic programming and object-oriented modeling and is formally grounded in the R^2L language which extends the standard syntax and semantics of Prolog with agent-like capabilities, including decisions, plans and actions, temporal reasoning, and constraints.

1.3.2.2 Encoding Clinical Guidelines in PRO*forma*

Like the GLIF model, PRO*forma* represents Guidelines as a directed graph in which the nodes are instances of a closed set of classes, called the PRO*forma* task ontology. Each Guideline in PRO*forma* is modeled as a plan consisting of a sequence of tasks.

The PRO*forma* task model (Figure 6) divides from the generic task (keystone) into four types: action, plan, decision, and enquiry. "Action" is a procedure to be carried out. This procedure may include presenting information or instructions to the user, sending email reminders, or calling other computer programs. "Plan" is the basic building block of Clinical Guidelines and may contain any number of tasks of any type, including other plans.

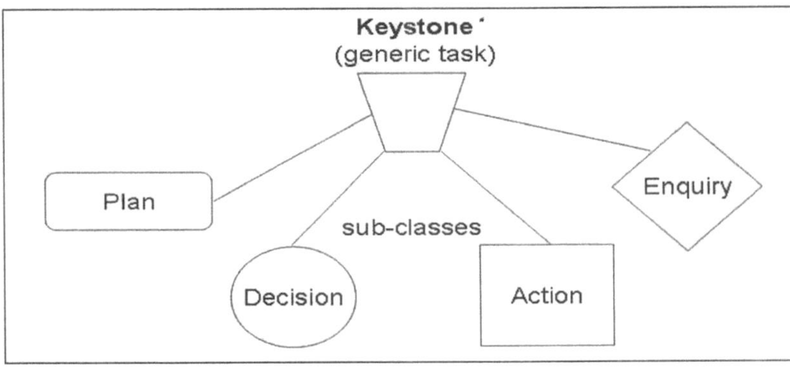

Fig. 6. Overall view of the PRO*forma* model.

"Decision" is a task presenting an option, *e.g.* whether to treat a patient or carry out further investigations, and "Enquiry" is a request for further information or data, required before proceeding with the application of the Clinical Guideline. All tasks share attributes describing goals, control flow, preconditions, and post-conditions. The simple task ontology should make it easier to demonstrate soundness and to teach the language to encoders.

1.3.2.3 The Graphical Editor "Arezzo"

The development environment for the Domino model consists of a graphical editor supporting the authoring process. An engine has also been developed to execute the Clinical Guideline specification as shown in Figure 7.

The "Composer" is used to create Guidelines, protocols and care pathways. The editor supports the construction of Clinical Guidelines in terms of the four task types described above. In the editor, logical and temporal relationships between tasks are captured naturally by linking them as required with arrows. Any procedural and medical knowledge required by the Guideline as a whole (or by an individual task) is entered using templates attached to each task. For each task, a current task state is defined, for example *Dormant* means that the task has not yet been started; *Requested* when an "Enquiry" task is activated and data values are sought for source data items. This is the default state for all tasks before the Guideline is started. All tasks and data items have attributes that define their properties and determine the behavior of the Guideline during enactment by the Arezzo Performer engine. The resulting instantiated graphical structure, as shown in Figure 8, is automatically converted into a database ready for execution.

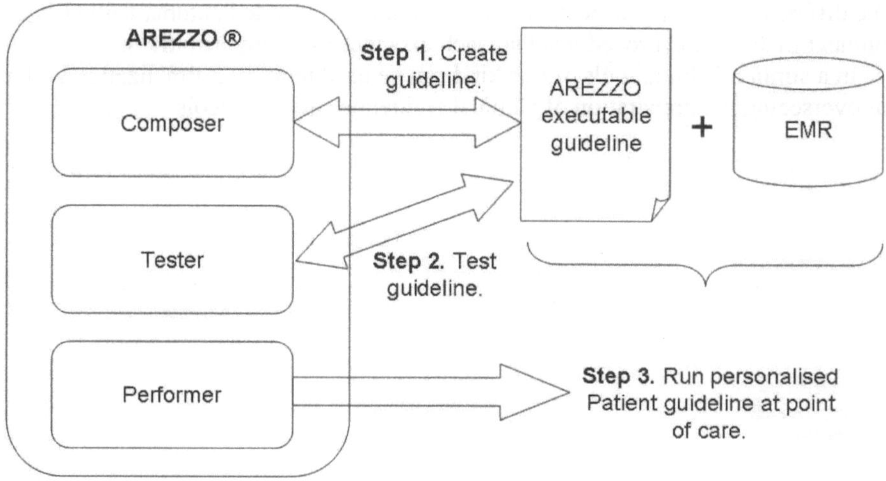

Fig. 7. Overview of Arezzo[1].

As an example, the top-level Cough Guideline is shown on the top left of Figure 8. The two inserts show nesting of the two plans of the top-level Guideline. The "Enquiry" task *(Initial assessment)* might request data about a patient's clinical signs. After this information is received, the "Action" *(Guideline is not appropriate)* or the "Plan" task *(CRX and initial treatment)* are handled. If the Clinical Guideline is appropriate, the "Plan" task is processed and the "Decision" task processes the data values.

Depending on which option the user chooses, the Guideline presents the appropriate "Action" task: *CRX first* or *CRX in parallel*. The scheduling constraint in the top-level Guideline states explains why the component *Investigations* will not be executed until the component *CRX and initial treatment* has been completed.

After the creation of the Guideline with the "Composer", the "Tester" (Figure 7) is used to test the Guideline logic before deployment. The engine can also be used as a tester during the application development phase. The "Performer" inference engine can then run the Guideline when making clinical decisions about a patient. This module also allows Guidelines to be embedded in existing Healthcare systems, linking seamlessly with local Electronic Medical Records and other applications to provide patient-specific assistance at the point of care.

As a conclusion, PRO*forma* offers a declarative interchange format for describing Clinical Guidelines together with a knowledge acquisition methodology and a tool set to simplify the composition and formal verification of applications.

PRO*forma* is the only approach which makes a distinction between a declarative language (*e.g.*, R^2L), used during the Guideline acquisition phase and a procedural language (*e.g.*, L_{R^2L}) that is processed by a general interpreter in an execution engine [23]. All other approaches require a custom-developed execution engine, in which

[1] http://www.infermed.com/arezzo/arezzo-components

the different procedural aspects of the Guideline are encoded automatically (*e.g.*, a number of Java or C procedures that each executes a certain primitive).

In a similar fashion, tools of this kind can be used to assist normalization bodies in overseeing the preparation of Clinical Guidelines and protocols.

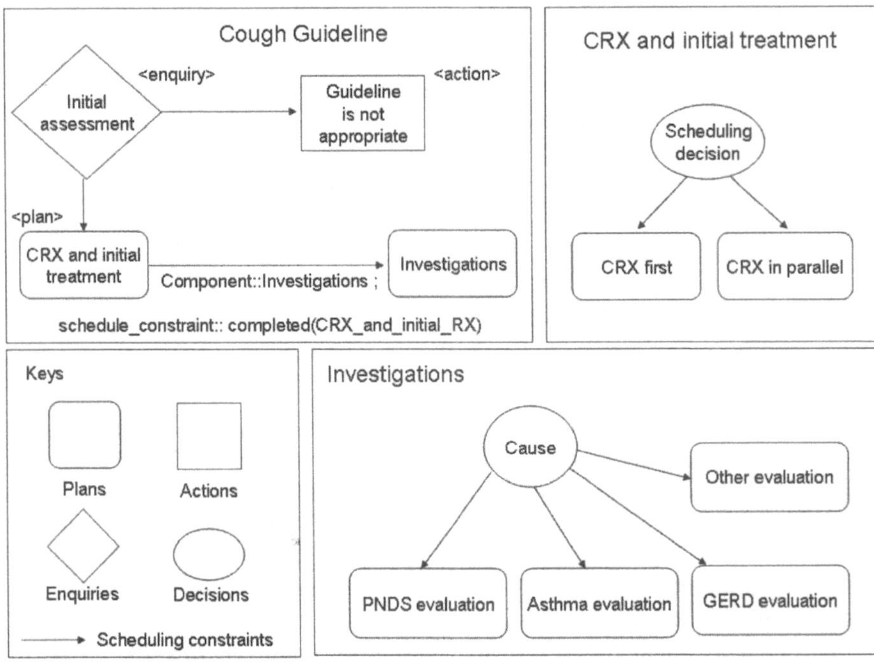

Fig. 8. Visualization of the Cough Guideline using Arezzo.

1.3.3 GUIDE

GUIDE is part of a Guideline modeling and execution framework being developed at the University of Pavia [17]. GUIDE aims to provide an integrated medical knowledge management infrastructure through a workflow called *careflow*.

1.3.3.1 Petri Nets for Representing Clinical Guidelines

GUIDE is based on Petri nets, a traditional formalism for modeling concurrent processes. The strength of the formalism, when applied to Healthcare, is its ability to support the modeling of complex concurrent processes (sequential, parallel and iterative logic flows) which are often part of Clinical Guidelines (see above).

In GUIDE, Petri nets have been extended to support the modeling of time, data and hierarchies. Clinical Guidelines could be represented directly through a Petri net, using a graphical editor which enables non-expert users to build a Petri net

(Figure 9). Considering the same example Clinical Guideline (Cough management) we can observe that it consists of a succession of ordered steps. Each step is triggered whenever the previous step is validated, and parallel or simultaneous steps can be represented corresponding to the temporal aspects of Clinical Guidelines. Petri net's computational properties have been largely used for workflow simulation, hence their use for simulating patients' management.

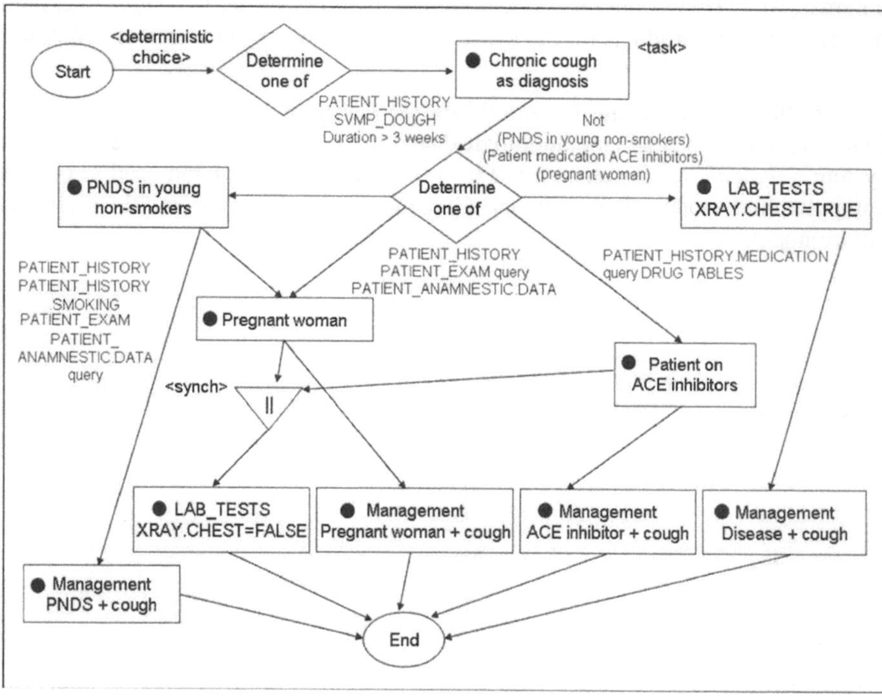

Fig. 9. The top-level GUIDE model of the Cough Guideline.

1.3.3.2 GUIDE's Workflow: the *Careflow* Approach

GUIDE is integrated into a workflow management system which is "a system that completely defines, manages, and executes workflow processes through execution of software whose order of execution is driven by a computer representation of the workflow process logic". It fully implements a Clinical Guideline and controls both its execution and outcome. The Workflow Management Coalition defines a workflow as: "The automation of a business process, in a whole or part, during which documents, information or tasks are passed from one participant to another for action, according to a set of procedural rules".

This definition can be transferred to the case of Clinical Guidelines. The promoters of GUIDE have coined the term *careflow* to refer to the workflow in the context of patient care. Quaglini et al. [17] have proposed a methodology for integrating knowledge representation tools with commercial workflow tools. The commercial tools are Income™ and Oracle Workflow™, used for *careflow* model simulation and *careflow* implementation, respectively.

GUIDE is thus an intermediate step, oriented towards medical experts, by means of which Clinical Guidelines may be formalized. From the Petri net objects, a translation into the Workflow Process Definition Language (WPDL which is the language recommended by the Workflow Management Coalition) is obtained automatically. They adopt this standard representation in order to be able to exploit different existing products for the subsequent phases of *careflow* implementation.

1.3.3.3 Clinical Guidelines Encoded into the *Careflow*

Figure 10 shows the main methodological steps to build a Guideline-based *careflow* system. *Medical* and *Organizational knowledge* are combined and used to build a computational model of the Clinical Guideline implementation within a clinical environment.

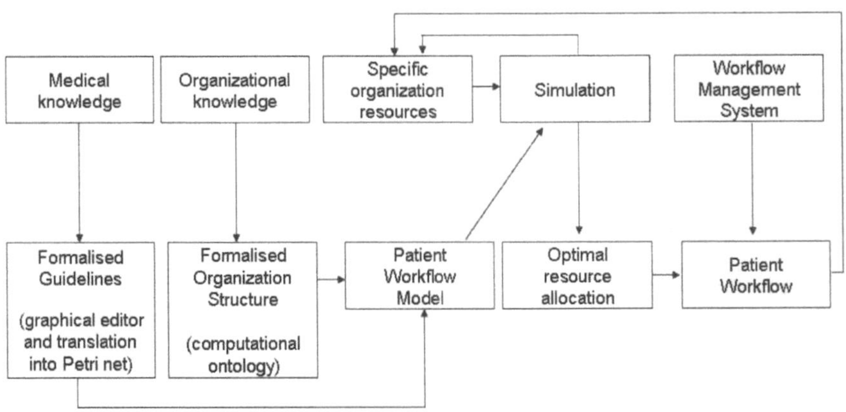

Fig. 10. A methodology for building a *careflow* management system.

Figure 10 above shows different kinds of feedback: the *Optimal resource allocation* is achieved by simulating different *Optimal resource allocations*, each arranged according to the previous simulation results.

GUIDE may also call external modules representing decisions as decision trees or influence diagrams that may take into account patient preferences, organizational preferences, and economic evaluations.

1.3.3.4 A New Approach for GUIDE

Recently, the GUIDE environment has integrated three main modules: the Guideline Management System (providing clinical decision support), the Healthcare Record System (providing access to patient data), and the Workflow Management System or Careflow Management System (providing organizational support) as shown in Figure 11 [24].

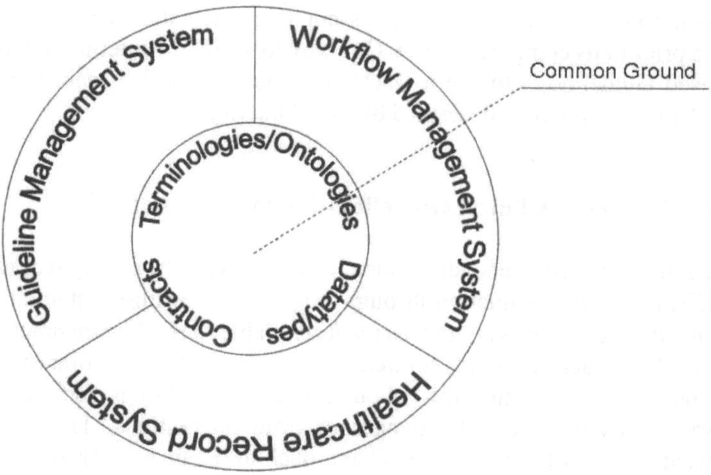

Fig. 11. The Pie model represents the separation of the three main modules.

This new approach is based on the separation between medical and organizational issues. Clinical Guidelines can be executed in three ways: (1) GUIDE can run a Clinical Guideline in simulation mode by simulating patient data; (2) it can simulate the effects of implementing a Clinical Guideline at a facility by translating a Clinical Guideline into Petri nets using the GUIDE editor, and augmenting the model with a knowledge base reflecting the facility's organizational structure; and (3) it can drive resource allocation and task management in clinical settings by using the Oracle™ Workflow tool.

A given Healthcare organization could perform some local adaptation of the GUIDE formalized Guideline. Revision could be performed both at local level and at global level with a feedback to the original Guideline authors in order to improve the original model. Several projects are in progress following this approach [24].

1.4 Disseminating Standardized Clinical Knowledge

The first approach for computerizing Clinical Guidelines has relied on rule-based systems. However, the developers who first implemented Clinical Guidelines found that many "published Guidelines suffer from unclear definition of specifications, incompleteness, and inconsistency, and these deficiencies compromise their value" [25]. Translation of "Guideline prose into computer executable statements by programmers is complex and arduous because Guideline developers do not plan for algorithmic implementation" [26]. As a result of the poor quality of Guideline structuring, Clinical Guidelines were often found not to "address all possible situations comprehensively, or provided alternative actions for the same antecedent" [26] when attempting to formalize it.

As a consequence, it has been found essential to verify the internal structure of a Guideline prior to its computerization. One way to verify the internal consistency of a text-based Guideline is to use a Decision Table [27] which makes explicit the different Clinical situations described by the Guideline.

1.4.1 Brief History of Clinical Guidelines Computerization

The first approach used to encode Clinical Guidelines electronically was developed for the HELP (Health Evaluation through Logical Processing) system at the LDH hospital in Utah [28]. This system was made available to Healthcare practitioners as early as 1975 in order to provide limited decision support at the point of care in the form of notification to clinicians "about events or conditions such as abnormal laboratory results or potentially dangerous drug interactions" [11]. The HELP system used the rules-based "if…then" approach to organize, represent and evaluate the contents of a Clinical Guideline.

At about the same time as the HELP system was developed, another rule-based approach to Clinical Guidelines computerization, the Regenstrief Medical Records System (RMRS) was created. It was developed to optimize information content and delivery to the medical practitioner. Consistent with this goal, the system was created with the ability to represent "current medical knowledge (text book information, published literature) in a codified and active form (*e.g.*, Guidelines) linked to specific patient states with the goal of improving clinical care and assess patient outcome" [11]. Today, this includes "a variety of computer-based informational feedback and interventions designed to change practitioner and/or patient behavior"[2].

1.4.2 The Arden Syntax

The Arden Syntax is perhaps the best known language for representing clinical knowledge required to create patient-specific DSS. The initial version of the Arden Syntax was based largely on the encoding scheme for generalized decision support used in the HELP system [29]. The Arden Syntax itself was developed in the 1980s and was "accepted as a standard by the ASTM in 1992" and then later by HL7[3]. The perceived modular independence of "if…then" rules led to the "development of the Arden Syntax for encoding MLM as a formalism for sharing medical knowledge used for making decisions" [30]. We may notice that in this case, the target user of the Arden Syntax is the clinician with little or no programming training. This is why it is not a full-feature programming language; for example, it does not include complex structures to preserve its readability and its proximity to natural language.

---

[2] www.regenstrief.org

[3] http://www.hl7.org

1.4.3 Medical Logic Modules and Clinical Guidelines

The Arden Syntax uses MLM to help providers make medical decisions, by using these models to generate alerts for abnormal laboratory results, drug interactions, diagnostic interpretations, etc. As a standardization tool, the Arden Syntax can be used to relate the contents of Clinical Guidelines to MLM embedding the standardized knowledge they convey. Each MLM is written to behave like a single rule, as instructions within a MLM execute sequentially until a specific outcome is reached.

Each MLM uses four main slots: an "evoke slot", a "data slot", a "logic slot" and an "action slot". The "evoke slot" acts as the trigger, and the "data slot" acts as a retriever of the relevant data from the database. The "logic slot" uses the data in the "if" part of the logic statement and the "action slot" executes the "then" piece of the statement to deliver a reminder or an alert based on the data (*e.g.*, to administer a follow-up preventive exam) or a specific Clinical Guideline recommendation (*e.g.*, dosage of medication). A triggering event can be as simple as the database entry of a diagnosis or another patient data variable (such as a lab test result).

1.5 Computational Tools Assisting Clinical Guidelines' Structuring

Clinical Guidelines are usually structured to highlight the various decision steps and the sequencing of therapeutic lines. This has induced substantial research in the use of computational tools assisting their structuring. The most comprehensive is the Guideline Elements Model (GEM) [31], which is an XML framework containing more than 100 mark up elements. This model facilitates the encoding of Clinical Guidelines and supports the automatic processing of marked up Clinical documents.

1.5.1 Guideline Markup Languages

Guideline Markup Languages became available after the widespread availability of HTML / XML browsers. Guideline Markup Languages use a flexible coding system that allows for mark up "tags" to designate concepts and relationships between concepts directly from a text-based Clinical Guideline. Once encoded, the hierarchical structure of markup languages allows the visualization of Clinical Guidelines at "different formats at various levels of detail according to the needs of the practitioner, while preserving their originally published form" [32]. This constitutes the essence of the mark up approach to Clinical Guideline representation, *i.e.* the ability to impose a structure that defines relationships between the data. With its flexibility and ability to define its own data elements (the definition takes place in a Document Type Definition, or DTD, attached to the mark up document), the markup language approach is designed to allow easy integration into any clinical information system.

1.5.2 Hypertext Guideline Markup Language

An example of a Guideline Markup Languages is the Hypertext Guideline Markup Language or HGML [32]. The HGML method of Guideline representation is "based on the markup concept for converting text-based Clinical Guidelines into a machine-operable form" by using the markup language ability to allow Guideline authors to mark up "document content and other relevant data (meta-data)" [32]. HGML is eXtensible Markup Language (XML) compatible, which allows for XML libraries and built-in user interface tools within a Web browser to allow the Guideline developer to simply "tag" the Guideline using the HGML structure. HGML uses the standard markup language format. Additional attributes can appear within the begin/end tag structure and are denoted using square brackets when they are optional.

Other advanced HGML tags are available to "facilitate inferences about the Guideline content, identifying levels of evidence for recommendations, and providing links to other documents or even decision theoretic models and simulations" [32].

In summary, HGML allows a textual Guideline to be tagged essentially to produce a structured version of the Clinical Guidelines. Markup language tags also allow representation of Guidelines in several alternative formats at differing levels of detail. The ability to define relationships between tags (or datatypes) is an important differentiation from rule-based languages.

1.5.3 Guideline Elements Model (GEM)

GEM [31] is another example of a Guideline markup language which uses XML to structure the heterogeneous knowledge contained in Clinical Guidelines. GEM is based on a hierarchy with 9 major branches as shown in Figure 12: *Identity*, *Developer*, *Purpose*, *Intended Audience*, *Method of Development*, *Target Population*, *Testing*, *Review Plan*, and *Knowledge Components*.

The *Knowledge Components* section represents recommendation's logic and constitutes "the essence of practice Guidelines". This section comprises the decision-making branch as it is used to represent the Clinical Guideline's recommendations, definitions, and algorithms. Each of the *Knowledge Components* uses "elements" (or tags) to describe specific terms that are defined by the National Guidelines Clearinghouse[4], a controlled vocabulary source.

[4] http://www.guideline.gov/

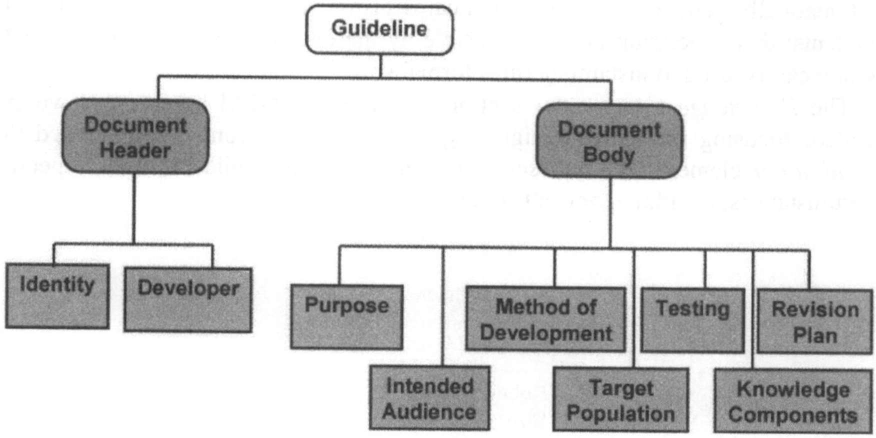

Fig. 12. Representation of the GEM hierarchy.

GEM is intended to facilitate the translation of natural language Guidelines into a standard, computer interpretable, format. One advantage of this format is that it can encode considerable information about Guideline recommendations in addition to the recommendations themselves, including the rationale for each recommendation, the quality of the evidence that supports it, and the recommendation strength assigned to it. GEM encoding of Guideline knowledge is possible through a mark up process that does not require programming skills. In particular, the GEM-Cutter[5] application is an XML editor that facilitates such Guideline mark up.

GEM is also intended for use throughout the entire Guideline life cycle, from Guideline authoring to their dissemination, implementation, and maintenance. In 2002, GEM became an international ASTM standard for the representation of Clinical Guidelines in XML format.

The GEM team is currently investigating reusable methods to facilitate Guideline authoring and implementation using GEM.

However, Guideline marking up has several limitations. Although it has been found comprehensive enough to model the information content of Clinical Guidelines, substantial variation is still observed in the creation of the GEM encoded instance of a given Clinical Guideline by different users [20]. As the model is simply an abstraction of the Guideline document, GEM alone does not support the resolution of ambiguities present in many textual Clinical Guidelines.

1.6 Extending the GEM Model to Generate a Rule Base System

As a preliminary research, we have proposed an extension of the GEM model refining the model's granularity through additional attributes [33]. The aim is to

[5] http://ycmi.med.yale.edu/GEM/

automatically generate a set of canonical decision rules from Clinical Guideline contents: this generation is made possible by the encoding of Guideline contents which can be used to instantiate rules formalisms.

The *Knowledge Components* section is one of the GEM aspects that we extended, focusing on elements signaling therapeutic decisions. We extended the *Conditional* element that represents recommendations applicable under specific circumstances, by adding new attributes to it (Figure 13).

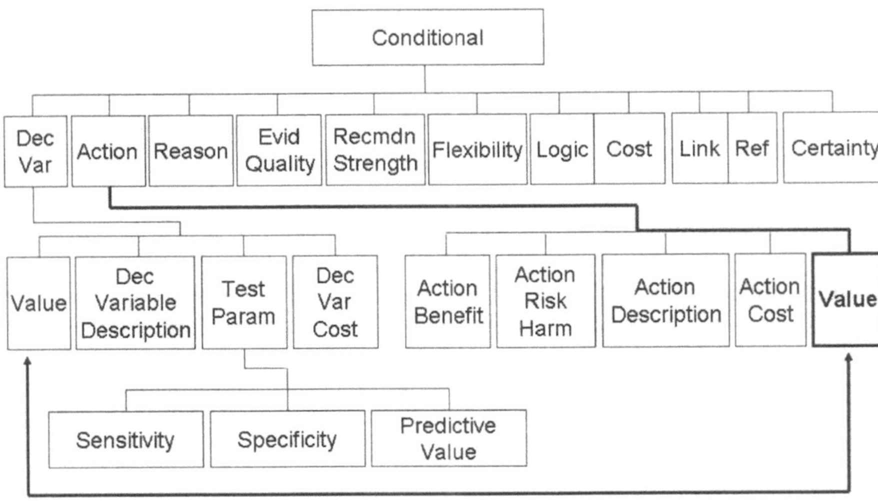

Fig. 13. The extended GEM DTD: the *value* sub-element (for the *action* element) bridges the gap between the decision variable and the action.

Only a few sub-elements are actually used: *decision.variable* (to describe elements of the decision), *action* (to describe the recommended therapy), *recommendation.strength* (to quantify the level of proof). In the GEM DTD, *Conditional* recommendations mainly rely on *decision.variable* and *action* elements. Decision variables are described by a *value*, a *description*, *test parameters* and a *cost*. Actions descriptions are structured through various fields, *i.e. benefit*, *risk*, *description* and *cost*, which can be grouped together into a single *action parameter* field.

The rationale for the generation of IF-THEN rules is the existence of decision variables in the Clinical Guidelines. More precisely, decision rules are represented as IF-THEN-WITH statements, where the condition (IF) part corresponds to a set of *decision.variable* elements of the GEM DTD, the action (THEN) part corresponds to a set of *action* elements, and the evidence (WITH) part corresponds to the *recommendation.strength* element [33]. To enable the generation of such rules from a GEM encoded instance, it has been necessary to modify the GEM encoding scheme to reflect the importance of decision variables, and obtain the same structure for both decision variables and actions in the DTD. This is why we first extended the original GEM DTD. We needed a homogeneous data model for *decision.variable* and *action* elements: as the decision variable contains a *value* sub-element, we added a similar field to the *action* element.

Even though this extension appears simple in terms of the additional categories introduced, its real power derives from the additional level of structuring which has a strong impact on the elicitation of rule content.

Another extension to the GEM model concerns the structure of actions, represented through the notion of therapeutic strategy (lines of treatment and level of intention). In the example of chronic diseases, therapeutic recommendations depend on the patient state and on her therapeutic history (*e.g.* inadequacy of previous treatment). To resolve Guideline ambiguities in the presentation of the chronological steps of the recommended therapy, we proposed a framework formalizing the therapeutic strategy for a given patient profile. A therapeutic strategy is represented by an ordered sequence of therapeutic lines; each therapeutic line is composed of a set of treatments ordered according to therapeutic levels of intention. Depending on a patient's clinical situation and her response to the ongoing therapy, the recommended treatment may either correspond to the next level of intention within the same therapeutic line or the first level of intention of the following therapeutic line [34].

We started by producing a new encoded instance for the Canadian Clinical Guidelines for hypertension management using our extension of GEM. We then developed a module to automatically derive decision rules from this GEM encoded instance. Finally, as a preliminary form of validation, the rule base automatically generated compared favorably with the manual generation of decision rules [35].

GEM already appears to facilitate the encoding of Clinical Guidelines, which support various aspects of Guideline computerization. Our proposed extension can further support the computerization of Clinical Guidelines through the various aspects of their life cycle, from production to consultation and use.

1.7 Development of Intelligent Editing Tools for Clinical Guidelines

An important aspect of Clinical Guidelines' computerization consists in assisting expert physicians in the production of Clinical Guidelines and their correct encoding in formats such as GEM. We observed several limitations during the manual encoding of Clinical Guidelines. Tools for facilitating the translation of text into a computable format have been developed but currently rely on a "manual" process as well, simply providing a graphical user interface. In the next section, we introduce a semi-automatic tool improving this process.

1.7.1 Supporting Knowledge Extraction from Clinical Guidelines

Our idea is to support the automatic process of knowledge acquisition from Clinical Guidelines (Figure 14) which is poised to play an important role in the Clinical Guidelines life cycle.

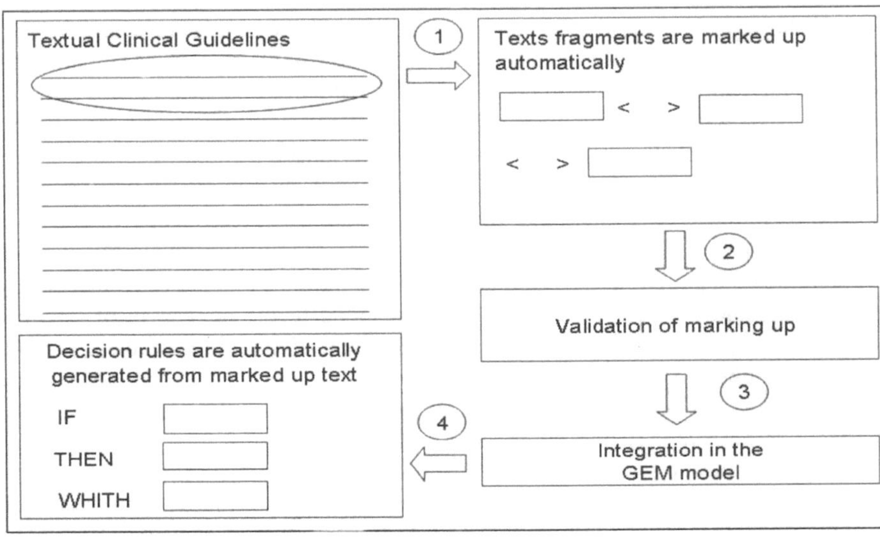

Fig. 14. Knowledge extraction from text: generation of decision rules.

This research may thus enhance existing tools such as GEM-Cutter which is a tool to facilitate the transformation of Clinical Guidelines information into GEM formats. But it still relies on a human step to paste text from Clinical Guidelines (containing appropriate knowledge) into the GEM markers. This is why we proposed to use text processing techniques to identify syntactic structures signaling GEM markers: because of the nature of the Guideline, these are referred to as *deontic operators*. Their automatic identification can support the development of intelligent editing tools for Clinical Guidelines.

1.7.2 Knowledge Extraction from Texts

Our source of inspiration was research in document processing, essentially for knowledge extraction from prescriptive texts similar to Clinical Guidelines but in other application domains. We based our work on the study of Moulin and Rousseau [36] describing a method to automatically extract knowledge from legal narratives texts based on "*deontic operators*". The following hypotheses have been raised by Moulin and Rousseau: "(i) some prescriptive texts, such as regulation texts, have a form and a content which can be transformed to create at least the kernel of knowledge bases; (ii) the statements of a regulation text can be analyzed in a systematic way in order to derive knowledge structures which are logically equivalent to the original text and which can be used by an inference engine; (iii) there is a similarity between the way a text is organized and the way a knowledge base can be structured".

In order to verify these hypotheses they developed a knowledge-acquisition system, which transforms a prescriptive text into a knowledge base that can be exploited by an inference engine.

Contents of prescriptive statements are specified by "normative propositions" which in the French texts studied by Moulin and Rousseau manifest themselves through verbs such as "pouvoir" *(be allowed or may)*, "devoir" *(should or ought to)*, "interdire" (*forbid*). The only category of statements whose syntactic form is, according to Kalinowski, typical of norms is deontic propositions. Kalinowski indicates that "whatever kind of norm we consider (moral, juridical, technical or other), the norm may be examined from the point of view of its syntactic structure on one hand, and, on the other hand, from the perspective of inferences in which they are eventually premises or conclusions" [37]. The three most frequent deontic modalities are thus introduced: obligation, interdiction and permission.

Moulin and Rousseau showed that knowledge extraction from legal texts based on deontic operators is a good way to resolve problems of knowledge acquisition from texts, without having to take into account the detailed meaning of recommendations.

1.7.3 Knowledge Extraction from Clinical Guidelines: a Succession of Steps

The first step consists in analyzing the regularities in Clinical Guidelines, *i.e.* concordances between verbs and expressions. This is done using a Concordance Program. In a second step, using results from the previous analysis, we defined Finite State Transition Networks (FSTN) to represent the surface presentation of deontic operators. We developed a system that runs FSTN to recognize syntactic expressions of deontic operators and automatically marks up Clinical Guidelines in terms of these operators.

1.7.3.1 Concordance in Clinical Guidelines

As a preliminary study, we used a corpus of 17 French documents such as Clinical Guidelines, consensus conference and medical teaching material (in the field of diabetes, hypertension, asthma, dyslipidemia, epilepsy, renal disease). This enables to collect examples of variability in the authoring of medical documents. We used the "Simple Concordance Program (4.07)[6]" to analyze these documents. This program provides scopes for each word in the corpus.

The aim of this step is also to verify Moulin and Rousseau's hypotheses in the case of Clinical Guidelines. We found several regularities specific to Clinical Guidelines which reproduced the patterns identified by Moulin and Rousseau. This

[6] http://asia.cnet.com/downloads/pc/swinfo/0,39000587,20043053s,00.htm

confirms that we may adapt the deontic logic approach to the processing of textual Clinical Guidelines.

Based also on our previous studies, we focused on verbs that produce decision rules and thus allow a selection of a sub-set of deontic operators. In order to consider deontic operators specific to medicine, we identified the following deontic operators in French: "devoir" (*should or ought to*), "pouvoir" (*be allowed or may).* However, we noticed that their syntax tends to be specific to the medical context. We observed that a deontic operator is most often followed by the auxiliary "être" (*be*) with a specific verb occurring in its past participle form. We categorized a sub-set of deontic operators associated to previously identified deontic operators. For example, in French "être recommandé" (*be recommended*), or "être prescrit" (*be prescribed*), "être conseillé" *(be advised)*, "être préféré" (*be preferred*). But this syntax is not the only one encountered. We thus collected a complete set of syntactic expressions for deontic operators to built FSTN that will mark up their occurrence in Clinical Guidelines.

1.7.3.2 FSTN for Marking Up Clinical Guidelines

We decompose the process of marking up in two stages. We first mark up deontic operators, and subsequently mark up their scope in the sentence. A scope that precedes a modal operator is called front-scope, whereas the back-scope corresponds to a scope which follows the operator.

Marking Up Deontic Operators

The first stage applies FSTN to mark up deontic operators in the sentence, as in the example shown in Figure 15.

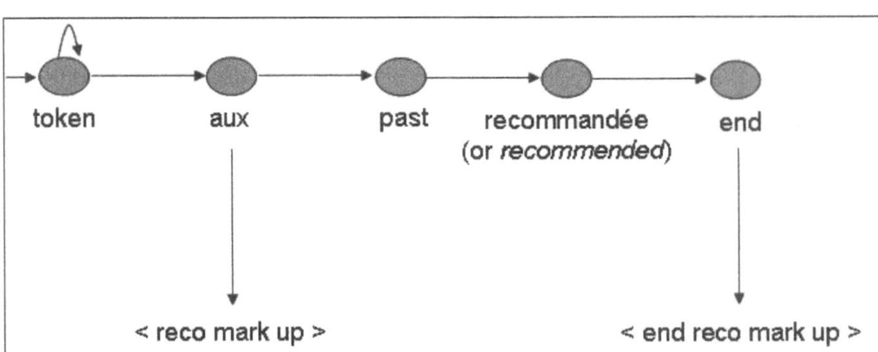

Fig. 15. FSTN for recognizing deontic operator.

We also sub-categorized deontic operators into monadic / dyadic operators, and active / passive forms of the sentence. This sub-categorization assists the marking up of front-scope and back-scope, and the correct identification of the type of information contained in each scope. We defined, as Moulin and Rousseau, an operator scope as the part of the sentence on which the modal operator is applied. Scopes thus correspond to the free text content of deontic expressions.

Marking Up Scopes

The second stage further applies FTSN to mark up scopes in the sentence, as shown in Figure 16, *i.e.* front and back scopes, by the simple processing of marked up operator types.

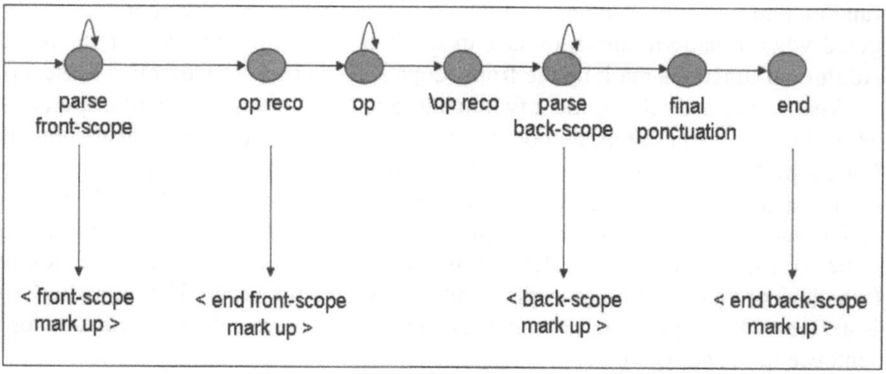

Fig. 16. FSTN for recognizing scopes.

1.7.3.3 Knowledge Extraction Based on FSTN

The system that we developed, based on FSTN as described above, leads to the automatic marking up of Clinical Guidelines. This system is structured as follows: (i) external files containing FSTN definition and syntactic elements corresponding to their nodes, and text to be tagged; (ii) the FSTN parser, implemented using generic functions.

FSTN Structure

The definition of FSTN is contained in an external file text. We adopt the following formalism: "[" indicates the beginning of the pattern, "]" its end, and "][" words that are ignored during parsing. For example, "est recommandé" (*is recommended*) corresponds to [[aux past]] (*aux* means auxiliary and *past* means past participle form) whereas "est généralement recommandé" (*is generally recommended*) corresponds to [[aux][past]]. This formalism has a simple structure and allows us to represent all patterns identified in the corpus.

Grammar

The grammar is also contained in an external text file. We identified terms, using our previous analysis with the concordance program. As an example, we present below some rewriting rules:

auxiliaire → est | sont	auxiliairy → is | are
deontic_operator → peut | peuvent	deontic_operator → may
infinitif → constituer | recommander	infinitive → constitute | recommend
participe_passé → constitué | recommandé	past → constituted | recommended

Internal Structure

We defined functions reading patterns, and rules according to current and previous context. We first generate FSTN from their definition files and then use these functions to parse the document. A function marking up deontic operators is triggered when a pattern corresponding to its FSTN definition has been recognized. Additional functions mark up the front-scope and the back-scope of that sentence.

We also defined rules to identify monadic and dyadic forms of deontic operators. Monadic and dyadic forms are not specific to deontic operators in medical contexts. For example, we defined passive forms whenever the "be" verb occurs after a deontic operator and an auxiliary occurs before the deontic operator. A dyadic form in active voice may be defined by the presence of an expression before and after deontic verbs; it can also be defined whenever expression such as a condition (whether) or an exception (except) occurs before deontic verbs. The monadic form is defined when a pronoun or an expression occurs before a deontic operator for a sentence in the active voice.

1.7.4 Example

Deontic Operator Considered

The deontic operator "est recommandé" in French (*is recommended*) is first automatically marked up, as in the example below. The process is based on the FSTN described in Figure 15. As an example, in French:

« Dans une quatrième étape du traitement, en cas d'échec de la bithérapie orale maximale, la mise à l'insuline **<Op Reco>** est recommandée **</Op Reco>**, sauf cas particuliers. »

For the fourth step of treatment, if optimal oral bitherapy is inefficient, insulin ***<Op Reco>*** *is recommended* ***</Op Reco>****, except for specific situations.*

Operator Scopes

The second step identifies scopes according to the previous marking up of deontic operators (cf. Figure 16), *i.e.* in this case "Dans une quatrième étape du traitement, en cas d'échec de la bithérapie orale maximale, la mise à l'insuline" (*For the fourth step of treatment, if optimal oral bitherapy is inefficient, insulin*) corresponds to the front-scope and ", sauf cas particuliers" (*, except for specific situations*) constitutes the back-scope. Hence the marked up text:

<Front Scope> Dans une quatrième étape du traitement, en cas d'échec de la bithérapie orale maximale, la mise à l'insuline **</Front Scope>** **<Op Reco>** est recommandée **</Op Reco>** **<Back Scope>**, sauf cas particuliers **</Back Scope>**.

<Front Scope> *For the fourth step of treatment, if optimal oral bitherapy is inefficient, insulin* ***</Front Scope>*** ***<Op Reco>*** *is recommended* ***</Op Reco>*** ***<Back Scope>****, except for specific situations* ***</Back Scope>****.*

1.7.5 Future Directions

We are currently developing a user-friendly interface to provide a more adequate tool for the interactive marking up of Clinical Guidelines. The development of this tool adopts the same approach as Moulin and Rousseau about ambiguous sentences in the text, *i.e.* where the system alerts the user and asks for confirmation of interpretation.

This automatic marking up can play a role through different steps of computerization of Clinical Guidelines. In a further study, we analyzed treatments according to scopes and deontic operators, and found that marked up treatments facilitate the translation into GEM markers.

One application of the semi-automatic marking up of texts is the generation of decision rules. The generation of decision rules itself can play an important role at various steps of the Clinical Guidelines workflow: DSS can be used to assess the consistency of textual Guidelines at the time of writing. From a different perspective, they can also assist the Guideline user at the point of care. In that sense the case study in automatic rule base generation we have presented is relevant to the overall problem of Guideline computerization.

1.8 Conclusion

In this chapter, we have reviewed several aspects of the computerization of Clinical Guidelines. As many studies have addressed the computerization of Clinical Guidelines, we tried to account for different standpoints on their computerization and their dissemination. As a synthesis of approaches that we described in this chapter, we may observe that the Arden Syntax and GLIF approaches focus on Clinical Guidelines standardization, and PRO*forma* and GUIDE on execution aspects. However, the representation model of the Arden Syntax differs from any other approach, as it is the only approach that models each Guideline as an independent modular rule. As a result, the Arden Syntax is most suitable for representing simple Guidelines such as alerts in reminder systems.

The GLIF, PRO*forma*, and GUIDE approaches all model Clinical Guidelines in a similar way, in terms of primitives (steps, tasks) that describe the control structure of a Guideline. GUIDE represents Clinical Guidelines through Petri nets integrated into a workflow; PRO*forma* relies on a task model to structure the Guidelines contents; GLIF defines different layers of abstraction, but uses flowcharts as a procedural representation of Guidelines contents.

All approaches have a formal syntax for their representation language: PRO*forma* uses BNF, GLIF uses UML, and GUIDE uses workflow process definition language.

However, we observed that the tools developed to assist the translation of Clinical Guidelines into computable format only operate manually. This is why our inspiration was driven from research in document processing, in particular techniques for information extraction from texts. In the FASTUS system [38], Hobbs et al. explain that in information extraction "generally only a fraction of the text is relevant, information is mapped into a predefined, relatively simple, rigid target representation; this condition holds whenever entry of information into a database is the task; the subtle nuances of meaning and the writer's goals in writing the text are of at best secondary interest". We thus adopted an approach based on surface structure, and on the study of Moulin and Rousseau, who have a compatible approach due to the fact that they have worked on prescriptive texts.

We claim this approach can improve existing tools such as GEM-Cutter. Clinical Guidelines show regularities in their authoring, and this is the reason why we follow Moulin and Rousseau in their use of deontic logic. Using our system, we are able to automatically mark up relevant information of Clinical Guidelines and translate automatically to a GEM encoding.

The computerization of Clinical Guidelines should address their entire workflow, from their production and encoding in document exchange formats, to their on-line consultation and their use for knowledge elicitation in DSS. Further work should also investigate the relations between their workflow and Health Information Systems.

References

1. Keckley PH. Evidence-Based Medicine in Managed Care: a Survey of Current and Emerging Strategies. Medscape General Medicine 6 (2004) 56.
2. McGlynn EA, Asch SM, Adams J, Keesey J, Hicks J, DeCristofaro A, and Kerr EA. The Quality of Health Care Delivered to Adults in the United States. The New England Journal of Medicine 348 (2003) 2635-2645.
3. Midwest Business Group on Health. Reducing the Costs of Poor-Quality Health Care Through Responsible Purchasing Leadership. Chicago, Il: Midwest Business Group on Health (2003).
4. Sackett DL, Straus SE, Richardson WS, Rosenberg W, and Haynes RB. Evidence-Based Medicine: How to Practice and Teach EBM. Edinburgh: Churchill Livingston (2000).
5. Grimshaw JM and Russel IT. Effect of Clinical Guidelines on Medical Practice: a Systematic Review of Rigorous Evaluations. Lancet 342 (1992) 1317-1322.
6. Cabana MD, Rand CS, Powe NR, Wu AW, Wilson MH, Abboud PAC, and Rubin HR. Why Don't Physicians Follow Clinical Practice Guidelines? A Framework for Improvement. The Journal of the American Medical Association 15 (1999) 1458-1465.

7. Medin DL and Ross BH. The Specific Character of Abstract Thought: Categorization, Problem Solving, and Induction. In: R.J. Sternberg, Ed. Advances in the Psychology of Human Intelligence. Hillsdale, NJ: Lawrence Erlbaum (1989) 189-223.
8. Patel VL, Arocha JF, Diermeier M, Greenes RA, and Shortliffe EH. Methods of Cognitive Analysis to Support the Design and Evaluation of Biomedical Systems: the Case of Clinical Practice Guidelines. Journal of Biomedical Informatics 34 (2001) 52-66.
9. Bennett JW and Glasziou PP. Computerised Reminders and Feedback in Medication Management: a Systematic Review of Randomised Controlled Trials. The Medical Journal of Australia 178 (2003) 217-222.
10. Lobach DF and Hammond WE. Computerized Decision Support Based on a Clinical Practice Guideline Improves Compliance with Care Standards. The American Journal of Medicine 102 (1997) 89-98.
11. Elkin PL, Peleg M, Lacson R, Bernstam E, Tu S, Boxwala A, Greenes R, and Shortliffe EH. Toward Standardization of Electronic Guidelines. MD Computing 17 (2000) 39-44.
12. Shiffman RN, Shekelle P, Overhage JM, Slutsky J, Grimshaw J, and Deshpande AM. Standardized Reporting of Clinical Practice Guidelines: A Proposal from the Conference on Guideline Standardization. Ann Intern Med 139 (2003) 493-498.
13. Tierney WM, Overhage JM, Takesue BY, Harris LE, Murray MD, Varco DL, and McDonald CJ. Computerizing Guidelines to Improve Care and Patient Outcomes: The Example of Heart Failure. Journal of the American Medical Informatics Association 2 (1995) 316-322.
14. Patel VL, Arocha JF, Diermeier M, How J, and Mottur-Pilson C. Cognitive Psychological Studies of Representation and Use of Clinical Practice Guidelines. International Journal of Medical Informatics 63 (2001) 147-167.
15. Ohno-Machado L, Gennari JH, Murphy SN, Jain NL, Tu SW, Oliver DE, Pattison-Gordon E, Greenes RA, Shortliffe EH, and Barnett GO. The Guideline Interchange Format: A Model for Representing Guidelines. Journal of the American Medical Informatics Association 5 (1998) 357-372.
16. Fox J, Johns N, and Rahmanzadeh A. Disseminating Medical Knowledge: the PRO*forma* Approach. Artificial Intelligence in Medicine 14 (1998) 157-81.
17. Quaglini S, Stefanelli M, Cavanelli A, Micieli G, Fassino C, and Mossa C. Guideline-Based Careflow Systems. Artificial Intelligence in Medicine 20 (2000) 5-22.
18. Hripcsak G, Ludemann P, Pryor TA, Wigertz OB, and Clayton PD. Rationale for the Arden Syntax. Computers and Biomedical Research 27 (1994) 291-324.
19. Peleg M, Tu S, Bury J, Ciccarese P, Fox J, Greenes RA, Hall R, Johnson PD, Jones N, Kumar A, Miksch S, Quaglini S, Seyfang A, Shortliffe EH, and Stefanelli M. Comparing Computer-Interpretable Guideline Models: A Case-Study Approach. Journal of the American Medical Informatics Association 10 (2003) 52-68.
20. Karras BT, Nath SD, and Shiffman RN. A Preliminary Evaluation of Guideline Content Mark-Up Using GEM - An XML Guideline Elements Model. Proceedings of the American Medical Informatics Association (2000) 413-417.
21. Peleg M and Kantor R. Approaches for Guideline Versioning Using GLIF. Proceedings of the American Medical Informatics Association (2003) 509-513.
22. Peleg M, Boxwala AA, Ogunyemi O, Zeng Q, Tu S, Lacson R, Bernstam E, Ash N, Mork P, Ohno-Machado L, Shortliffe EH, and Greenes RA. GLIF3: The Evolution of a Guideline Representation Format. Proceedings of the American Medical Informatics Association (2000) 645-649.

23. Fox J, Beveridge M, and Glasspool D. Understanding Intelligent Agents: Analysis and Synthesis. Ai Communications 16 (2003) 139-152.
24. Ciccarese P, Caffi E, Boiocchi L, Quaglini S, and Stefanelli M. A Guideline Management System. In: M. Fieschi et al., Eds. IOS Press. Proceedings of International Medical Informatics Association (2004) 28-32.
25. Shiffman RN and Greenes RA. Improving Clinical Guidelines with Logic and Decision-Table Techniques: Application to Hepatitis Immunization Recommendations. Medical Decision Making 14 (1994) 245-254.
26. Shiffman RN, Brandt CA, Liaw Y, and Corb GJ. A Design Model for Computer-based Guideline Implementation Based on Information Management Services. Journal of the American Medical Informatics Association 6 (1999) 99-103.
27. Shiffman RN. Representation of Clinical Practice Guidelines in Conventional and Augmented Decision Tables. Journal of the American Medical Informatics Association 4 (1997) 382-393.
28. Kuperman GJ, Gardner RM, and Pryor TA. The HELP System. Springer-Verlag, New York (1991).
29. Gardner RM, Pryor TA, and Warner HR. The HELP Hospital Information system: update 1998. International Journal of Medical Informatics 54 (1999) 169-182.
30. Pryor TA and Hripcsak G. The Arden Syntax for Medical Logic Modules. International Journal of Clinical Monitoring and Computing 10 (1993) 215-224.
31. Shiffman RN, Karras BT, Agrawal A, Chen R, Marenco L, and Nath S. GEM: A Proposal for a More Comprehensive Guideline Document Model Using XML. Journal of the American Medical Informatics Association 7 (2000) 488-98.
32. Hagerty CG, Pickens D, Kulikowski C, and Sonnenberg F. HGML: A Hypertext Guideline Markup Language. Proceedings of the American Medical Informatics Association (2000) 325-329.
33. Georg G, Séroussi B, and Bouaud J. Extending the GEM Model to Support Knowledge Extraction from Textual Guidelines. International Journal of Medical Informatics (2004) In Press.
34. Georg G, Séroussi B, and Bouaud J. Interpretative Framework of Chronic Disease Management to Guide Textual Guideline GEM-Encoding. Studies in Health Technology and Informatics 95 (2003) 531-536.
35. Georg G, Séroussi B, and Bouaud J. Does GEM-Encoding Clinical Practice Guidelines Improve the Quality of Knowledge Bases? A Study with the Rule-Based Formalism. Proceedings of the American Medical Informatics Association (2003) 254-258.
36. Moulin B and Rousseau D. Knowledge Acquisition from Prescriptive Texts. Proceedings of the Association for Computing Machinery (1990) 1112-1121.
37. Kalinowski G. La Logique Déductive. Presses Universitaires de France (1996).
38. Hobbs JR, Jerry R, Appelt DE, Bear J, Israel D, Kameyama M, Stickel M, and Tyson M. FASTUS: A Cascaded Finite-State Transducer for Extracting Information from Natural-Language Text. In E. Roche and Y. Schabes, Eds. Finite State Devices for Natural Language Processing, MIT Press, Cambridge, Massachusetts (1996) 383-406.

2 Case-based Medical Informatics

Stefan V. Pantazi[1], José F. Arocha[2], Jochen R. Moehr[1]

[1] School of Health Information Science, University of Victoria, HSD Building, Room A202, Victoria, BC, Canada, V8W 3P5

[2] Department of Health Studies and Gerontology, University of Waterloo, BMH, Room 2319, 200 University Ave. W., Ontario, Canada, N2L 3G1

Summary

The "applied" nature distinguishes applied sciences from theoretical sciences. To emphasize this distinction, we begin with a general, meta-level overview of the scientific endeavor. We introduce the notion of *knowledge spectrum* and four interconnected modalities of knowledge. In addition to the traditional differentiation between implicit and explicit knowledge, we outline the concepts of general and individual knowledge. We connect *general knowledge* with the *"frame problem,"* a fundamental issue of artificial intelligence, and *individual knowledge* with another important paradigm of artificial intelligence, *case-based reasoning*, a method of individual knowledge processing that aims at solving new problems based on the solutions to similar past problems.

Further, we outline the fundamental differences between Medical Informatics and theoretical sciences and explain why Medical Informatics research should advance individual knowledge processing (case-based reasoning), why natural language processing research is an important step towards this goal and why the goal individual knowledge processing may have deep ethical implications for patient-centered health medicine.

In order to support our explanations, we focus on fundamental aspects of decision-making, which connect human expertise with individual knowledge processing. We continue with a knowledge spectrum perspective on biomedical knowledge and show that case-based reasoning is the paradigm that can advance towards personalized healthcare and that can enable the education of patients and providers.

Our discussion on formal methods of knowledge representation is centered on the frame problem. We propose a context-dependent view on the notion of "meaning" and advocate the need for case-based reasoning research and natural language processing. In the context of memory based knowledge processing, pattern recognition, comparison and analogy-making, we show that while humans seem to naturally support the case-based reasoning paradigm (memory of past experiences of problem-solving and powerful case matching mechanisms), technical solutions are challenging.

S.V. Pantazi, J.F. Arocha and R. Moehr: *Case-based Medical Informatics*, StudFuzz **184**, 31–31 (2005)
www.springerlink.com

Finally, we present and propose solutions to the major technical challenges of individual knowledge processing: case record comprehensiveness, organization of information on similarity principles, development of advanced data visualization techniques and of pattern recognition in heterogeneous case records, and solving ethical and privacy and confidentiality issues.

2.1 A meta-level view of Science

Placing Medical Informatics in the context of other sciences and bringing coherence in its formal education will necessarily place the discussion at a meta-level view of science, which traditionally was the concern of philosophers [1]. From such a general perspective, science could be defined as "the business of eliciting theories from observations in a certain context, with the hope that those theories will help to understand, predict and solve problems." Also revolving around the "business of creating theories," R. Solomonoff's ideas [2], summarized in [3], contribute to the basis of Algorithmic Information Theory (AIT) [4], a relatively new area of research initiated by A. Kolmogorov, R. Solomonoff and G. Chaitin, and regarded as the unification of Computer Science and Information Theory. According to Solomonoff's view, a scientist's theories are compressions of her observations (i.e., her experimental data). These compressions are used to explain, communicate and manage observations efficiently and, if valid, to help solving problems, understanding and predicting. Intuitively, the higher the compression achieved by the theory, the more "elegant" that theory and the higher its chances of acceptance. This very general perspective of the scientific endeavor also makes science to appear twofold: it comprises the creation of theories (i.e., theory elicitation) as well as their subsequent use in understanding, predicting and solving problems (i.e., theory application). Therefore, science seems to be driven by two opposite forces: that of creating theories, and that of applying those theories to practical applications.

The four-dimensional space-time continuum we live in (i.e., our universe) forms the *reality* (i.e., the *context*) of all scientific observations. The compression of the immense complexity and dynamicity of this reality in concise "theories of everything" was already demonstrated by Zuse [5] and recently Schmidhuber [6]. These results of theoretical computer science demonstrate the power of human theory elicitation and provide important answers to old questions of science and philosophy. They also fuel SciFi literature and have a high impact on popular science given by the nature of the questions investigated (e.g., "is God a computer?"). However, their unfeasibility when applied to practical problems, which would be equal to building computing devices capable of running precise simulations of our reality, also widens the gap between theoretical research and practical sciences. For the time being, humanity still needs to divide science and define human knowledge as a collection of individual theories elicited from scientific observations. The immense number of theories that comprise the collective human knowledge about every possible subject, as well as its extraordinary dynamics, have forced us to divide it into what we commonly refer to as *knowledge domains*, thereby reducing the contexts of our observations to smaller space-time continuums. The attempts to process with computers the knowledge in a domain have taught us that we need to recognize the reality of the "knowledge acquisition bottleneck" [7] and to not underestimate the importance of common-sense knowledge (see [8] and [9-11]). The particularities with regard to the context retention, acquisition, representation, transferability and applicability of domain knowledge, causes us to distinguish between different modalities of domain knowledge, and place them on what we refer to as the *knowledge spectrum*.

2.2 The knowledge spectrum

The knowledge spectrum (Figure 2.1) spans from a *complex reality* (the source of experimental data and information gathered from observations and measurements) to *high-level abstractions* (e.g., theories, hypotheses, beliefs, concepts, formulae etc). Therefore, it comprises increasingly lean modalities of knowledge and knowledge representations media and the relative boundaries and relationships between them. Two forces manifest on the knowledge spectrum: that of creating abstractions and that of instantiating abstractions for practical applications. The former is the theory elicitation and is synonymous to processes of context reduction and knowledge decomposition. The latter, theory application, equates to context increase and knowledge composition processes. The engines behind the two knowledge spectrum forces are the *knowledge processors*, natural or artificial entities able to create abstractions from data and to instantiate abstractions in order to fit reality.

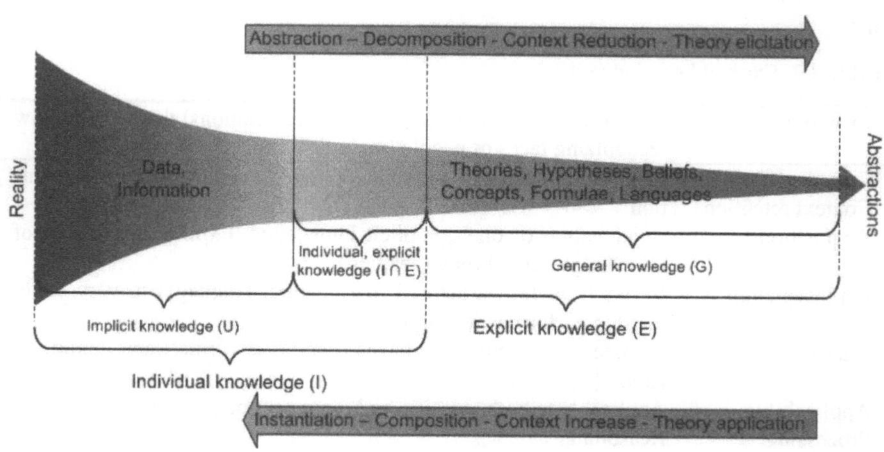

Fig. 2.1. The knowledge spectrum

Knowledge is traditionally categorized into *implicit* and *explicit* (Tables 2.1, 2.2) and ranges from rich representations grounded in a reality, to highly abstracted, symbolic representations of that reality. The classical distinction between data, meta-data, information, knowledge and meta-knowledge is simplified by our subscription to the unified view of Algorithmic Information Theory (AIT) [4], which recasts all knowledge modalities and their processing into a general framework requiring a Universal Turing Machine, its programs and data represented as finite binary sequences. From this perspective a precise distinction between these modalities becomes unimportant.

Table 2.1. Implicit knowledge (U)

Example	The implicit knowledge used to recognize the face of a specific person.
Complexity, Context retention	Rich, grounded in reality. High retention of context in form of salient features.
Acquisition	Detection, learning of correlations and regularities of environment.
Representation	Unstructured, present implicitly in data recordings of the environment (e.g., image of a person).
Transferability	Transferable only in implicit form through the data recordings (i.e., representations) of the environment.
Applicability	Very well applicable to specific problem instances.
Processing mechanisms	Pattern recognition, feature selection, associative memory.

Implicit knowledge (U, from unobvious, unapparent) is the rich, experiential, sensorial kind of knowledge that a knowledge processor acquires when *immersed into an environment* (i.e., grounded in an environment), or presented with detailed representations of that environment (e.g., images, models, recordings, simulations). It is very well applicable to specific instances of problems and relies on processing mechanisms such as feature selection, pattern recognition and associative memory.

Table 2.2. Explicit knowledge (E)

Example	The explicit knowledge (e.g., textual descriptions) that would allow recognizing faces of people (including a specific person).
Complexity, Context retention	Lean, more abstract, symbolic. Variable amount of context retention.
Acquisition	Explicitation of one's implicit knowledge. Explicit acquisition of knowledge (e.g., through reading).
Representation	Varies from less structured (e.g., natural language) to very structured (e.g., formal descriptions).
Transferability	Transferable through languages (natural or formal) and communication (e.g., verbal).
Applicability	Applicable to both, specific and more generic problems.
Processing mechanisms	Reasoning.

Explicit knowledge (E) is the abstract, symbolic type of knowledge present explicitly in documentations of knowledge such as textbooks or guidelines. It requires a representation language and the capability of a knowledge processor to *construe the meaning of concepts* of that language. It is applicable to both specific and generic problems and relies on explicit reasoning mechanisms.

The distinction between implicit and explicit knowledge are useful to characterize the nature of human expertise, but become problematic when one wants to describe fundamental differences between theoretical and applied sciences: many applied sciences, especially knowledge intensive ones, in addition to general theories of problem solving, also make use of explicit knowledge in order to describe, with various degrees of precision, particular instances of problem solving and theory application. This represents the rationale for further dividing the knowledge spectrum into *general and individual knowledge* (Tables 2.3, 2.4).

Table 2.3. General knowledge (G)

Example	Explicit general propositions, rules, algorithms, guidelines and formal theories for recognizing faces of people (e.g., a formal theory of human face recognition).
Complexity	Very lean, abstract, symbolic.
Acquisition	Identical to acquisition of explicit knowledge.
Representation Transferability	Very structured, highly transferable, explicitly as general propositions, rules and guidelines.
Context retention Applicability	Does not retain context. Easy applicable to generic problems, difficult to apply to specific problem instances (e.g., recognition of the face of a specific person).
Processing mechanisms	Logic reasoning.

Table 2.4. Individual knowledge (I)

Example	The implicit knowledge used to recognize and the explicit knowledge (e.g., textual description) that would allow recognizing the face of a specific person.
Complexity	Varies from rich to lean.
Acquisition	Identical to acquisition of both implicit and explicit knowledge.
Representation Transferability	Varies from unstructured to less structured. Transferable in both implicit and explicit form.
Context retention Applicability	Retains context. Well applicable to specific problem instances, especially if context retention is high.
Processing mechanisms	Pattern recognition, feature selection, associative recall, case-based reasoning.

2.2.1 General knowledge and the frame problem

General knowledge (G) (Table 2.3) is the explicit, abstract, propositional type of knowledge (e.g., guidelines), well *applicable to context-independent, generic problems*. However, it is more difficult to use in specific contexts because of the gap between the general knowledge itself and a particular application context. This knowledge gap translates into *uncertainty* when a general knowledge fact is instantiated to a specific situation. For example, knowing generally that a certain drug may give allergic reactions but being uncertain whether a particular patient may or may not develop any, is an example of what we consider the uncertainty associated with general knowledge. The creation of general knowledge (i.e., abstraction, generalization, context reduction, theory elicitation) is a *relevance-driven process* done by "stripping away irrelevancies" [8]. This causes general knowledge to have a lower complexity and be more manageable: "generalization is saying less and less about more and more" [8].

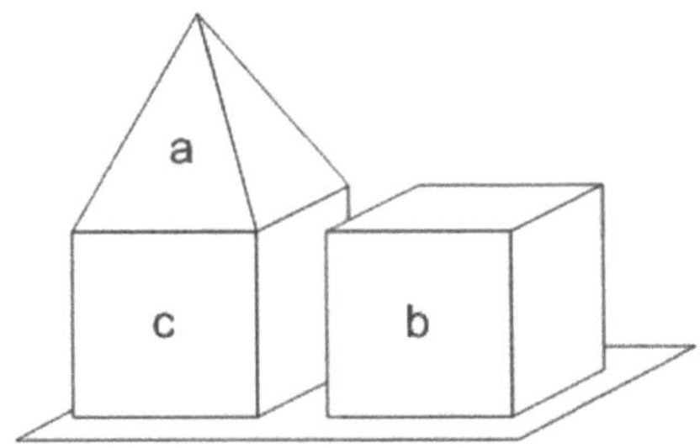

Fig. 2.2. A blocks world example[1]

Formal representations of explicit knowledge have been common in early artificial intelligence (AI) applications in the context of expert system development. They operated under the "closed world assumption" and were meant to make the representation of knowledge manageable, reproducible and clear. However this assumption also rendered the expert systems "brittle" or completely unusable when applied to real world problems [12]. The completeness necessary for automatic reasoning using explicit reasoning mechanisms can be illustrated with the following formal definition of the concept of "a brick" in a limited, hypothetical world, containing only simple geometric objects such as bricks and pyramids (Figure 2.2)(adapted from [13]): "being a brick implies three things:

1. First, that the brick is on something that is not a pyramid;
2. Second, that there is nothing that the brick is on and that is on the brick as well; and
3. Third, that there is nothing that is not a brick and the same thing as the brick."

This definition could have the predicate calculus representation in (1). It follows closely the natural language description and reads: "for all X, X being a brick implies three things:

1. There exists Y such that X is on Y and Y is not a pyramid,
2. There exists no Y such that X is on Y and Y is on X (at the same time)
3. There exists no Y such that Y is not a brick and Y is the same as X (at the same time).

[1] In this particular example expressions such as: on(a,c), on(c, table), on(b,table), pyramid(a), brick(b), brick(c), ¬same-as(a,c), same-as(b,c), etc., are true.

$$
\begin{aligned}
&\forall X\,(\text{brick}(X)\rightarrow \\
&[(\exists Y(\text{on}(X,Y) \wedge \neg\text{pyramid}(Y))) \wedge \\
&(\neg\exists Y(\text{on}(X,Y) \wedge \text{on}(Y,X))) \wedge \\
&(\neg\exists Y(\neg\text{brick}(Y) \wedge \text{same-as}(Y,X)))]
\end{aligned}
\tag{1}
$$

This representation shows that an intelligent agent who has no implicit knowledge of the hypothetical physical world and no capacity of generalization or analogy making, must be explicitly provided with all knowledge necessary to reason about "bricks" in that limited reality. Such approaches are known to suffer from a fundamental shortcoming, the "frame problem."

Daniel Dennett was the first philosopher of science who clearly articulated the "frame problem" and promoted it as one of the central problems of artificial intelligence [14] (also see [15]). Janlert [16] identifies the frame problem with "the problem of representing change." In [12] the frame problem is defined as "the problem of representing and reasoning about the side effects and implicit changes in a world description." In order to articulate and circumvent the abstract nature of its definition, Dennett has invented a little story involving three generations of increasingly sophisticated robots. These fictitious robots are products of early artificial intelligence (AI) technology that use automated reasoning based on formal representations similar to the brick example. These particular robots are specifically designed to solve a problem consisting of the retrieval of their life-essential batteries from a room, under the threat of a ticking bomb set to go off soon. Although increasingly sophisticated in their reasoning, all three successive versions of the robot fail:

- The first robot fails by *missing a highly relevant side effect* of pulling the wagon with the batteries out of the room: the ticking bomb sitting on the same wagon was also retrieved, together with the batteries.
- The second robot did not finish its *extensive, irrelevant side-effect reasoning procedures* before the bomb goes off. As Dennett ironically puts it, the robot "had just finished deducing that pulling the wagon out of the room would not change the color of the room's walls and was embarking on a proof of the further implication that pulling the wagon out would cause its wheels to turn more revolutions than there were wheels on the wagon – when the bomb exploded."
- The third robot failed because it was "*busily (i.e., explicitly) ignoring some thousands of implications it has determined to be irrelevant*" and its batteries were therefore lost in the inevitable explosion.

The frame problem can therefore be recast as *a problem of relevance* [15] (see preface), which is compounded by time constraints. It demonstrates that relevance judgment mechanisms based on general knowledge are time consuming and cause the failure to solve time-constrained decision problems. *It is a problem only because in the real world we do have time constraints.*

2.2.2 Individual knowledge and case-based reasoning

Individual knowledge (I) (Table 2.4) or instance specific knowledge, on the other hand, is a knowledge modality very well applicable to real problems, because it *identifies uniquely and matches precisely an application context.* The knowledge gap and uncertainty are reduced but still exist because of our changing reality (time dimension), which may render individual knowledge about a patient collected in the past (e.g., value of blood pressure from a month ago), less applicable in the present or future. Because it preserves context (i.e., it is more grounded), individual knowledge has a higher complexity than general knowledge and hence is more difficult to manage (i.e., has high memory requirements). For example, knowing the drugs and the precise description (e.g., numeric, textual, visual) of the allergic reactions that they caused in a certain person, as well as many other particular knowledge facts about individual, is what we call individual knowledge. The uncertainty and knowledge gap related to the application of such knowledge to future instances of decision making involving that individual are reduced: individual knowledge is supposed to fit very well the application context where it was originally captured.

Individual knowledge captured from a very specific context (e.g., diagnosing a particular patient with a particular disease) can be extrapolated to similar contexts. The higher the similarity between contexts, the smaller the knowledge gap and instantiation uncertainty and the higher the chances for a successful solution to a new problem. For this reason, individual knowledge processing has become increasingly important for artificial intelligence applications and is defined as the approach to solving new problems based on the solutions of similar past problems [12, 17-19]. It has several flavors (e.g., exemplar-based, instance-based, memory-based, analogy-based) [19] which we will refer to interchangeably, through the generic term of "case-based reasoning" (CBR).

There are four steps (the four "RE") that a case-based reasoner must perform [12, 18, 19]:

1. RETRIEVE: the retrieval from memory of the cases which are appropriate for the problem at hand; this task involves processes of analogy-making or case pattern matching;
2. REUSE: the decomposition of the retrieved cases in order to make them applicable to the problem at hand;
3. REVISE: the compositional adaptation and application of the knowledge encoded in the retrieved cases to the new problem; and
4. RETAIN: the addition of the current problem together with its resolution to the case base, for future use.

CBR entails that an expert system has a rich collection of past problem-solving cases stored together with their resolutions. CBR also hinges on a proper management of the case base and on appropriate mechanisms for the matching, retrieval and adaptation of the knowledge stored in the cases relevant to a new problem. Ideally, the individual knowledge in a case-base will progress asymptotically towards an exhaustive knowledge base, which represents the "holy grail" of knowledge engineers. From a learning systems point of view, similarly to artificial neural networks [20, 21] and inductive inference systems [22] that learn from training examples, a CBR system acquires new knowledge, stores it in a case base and makes use of it in new problem solving situations.

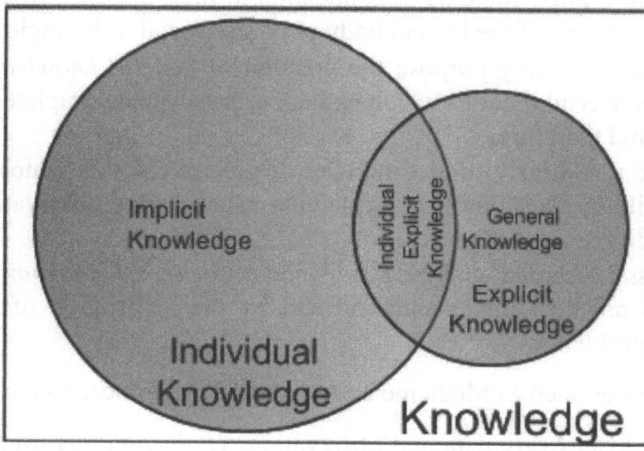

Fig. 2.3. The relationships between the knowledge modalities

The absolute positions and shapes of boundaries between the four knowledge modalities, although admittedly not as precise as drawn on the knowledge spectrum in Figure 2.1, are not of importance for this discussion. However, the relative relationships between knowledge modalities are, and can be represented formally as a Venn diagram (Figure 2.3), which implies that:

- Individual knowledge has a higher complexity than the explicit knowledge elicited from the same context (i.e., $C(I) > C(E)$). This is equivalent to stating that, for example, the picture of a person encodes more knowledge than the textual description of that person's appearance.
- Implicit knowledge is a subset of the individual knowledge (i.e., $U \subset I$).
- General knowledge is a subset of the explicit knowledge (i.e., $G \subset E$).
- The set of individual knowledge represented explicitly formed by the intersection of individual knowledge with explicit knowledge is a nonempty set (i.e., $I \cap E \neq \varnothing$). This is equivalent to stating that it is possible, for example, for an explicit textual description to identify a context uniquely (e.g., the complete name and address of a person at a specified moment in time).

2.3 A meta-level view of Medical Informatics

The meta-level overview of sciences and the definitions and properties of the knowledge spectrum and knowledge modalities enable us to draw some fundamental differences between theoretical sciences and applied sciences such as

Medicine [23] and Medical Informatics. From this perspective, theoretical sciences (e.g., theoretical computer science):

- Make use of observations which are highly abstract symbolisms and create far more limited contexts of application of their theories, when compared to the complexity of the human body or of any social or biological system,
- Have as a primary purpose the creation of *general knowledge* comprising valid, powerful theories which explain precisely and completely the observations, and therefore,
- Include a relatively limited number of precise theories which are evaluated primarily by their power of explaining experimental observations, elegance, generality, and
- Are less concerned with the acquisition of the *individual knowledge* required by the practical implementation and by the application of results to real world problems.

Applied sciences such as Medicine and Medical Informatics, on the other hand:

- Gather extensively data and observations (*individual knowledge*) from very complex systems [8, 24] (e.g., human body), which are characterized by high individual variation and randomness;
- Have as a primary purpose not only distilling data and observations into *general knowledge,* but are also concerned with the implementation details and with the application of theories to individual problem solving (e.g., diagnosis and treatment of real patients),
- May lack the incentive to refine existing theories which are objectively wrong as long as practical success is achieved [23],
- Contain very few simple, "elegant" theories (*general knowledge*) that can solve individual problems completely or explain and predict accurately [25], because of the complexity of the human body and its individual variation and, therefore,
- May pursue the application of a multitude of mutually contradictory, poorly grounded, general theories (e.g., the general theory of medical reasoning and the concepts of "diagnosis" and "symptom") [1, 23],
- Abound in general theories (e.g., guidelines) which are "lossy" (i.e., ignore individual context variation) and which are evaluated statistically by their practical success relative to existing ones (e.g., cancer therapy),
- Attempt to make up for the *knowledge gap* between general knowledge and the reality where knowledge is applied, by employing experienced clinicians who require extensive training and information technology (e.g., decision support), and, in addition,
- Are compounded by time-constrained circumstances and largely unsolved ethical issues (e.g., privacy and confidentiality, genomics research).

Given the special circumstances of our applied science in the context of other sciences and the increasing recognition of the importance of knowledge processing to Medical Informatics [26], it follows logically that Medical Informatics should complement the traditional quest for general biomedical knowledge with the advance of acquisition, storage, communication and use of individual knowledge. By doing so, Medical Informatics will provide a solution to the problems that arise during the use of general knowledge and, in the same time, will enable clinical research as well as advanced decision support and education of both healthcare providers and patients.

Individual knowledge processing equates to a CBR approach that employs collections of patient cases. Currently, such collections are the focus of research on Electronic Health Records (EHR). Envisioned as "womb to tomb" collections of patient-specific data, EHR contain a wealth of data that could be used to support case-based decisions. If EHR are to be used in a CBR context, the issues pertinent to the design of case-bases automatically become pertinent to the EHR design, and the CBR paradigm becomes important to Medical Informatics.

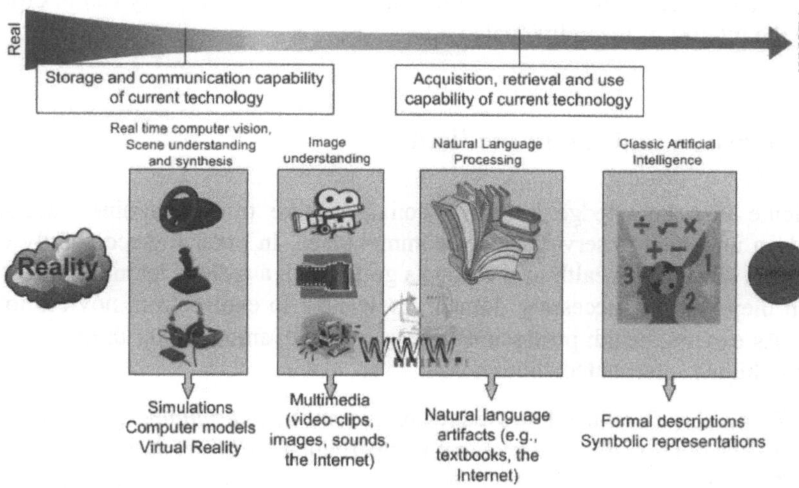

Fig. 2.4. Knowledge representation media on the knowledge spectrum[2]

The overall *knowledge processing capacity* of healthcare systems is distributed between two sources: human resources (i.e., healthcare professionals) and information technology (Medical Informatics). An ideal CBR approach would increase this knowledge processing capacity by allowing for the automatic processing (acquisition, representation, storage, retrieval and use) of individual knowledge present in increasingly rich knowledge media such as natural language artifacts, images, videos and computer simulations of reality (Figure 2.4). The storage and communication of knowledge are well advanced by current information technology. However, most of the acquisition, retrieval and knowledge use are, and will continue to be the task of professionals until advanced processing (e.g., real-time

[2] The storage and transmission of knowledge are more advanced compared to the knowledge acquisition, retrieval and use capability of current technology.

computer vision, scene understanding and synthesis, image understanding, robotics, natural language understanding) are applicable. Given the widespread use of natural languages as knowledge representation and communication media, it follows that natural language processing (NLP) research is a very important component of Medical Informatics, required to advance the organization and processing of individual knowledge in reusable case-bases. Further, the goal to advance processing of increasingly complex knowledge representations (e.g., natural language, sounds, images, simulations) and create intelligent machines that can hear, see, think, adapt and make decisions, brings Informatics even closer to what traditionally was the concern of Artificial Intelligence (AI).

Finally, because the knowledge processing capacity of human resources tends to remain relatively constant, moving towards the ideal of individual knowledge processing, no matter how slowly, may also have *ethical implications* because it proves that medical informaticians are trying to do everything they can in order to serve the interest of the individual.

2.4 Decision making in medicine

Medicine is a knowledge intensive domain where time-constrained decisions based on uncertain observations are commonplace. In order to successfully cope with such situations, health professionals go through a tedious learning process in which they gain the necessary domain knowledge to evolve from novices to experts. As experts, health professionals have attained, among other things, two important, highly interrelated abilities:

- To be able to reduce knowledge complexity by *determining efficiently what is relevant* for solving a problem in a particular situation, and,
- To be able to reduce the knowledge gap between knowledge facts and reality which translates into being able to *reduce the uncertainty of knowledge* instantiation to a particular context.

For example, both the presence and the absence of a past appendectomy are relevant and contribute (potentially unequally) to reducing the uncertainty of instantiation of the biomedical knowledge of an expert to a particular context of a patient with right lower abdominal pain. Fundamental to decision making, relevance judgments and uncertainty reduction seem both closely connected with the quality and quantity of knowledge available for solving a problem as well as with the nature of knowledge processing mechanisms. Studies of expert-novice differences in medicine [27] have shown that the key difference between novices and experts is the highly organized knowledge structures of the latter, and not the explicit strategies or algorithms they use to solve a problem. This is supported by expert system development experiences, which showed that a system's power lies in the domain knowledge rather than in the sophistication of the reasoning strategies [12]. Studies of predictive measures of students' performance indicate tests that measure the acquisition of domain knowledge to be the best predictors [28]. The work on naturalistic decision-making (NDM) and the development of psychological models of "recognitional decision-making" such as the Recognition-Primed Decision (RPD) [29-31], suggest the heavy dependence of decision makers on their previous experience of problem-solving and also on their ability to perform mental simulations.

The discussion around the amount of problem solving experience of a decision maker becomes critical in time-constrained decision circumstances. The exhaustiveness of the knowledge base and the efficiency of retrieval mechanisms now become paramount to the decision speed. Empirical evidence that shows the existence of "systematic changes of cognitive processes" related to time stress, comes from the studies on the psychology of decision-making under time constraints [32]. Although most of these studies attest the overall negative effect of time stress on the "effectiveness of decision-making processes" [33], others [29, 31] argue that even extremely time-constrained situations could be handled successfully by human subjects, given enough expertise (i.e., enough problem solving experience).

Since humans are able to make sound relevance judgments and reduce instantiation uncertainty of knowledge most of the times, the following questions arise: What is their strategy for increasing the exhaustiveness of their knowledge base while managing its exponential complexity? How do they represent and organize their knowledge and how do they manage time-constrained situations? At least some of these questions have been under intense scrutiny that has resulted in important empirical work on naturalistic decision-making [30, 31, 34, 35]. Important insights have been gained at the individual but also at the organizational and social levels. Coherent with the importance of the social aspects of decision-making, Armstrong[3] builds an interesting argument about the Darwinian evolution, social networking and the drive for knowledge discovery of the humanity as being some of the reasons that contribute to the human decision making potential.

[3] In an online essay no longer available unfortunately, Eric Armstrong proposes Darwinian evolution, social networking and the drive for knowledge discovery as explanations for the human potential to solve frame problems.

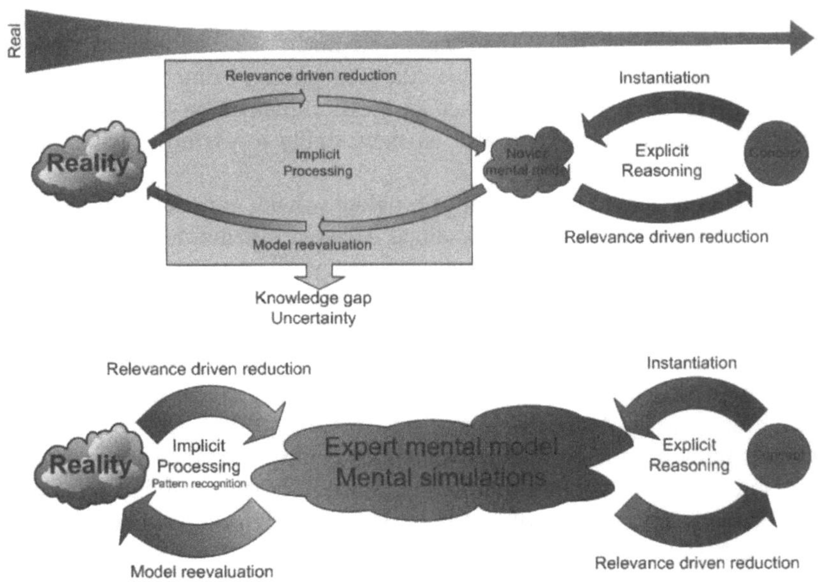

Fig. 2.5. Knowledge representation and processing in novices and experts

From the perspective of the knowledge spectrum, it seems reasonable to associate expert decision makers with individual knowledge and novices with the more abstract general knowledge about a subject, available in explicit knowledge artifacts (e.g., textbooks, guidelines). It is also conceivable that mental models of experts span a great length of the knowledge spectrum, causing them to efficiently perform implicit processing (feature selection, pattern recognition, associative recall) and also just-in-time explicit reasoning (Figure 2.5). The ability to move freely across the knowledge spectrum causes experts to efficiently reduce data to abstractions and to create hypotheses and micro-theories through sound relevance judgments. The powerful mental simulations that experts can perform allow them to construe the appropriate meanings of concepts and to verify their hypotheses against contexts of reality.

Novices, on the other hand, have limited mental models of reality situated towards the abstract region of the spectrum. This causes them to have difficulties with construing appropriate meanings of concepts due to the wider knowledge gaps between their mental models and reality. Novices are therefore unable to make sound relevance judgments and limited in their ability of interpreting data and of creating abstractions. They are also usually overwhelmed by the explicit, general knowledge present in textbooks and guidelines and unable to fully construe the meanings of concepts present in such knowledge artifacts.

In conclusion, in information and knowledge intensive domains such as medicine, explicit reasoning is important but individual knowledge acquisition (i.e., experience) and processing (i.e., CBR) are crucial for decision-making. Because the nature of expertise seems largely connected with individual knowledge processing, it follows that the evolution of novices into experts is unattainable only by the provision of extensive general knowledge. In addition, not only the individual learning but also the collective sharing of experiences (e.g., case records, personal stories, etc.) between individuals and between generations, contribute to the way humans deal with decision problems.

2.5 Patient-centered vs. population-centered healthcare

The major driving force of science is universally applicable knowledge (i.e., general knowledge). While creating and communicating new knowledge, scientists move across the knowledge spectrum from the data that captures the reality of their experiments and observations towards abstract representations that allow them to communicate their theories. In biomedical research, such an example is the randomized controlled trial (RCT), currently regarded as the gold standard for knowledge creation. The correct design of an RCT is crucial for the validity of the medical evidence obtained. A correct randomization process in RCTs will limit the bias and increase the chance for applicability of the evidence obtained, to a specifically selected group of patients (e.g., "women aged 40-49 without family history of breast cancer"). However, at the same time, the randomization process removes the circumstances of individual cases and creates a knowledge gap between the RCT evidence and future application instances. As with any statistical approach, the RCT-based evidence is best applicable at the population level rather than at the individual level.

This depersonalization of medical knowledge and evidence was also noted by others [36, 37] and could also be illustrated by the observation that most patients feel relieved when told that the chances of being successfully treated for a certain condition are 99%, for example. Although this is psychologically very positive, the patients should not necessarily be relieved, as they could very well happen to fall among the 1%, for whom things could go wrong and for whom, usually, the RCT-based evidence does not provide additional information. An experienced physician and, from a CBR perspective, a highly efficient case-based reasoner, is most of the times able to individualize the medical decision for a particular patient for whom things are likely to go wrong and fill in the knowledge gap between the RCT evidence and the medical problem at hand. This could lead to avoiding a therapeutic procedure recommended by the medical evidence. The individual knowledge that this decision is based on is usually not provided by the RCT, but is acquired through a tedious process of training. This decision is often so complex that it cannot be easily explained as it becomes heuristic in nature and is motivated by the individual knowledge that a decision maker possesses.

Others [38] have also pointed out that when physicians manage their cases (e.g., diagnosis and treatment), their previous experience allows them to make informed decisions based on heuristics rather than on a sound, complete and reproducible reasoning, such as logical inference based on a predicate calculus representation of a problem. In addition, human experts often disregard probabilistic, RCT-type of evidence and consistently detach themselves from the normative models of classical decision theory (e.g. probability theory, Bayes theory) in favor of heuristics-based approaches. Although prone to occasional failures, heuristics-based decisions are much more efficient in time-constrained and uncertain situations [31].

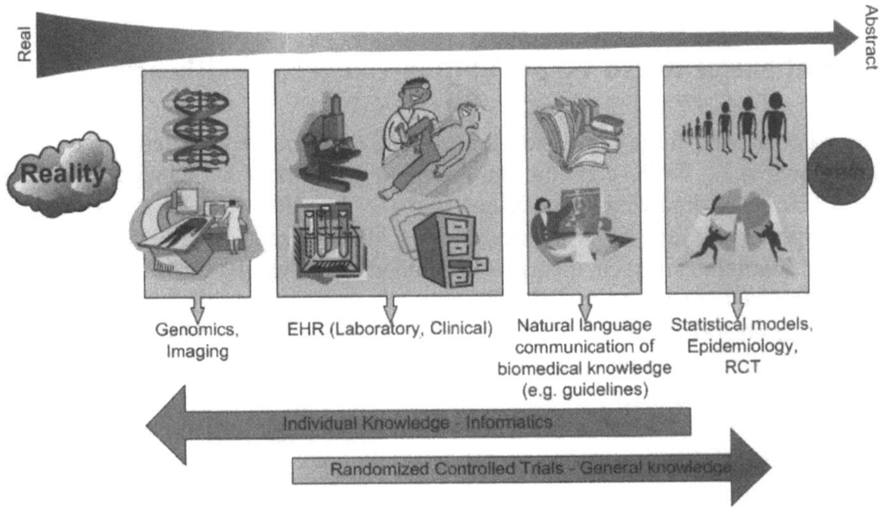

Fig. 2.6. Biomedical knowledge on the knowledge spectrum

From the perspective of the knowledge spectrum, the driving forces of Health Informatics and RCT methodology seem to have opposite directions: while Informatics aims towards *individual knowledge and personalized health care*, the general knowledge gained through populational studies (e.g., RCTs) targets *the ideal of universal applicability* (Figure 2.6). The value of a single bit of data (e.g., a Yes/No answer to a specific question such as a past appendectomy) can be very relevant in a decision-making context if it reduces the overall uncertainty of knowledge. However, such individual bits of data are inevitably lost during the creation of general knowledge.

Rigorously and expensively collected, general, populational level knowledge is useful only in situations where individual knowledge lacks (e.g., new drugs), providing the decision makers have access to it and are able to apply it to specific situations. However, general knowledge is unlikely to be used as such in many naturalistic decision-making processes, because it does not support the way expert decision makers think. The knowledge gap and inherent instantiation uncertainty manifested in the application of general knowledge does not fully enable the education of providers and patients who would benefit from the additional knowledge in individual contexts of successful or unsuccessful application instances. Informatics, on the other hand, by advancing individual knowledge processing, provides an alternative solution to the problems that arise from the use of general knowledge that targets universal applicability. An integral part of individual knowledge, genomic data is already recognized [36, 37] as being of extreme importance for a solution to the problems of general knowledge.

2.6 Knowledge representation

Knowledge representation is a central problem of informatics. Knowledge representation modalities vary from abstractions based on formal languages and situated on the abstract side of the knowledge spectrum, to data rich, multimedia-like representations of knowledge that can be mapped closer to the reality side of the knowledge spectrum.

2.6.1 Formal languages

As we mentioned earlier, the application of formal knowledge representations to real problems suffers from a fundamental shortcoming: the frame problem. Given the capability of relatively effortless human relevance judgment, the frame problem seems a rather "artificial" creation, difficult to grasp and which usually goes unnoticed. In order to circumvent its abstract nature, Dennett uses a story-telling approach. However, the frame problem also applies to and could be illustrated from the perspective of humans, who in their first years of life, learn and can easily and efficiently reason about the side effects and the implicit changes of the complex four-dimensional spatio-temporal physical world in which they live. As this learning gradually becomes common sense knowledge, it causes us to efficiently determine the relevant implicit changes while ignoring the non-relevant ones for a given situation. For example, such facts as that the clothes we are wearing are moving with us while walking or traveling are most of the times irrelevant given the context of a planned trip. However, if the trip involves some rapid movement through the air such as riding a motorbike, suddenly, wearing a sombrero becomes a relevant fact. As experts at managing our physical world, we are able, through an effortless but powerful mental simulation, to determine the relevance of such a particular fact. The recall of our personal experiences of moving fast through the air and of the dragging force of the air becomes paramount. Therefore, intelligent agent must be endowed with efficient mechanisms for determining the relevance of particular facts for a decision.

We suggest that what made the robots vulnerable was their creators' choice for knowledge representation and reasoning: the robots did not have quick access to implicit knowledge about the relevance of particular facts (i.e., records of problem solving instances), but only to explicit facts stored in frames which had to be employed in time-consuming, immense number of explicit relevance judgments about the effects of particular actions. Although they were supposed to be experts at their task, the robots were behaving like novices. The frame problem is not a problem of the knowledge representation per se, but a problem of the choice for representation of knowledge needed to solve time-constrained decisions. In other words, formal representations and logic reasoning work, but not in time constrained, complex situations.

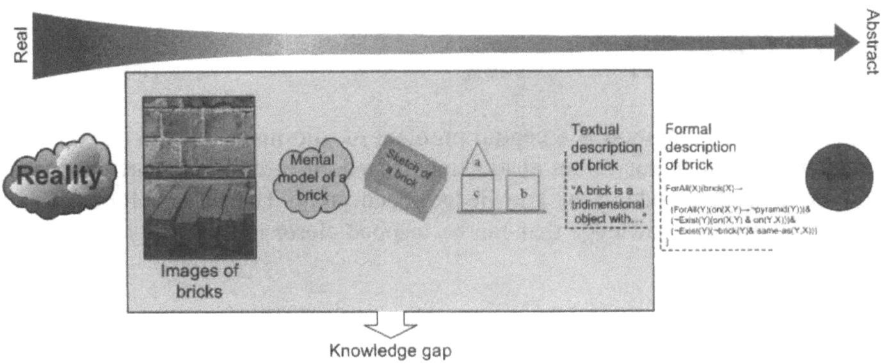

Fig. 2.7. Representations of "brick" on the knowledge spectrum[4]

From the perspective of our knowledge spectrum, explicit, formal representations sit on the abstract side of the spectrum (Figure 2.7). The retrieval of explicit knowledge representation is currently the subject of the increasingly important research in information retrieval (IR). It is commonly accepted that IR is strongly coupled with the notion of *intended meaning of concepts*: a retrieved document is considered to be relevant to a query if the intended meanings of the authors of a document are relevant to the intended meaning of that query. We propose that "meaning," a property that characterizes all concepts present in explicit knowledge, is intimately connected (if not identical) with the *notion of context*. According to this rather paradoxical view, meaning, a property that characterizes the abstract side of the knowledge spectrum, is strongly coupled with context which, by definition, is a feature of the reality side of the knowledge spectrum. Therefore, in order to construe meaning appropriately one needs to be able to efficiently move from abstractions towards richer representations of reality. This movement on the knowledge spectrum is necessary in order to fill the knowledge gap between abstract concepts and the richer mental representations required for construing their meaning.

Explicit, formal representations attempt to capture general truth and generally applicable problem solving strategies, but become too abstract in nature. Through the abstraction process, which is essentially a reduction driven by the relevance judgments of knowledge creators, the context of a problem is lost. Losing context creates difficulties with construing meaning (which is context-dependent by definition) and widens the knowledge gap between the representation itself and the reality of a future problem-solving instance. The knowledge gap translates into the instantiation uncertainty that characterizes the application of general knowledge to specific problems (e.g., one may utter the word "brick," but what particular shape,

[4] Such representations range from rich (e.g., images, mental models) to less complex (sketches and diagrams) and to symbolic descriptions (textual, formal and conceptual).

dimension, kind, type, material, make, color etc. do they mean exactly to use in the construction of a particular brick wall?). Making up for the knowledge gap through explicit relevance reasoning becomes time consuming and consequently takes its toll on the applicability of the representation. In sensitive applications such as medical decision-making and health research, general knowledge may potentially be harmful (e.g., prescribing an highly recommended drug to which a patient has a undocumented allergy). In addition, abstractions and general methods and theories of problem solving and decision-making (e.g., guidelines) do not fully enable the education of individuals and the learning from successes and mistakes. For example, knowing that an anonymous patient developed some allergy to an unknown drug is nearly useless compared to knowing that a specific patient, with a detailed health record which may include a genomic profile, developed a particular kind of allergic reaction, at a certain time, to a specific type, brand of a drug form a particular batch. The latter not only can help the research, but also could enable the prediction of future allergic reactions in that patient or in patients that exhibit similarities with that individual case.

Knowledge representation approaches must therefore preserve to the extent possible, the context of a problem-solving instance. By efficiently recalling similar past instances of problem solving and their contexts, intelligent agents are immediately provided with implicit knowledge about relevance, encoded in the retrieved contexts and, in the same time, with more possibilities to reduce the instantiation uncertainty of general knowledge when applied to specific problems. To enable this, informatics research must advance the processing of rich representations of the knowledge encoded in past problem solving cases: this is the definition of CBR research.

2.6.2 Natural languages

Similar to formal specifications (e.g., predicate calculus), natural languages use abstractions, i.e., concepts. However, their richness and power of expression place them on the knowledge spectrum to the left side of formal specifications, but to the right side of rich descriptions consisting of images, sounds, video-clips and simulations of reality (Figure 2.4). Natural languages have power of expression but loose semantics and inherent ambiguity. However, despite their abstract nature, they remain the indispensable, main knowledge representation and transfer media between humans.

In order to illustrate our point about ambiguity, we direct the reader to the previous natural language definition of the concept of "a brick." Although the definition may look unequivocal, there are subtle ambiguities that make a difference in the predicate calculus representation. The first condition of an object to be "a brick" (i.e., "the brick is on something that is not a pyramid," highlighted in the equations 2 and 3) is an ambiguous natural language construction and could have slightly different formal representations:

$$\begin{aligned}&\forall X\,(\text{brick}(X)\rightarrow[\\&\boxed{(\forall Y(\text{on}(X,Y)\rightarrow \neg\text{pyramid}(Y)))} \wedge\\&(\neg\exists Y(\text{on}(X,Y) \wedge \text{on}(Y,X))) \wedge\\&(\neg\exists Y(\neg\text{brick}(Y) \wedge \text{same-as}(Y,X)))]\end{aligned} \tag{2}$$

$$\begin{aligned}&\forall X\,(\text{brick}(X)\rightarrow[\\&\boxed{(\exists Y(\text{on}(X,Y) \wedge \neg\text{pyramid}(Y)))} \wedge\\&(\neg\exists Y(\text{on}(X,Y) \wedge \text{on}(Y,X))) \wedge\\&(\neg\exists Y(\neg\text{brick}(Y) \wedge \text{same-as}(Y,X)))]\end{aligned} \tag{3}$$

In (2) this condition has been interpreted as: "the brick being on something IMPLIES that that something is not a pyramid" and was therefore represented as "for all Y, if X is on Y, this implies that Y is not a pyramid." In (3), which is identical to (1) but is repeated to the benefit of the reader, this condition was interpreted as "the brick MUST BE (or is always) on something that is not a pyramid" and that was represented as "there exists Y such as X is on Y and Y is not a pyramid."

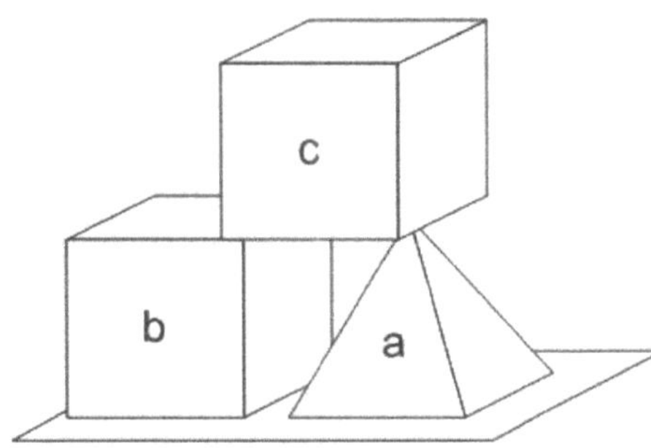

Fig. 2.8. A blocks world example[5]

The first definition is therefore more "relaxed" as it allows the possibility that a brick sits on nothing. The second definition is more restrictive, because it requires the brick to be on something that is "not a pyramid" or otherwise X is not a brick anymore. Therefore, the first definition is more general and defines the concept of "a brick" in such a way that the definition would be true even in a world with no gravity (i.e., the brick is on nothing). In addition, definition (3) does not reject the possibility that an object sits on both another brick and a pyramid, at the same time (Figure 2.8).

The point is that, most often, humans receive and transmit knowledge without the deep understanding and completeness required by an exact mathematical rep-

[5] In this particular example, indicated in a review of our work by Dr. Stefan Schulz, brick(b), brick(c), pyramid(a), on(c,b), on(c,a) are true and therefore not rejected by definition (3): the condition that "c" MUST sit on something that is not a pyramid in order to be a brick is met by on(c,b).

resentation of the knowledge to be transmitted. This shallowness has also been recognized by others [39] who are trying to draw natural language processing researchers' attention to the fact that humans are rather superficial in their knowledge acquisition and processing and often make use of "underspecified" representations. Although, since the early days of science, scientists have fallen in love with the pure reasoning approaches, as they were reproducible, unambiguous means to express new knowledge, the problems with the use of classical predicate calculus as a knowledge representation method and of the classical logic inference as a reasoning strategy are discouraging. This is due to the requirements of complete, unequivocal representations, which prevents them from dealing with the messiness of the real world problems.

If possessing the necessary knowledge, humans are able to effortlessly fill the knowledge gaps between natural language representations and their richer representations of reality (i.e., mental models), and to easily construe the appropriate meaning of potentially ambiguous concepts. Although current technology allows for its storage, knowledge present in richer media (e.g., images, videos, simulations) is currently very difficult to process (e.g., real-time computer vision, scene understanding and synthesis, image understanding) using today's technology.

Because natural languages are used by people universally and allow rich representations that no other language specification can attain, natural language processing (NLP) research is a first step that Informatics should take in order to advance the organization and processing of individual knowledge in case-bases that can be reused. The insights gained will advance knowledge processing towards richer knowledge representation media, will reduce the knowledge processing gap and consequently increase the knowledge processing capacity currently supported largely by human knowledge processors.

2.7 Knowledge processing

Knowledge processing is accomplished by knowledge processors, natural or artificial entities able to create abstractions from data and to instantiate abstractions in order to fit reality. Regardless of their nature, two important features of such processors are their memory and their processing mechanisms.

2.7.1 Memory-based processing

It is accepted that storage and manipulation of information are necessary for complex cognitive activities in humans [40]. Memory is also considered crucial for both the "situation recognition" and mental modeling processes that are part of naturalistic decision models [31].

From a computational point of view, one could easily argue that without a random access memory structure there can be no effective processing. In the context of "the computational architecture of creativity," this argument is clearly outlined in [41]. It is based on the examination of the classes of computational devices, in the ascending order of their computational power, ranging from finite-state machines to pushdown automata and linear automata. These are paralleled by their corresponding grammars, arranged similarly in the Chomsky hierarchy, consisting of regular grammars, context-free grammars, context-sensitive grammars and of the unrestricted transformational grammars for machines with random access memory [41].

Recent natural language processing (NLP) research stresses the importance of memorization of individual natural language examples [42]. The importance of memory is also emphasized in earlier [43] and more recent models of language processing in humans [44, 45]. These converge on the idea that natural language processing, regardless of the processor, is memory-based (i.e., case-based). Additional evidence comes from the fact that most language constructs (e.g. words, phrases, sentences, etc.) have very low frequencies and form a highly dimensional but very sparse pattern space. In fact, the very low frequency of most words in the English language (i.e., Zipf's law) is known from the 1940s since Zipf's famous book "Human Behavior and the Principle of Least Effort" [46] which is discussed in [47]. The main implication of "Zipf's law" is that purely statistical approaches or language processing algorithms that do not memorize training examples will either lose important information or may need extensive data (potentially impossible to collect) in order to be able to retain important features which have extremely low frequencies [48] and which may be crucial for construing the appropriate meanings of a language's concepts.

The tradeoff between learning effort and communication efficiency seems to be biased naturally towards memorization rather than towards logical reasoning. The processing complexity of natural language might therefore not be an intrinsic quality of the algorithms, but rather a function of the memorization capabilities of the language processor. By analogy, the advanced knowledge processing in humans might not be the result of very sophisticated reasoning strategies, but rather the utilization of a limited reasoning apparatus on a huge knowledge base, consisting of rich representations of one's experience. The limitations in reasoning are balanced by complex spatio-temporal pattern recognition capabilities operating on a case base built from years of experience. This case base includes common-sense knowledge.

Furthermore, people and computers memorize information differently. Both have a short term, working memory and long-term memory for storing data and information. However, the memory access is carried out in different ways. Computers can reliably store large streams of data, which most of the times have a very well defined spatial and temporal structure (e.g., a movie clip). In contrast, people can only store information and knowledge rather than data and their storage is unreliable, temporally fragmented and spatially incomplete. Computers have very reliable memories capable of error checking at the bit level while the human memory supports only a high-level semantic consistency check. Finally, computers access their memory in a random seek fashion, being able to position their "reading heads" at any position in the data streams in order to extract a certain block of data. People can access their memory by content, by being provided with an incomplete description of a potentially complex, spatio-temporal pattern serving as a retrieval key. Therefore, one of the main differences between computers and humans is that computers have *address-based random access memories*, while humans possess *content-addressable memories*.

In conclusion, from a case-based reasoning perspective, humans seem to be naturally endowed with the necessary structures for efficient case base acquisition, organization and retrieval while computers do not directly support this way of processing information and knowledge.

2.7.2 Pattern recognition, comparison and analogy making

Pattern recognition is an undisputed feature of human cognitive abilities and a research area in its own right. However, it does not seem to be as pervasive as it should, in the information processing systems in current use. Natural language, as a product of human cognition, offers compelling evidence that people are naturally inclined toward processing information using pattern recognition and similarity principles. This evidence is supported by the widespread use of language devices such as the *simile* and the *metaphor*. These are examples of comparison and analogy making that humans perform without effort, in contrast to the difficulty of implementing them in the artificial information processing systems [49]. Analogy making is essential to generating new knowledge and new artifact designs [50], as well as to problem solving and inductive reasoning [51, 52]. In a case-based reasoning context, the essential tasks of case matching and retrieval rely on pattern recognition, comparison and analogy making. In a decision making process, these mechanisms provide the immediate, implicit access to information about relevance stored in the contexts of similar instances of problems solving.

The patterns and analogies that humans are able to handle are often represented by complex spatio-temporal events with a potentially multi-sensorial impact. For example, while humans have no difficulty in understanding a metaphor like "the computer swallowed the disk," an artificial information processing system that has no visual input sensors and which lacks the capability of image understanding, would probably never be able to perceive this particular analogy with the same speed, because of the extensive reasoning and amount of explicit knowledge needed to bring the swallowing process, as it occurs in living things, close to the action of inserting a disk into a computer's disk drive.

In addition to operating on high dimensional, complex spatio-temporal patterns, analogy making in humans may also possess a dynamic component that could yield different relevance judgment outcomes, depending of context. A very illustrative example is given by French and Labiouse in [53], using the concept of a "claw hammer." According to its designed purpose, the "claw hammer" is semantically close to other concepts like "nail," "hit" and "pound." However, it may be dynamically "relocated" in the semantic space, through a mental simulation and analogy-making process, to the dynamically created class of "back-scratching devices," in the semantic neighborhood of the "itch," "scratch" and "claw" concepts. Similarly, one could think about the concept of a wooden decoy duck, which inherits properties from at least the "wooden object", "animal duck", "toy" and "hunting gear" classes. This concept may also be dynamically relocated into the semantic neighborhood of any of the classes, depending on the context of use that may be focused on themes such as "combustibles" or "hunting" for example. In the medical domain, the contextual dependence of relevance judgments, classifications and analogies is even more important, as these are often based on uncertain information and may be dynamically reevaluated in the light of new information about the patients or about their diseases.

Polyhierarchy and multiple inheritance are indisputable desiderata of terminology systems [54]. However, building multiple inheritance mechanism using current technology seems very difficult, simply because the number of possible alternative classifications increases exponentially with the number of concepts. It is very unlikely that this kind of taxonomic dynamicity (e.g., the claw hammer circumstantially classified as a back-scratching-device) of the human semantic space could work on such fixed conceptual structures which are constructed beforehand through learning, in human semantic memory. A more plausible hypothesis is that such ad-hoc classifications are circumstantially created using mechanisms that are closer to a distance calculation between high dimensional, distributed, vector representation of concepts. This is in agreement with neurolinguistic evidence from functional brain imaging studies of the human semantic memory. These studies suggest the existence of distributed feature networks for the representation of object concepts [55] and help the case for less structured approaches to capturing and representing semantics such as compositional terminology schemes (e.g. as in GALEN [56] and SNOMED [57]), latent semantic indexing (LSA) [58-62] and connectionist models [45, 63]. These approaches allow for a multidimensional semantic space where concept features can vary in importance, evolve or change dynamically, accounting for the exponentially many possible classifications and subtle variations of concept meaning. Such variations include new concepts meanings, as well as other less plausible but potentially humorous meanings that have the power to evoke laughter. This contrasts with the fixed or highly structured semantic representation schemas (e.g. fixed knowledge frames, semantic networks, ontologies), which fail to capture concept semantics in a way that provides richness, dynamicity and reusability.

The dynamicity of concept meanings and relevance judgments may offer at least one of the reasons why fixed classification schemes, controlled terminology systems or open domain ontologies have not turned out satisfactory. It may also explain why existing lexical databases based on carefully handcrafted knowledge such as WordNet [64] often contain either too fine-grained or too coarse-grained, "static" semantic information [58]. In information intensive domains like medicine, concept dynamicity may account for why the development of a universal (i.e., one size fits all) clinical terminology system is so difficult [65].

From a case-based reasoning perspective, humans are naturally equipped with powerful pattern matching and classification capabilities which allow them to cope with complex, time-constrained relevance judgments, to easily construe meaning of concepts and to tolerate the ambiguity of natural language. Only relatively recently have computers come close to this functionality with the introduction of data mining and machine learning techniques such as self organizing maps and clustering algorithms based on similarity metrics [66]. In such machine learning approaches, the important problem of feature selection equates to a problem of relevance.

2.8 Challenges and solutions

CBR approaches, devised originally as a solution to automated planning tasks [67], have been since used in various applications including healthcare, legal and military (e.g., battle planning) [19]. This already shows a particularly good fit of a medical decision support based on CBR with its human users, the healthcare professionals.

Medicine has always and will always be a case oriented profession. Medical Informatics has recognized this early through the works of various researchers who pioneered the area of decision support systems [68]. Relevant to CBR work are also the attempts to enhance early decision support systems with domain knowledge from simulated patient cases [69].

One very effective form of medical education is the retrospective analysis of case records where health professionals, both experienced or novices, learn from their own and from others' successes and failures [70]. Providing that legal and ethical implications such as provider and patient protection are dealt with appropriately, the efficacy of this teaching method can be improved if case records are continuously created, enriched, accumulated and organized on similarity principles. This is possible through a CBR approach of the EHR which, from this perspective, could serve as a comprehensive case base of managed patients that will evolve asymptotically towards an exhaustive knowledge base.

The exploration of CBR in medical contexts is increasing [71-76]. Regardless of the problem nature, the most important technical components of a CBR expert system are the case base (i.e., the memory of past problem-solving instances) and the case matching or pattern matching procedure that retrieves relevant cases for a certain problem. While humans seem to possess a natural support for these two components, there is a lot of work to be done in order to make the computer support this kind of knowledge acquisition and processing. We envision four important challenges in advancing case-based medical informatics:

1. Case record comprehensiveness,
2. Organization of information on similarity principles,
3. Development of advanced data visualization techniques,
4. Development of pattern recognition in heterogeneous case records, and
5. Solving ethical issues and provision of privacy and confidentiality.

2.8.1 Case record comprehensiveness

Record comprehensiveness is needed because the exhaustiveness of a case base is not only a function of the number of records but also of the richness of each case record. Current technology limits the acquisition and especially the processing of comprehensive EHR records which incorporate structured data, images, video-clips, bio-signals, genomic data, unstructured textual data covering clinical findings, detailed patient history, etc. However, as technology advances and knowledge acquisition bottlenecks are overcome, it may be possible to subdue the sparse and heterogeneous nature of the EHR and to allow the creation of representative case-bases organized on principles that facilitate similarity-based retrieval.

Temporal knowledge is a good example of a heterogeneously represented type of knowledge in the form of potentially non-interoperable standards for dates and times and in the form of temporal knowledge with various degrees of precision, embedded in knowledge facts such as "soon after receiving the drug, the patient developed a rash." Currently, for many people, the problem may seems to boil down to devising yet another standard which encompasses all the different temporal representations of dates, times and temporal concepts into a unified, common representation. From a knowledge engineering standpoint, and again currently for many researchers, this equates to the creation of a comprehensive ontology of temporal knowledge. However, the problem of representing time starts to look like a somewhat limited version of another burning problem of Medical Informatics: that of medical terminologies. The fact that all these issues remain largely unsolved, can only help the case for CBR and for adaptive, empirical methods and approaches to knowledge processing. Such approaches have the potential to cope and overcome the problems with redundant, possibly ambiguous representations, possessing variable degrees of precision.

2.8.2 Organization of information on similarity principles

Similarity based retrieval is difficult with current database technology. For example, queries to retrieve cases which are similar to a textual description of a given case are difficult to answer. The comprehensiveness of EHR must be complemented with the possibility of indexing its heterogeneous case records on similarity principles. Conceptually, the functionality of EHR will become that of an associative memory of case records that will enable the CBR paradigm.

2.8.3 Development of advanced data visualization techniques

The organization of case-bases must be complemented by the development of advanced data visualization techniques that comply with the principles of organization of information by similarity. One example of such data visualization techniques is the self-organizing map [66]. These models are able to perform cluster analyses on high dimensional data sets and provide a visual display, which can help with the navigation through and retrieval of similar cases. For instance, the self-organizing map obtained from the analysis of the Wisconsin Breast Cancer Dataset [77] used to cluster and classify cases based on their similarity in [78], could also be used for data visualization and navigation purposes, in a CBR context (Figure 2.9). It also demonstrates how high level abstractions (i.e., benign tumors forming the green cluster on the map) can be derived through an entirely automatic, data driven approach.

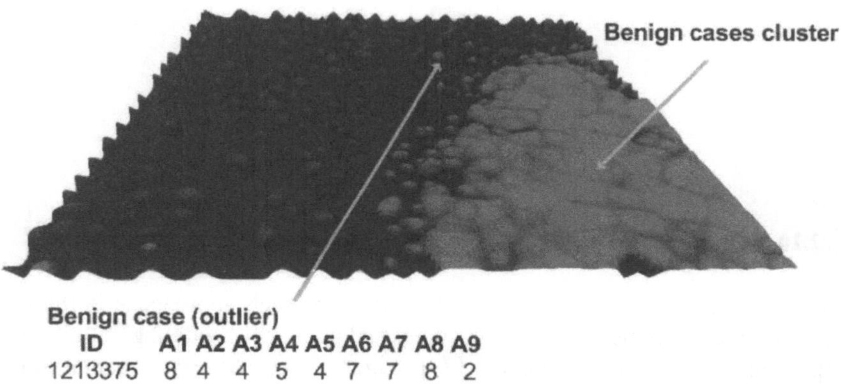

Fig. 2.9. Example of self organizing map (associative memory)[6]

2.8.4 Development of pattern recognition in heterogeneous case records

CBR relies on the proper management of the case base and on appropriate mechanisms for matching and retrieval of these case records. All similarity retrieval mechanisms are based on some sort of distance calculation between the problem at hand and the records in the case base, followed by the retrieval of the most relevant ones. Clinical narratives and other EHR components containing unrestricted text represent a particularly difficult challenge for semantic similarity measures. The development of terminology systems based on less structured (e.g., latent semantic indexing, connectionist models) and data-driven approaches will provide the semantic richness, dynamicity and reusability needed for such complex tasks.

[6] Each one of the 9-dimensional (A1-A0) 683 individual cases, is associated with (mapped on) a region on the 2-dimensional map and highlighted using a 3rd dimension (an "activation bubble" with elevation and color). The organization of individual descriptions of cases obeys similarity principles: similar cases are closely mapped and very similar cases form clusters (e.g., the green area contains most of the benign cases).

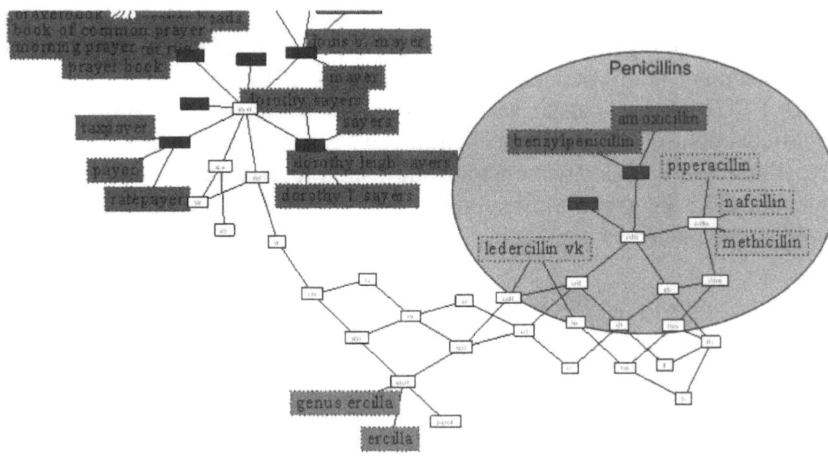

Fig. 2.10. Example of similarity based retrieval and knowledge induction[7]

A concrete example for the potential feasibility of such approaches is the automated knowledge induction based on contextual similarity modeling, ranging from morphological to sentential context [79] (Figure 2.10). An experimental knowledge processing system can induce automatically the new knowledge fact that *Ayercillin*, an item unknown to the system and hence not appearing in Figure 2.10, is most likely to be a drug, precisely a penicillin. The decision is based on morphological (e.g., "-cillin"), semantic (e.g., six of the similar items are known to be drugs, precisely, penicillins) and pragmatic (e.g., the six, semantically similar items are consistent with the use in a medical context) similarities that help in filtering out the non-relevant information (e.g., book of common prayer). On the same basis, the system can also induce that surgical procedures ending in "-tomy" (e.g., perineotomy, valvulotomy, myringotomy, strabotomy) are usually incisions while those ending in "-ectomy" (e.g., myringectomy, tonsillectomy, splenectomy, nephrectomy) are usually removals, that concepts containing the morpheme "leuco" (e.g., leucocyte, leucothoe, platalea leucorodia) are usually associated with color white while those containing "eryth" (e.g., erythroblast, erythema, erythrina) with color red.

However, despite such proof-of-concept applications and other progress in data mining and knowledge extraction from heterogeneous databases, case matching remains largely an open research question.

[7] Ayercillin, a relatively new drug, unknown to the automated system, is likely to be a penicillin because of its high contextual similarities with known penicillines.

2.8.5 Solving ethical issues and provision of privacy and confidentiality

Out of the four challenges, solving ethical issues and the provision of privacy and confidentiality measures is perhaps the most important because of its potential to become a major obstacle to individual knowledge processing. The very fact that individual knowledge has the capacity to contribute to solving future problem instances, raises the important ethical issue whether such knowledge should be made available to decision makers and researchers. Because the very definition of individual knowledge implies the possibility to match it in time and space with an application context, i.e., with a real patient, sharing individual knowledge is counterbalanced by the needs for privacy and confidentiality. In addition, to further complicate matters, it may turn out that some of the most useful cases for future instances of decision making are instances of medical errors or other unexpected events that are unique in their course of events and therefore easily identifiable together with their contexts (e.g., patients, providers, family members, etc.).

The high complexity of individual knowledge renders explicit, manually controlled access to individual knowledge cases and their components unfeasible. The only solution to this problem seems to be of technological nature. Current privacy and confidentiality measures which include de-identification, de-nominalization and scrambling of the unique personal identifiers automated or semi-automated seem insufficient to counteract the potential to identify patients from unique, individual knowledge patterns. Fortunately, the provision of privacy and confidentiality could be regarded just as a special case of *knowledge processing*, which involves knowledge about the proper use (e.g., access, modification, transfer) of individual knowledge. Because the object of such processing is "*knowledge about knowledge*," the provision of privacy and confidentiality measures becomes a form of meta-knowledge processing. This potentially complex, particular case of meta-knowledge processing could be implemented and managed using the very principles of CBR paradigm itself, by building case-bases with examples of both proper and improper (simulated, not necessarily real) individual knowledge accesses and that can be compared with future access instances. Therefore, overcoming this important challenge also hinges on the advancement of knowledge processing on CBR principles.

2.9 Outlook

The natural integration of learning with reasoning and the CBR resemblance to the cognitive models of human decision-making hold the promise to overcome the "brittleness" and "knowledge acquisition bottleneck" of classical expert systems. The CBR applications to the medical field have the potential to offer the training and decision support needed by health professionals and the means towards a true patient-centered healthcare. If successful, CBR research may also fulfill a long-standing need for intelligent information processing.

Challenges on the way to accomplish this include the increasing complexity, ethical issues as well as the paradigm shift that our current computing devices must undergo in order to support knowledge processing on similarity principles. This calls for further investigation of information processing models that, similarly to human experts, are capable to efficiently move across the knowledge spectrum. One class of such models is represented by artificial neural networks [21], some highly adaptive information processing models able to create high-level abstractions from raw data, completely automatically [66] and "learn by themselves" new information processing functions from data. From this perspective, Informatics aligns closely to the goal of creating intelligent machines that can hear, see, speak, think, adapt and make decisions.

Acknowledgements

We whish to thank Dr. André Kushniruk, Scarlette Verjinschi, Dr. Jim McDaniel, Dr. Yuri Kagolovsky, Dr. Stefan Schulz and Dr. James Cimino for their comments on earlier, various versions of this work. Also, special acknowledgements are addressed to Dr. Mahmood Tara for observations and interesting discussions on many aspects and ideas introduced in the paper. We also want to thank other individuals who provided informal feedback on the initial stages of the knowledge spectrum idea.

References

1. Moehr JR, Leven FJ, Rothemund M: **Formal Education in Medical Informatics. - Review of Ten Years' Experience with a Specialized University Curriculum.** *Meth Inform Med* 1982, **21**:169-180.
2. Solomonoff RJ: **A FORMAL THEORY OF INDUCTIVE INFERENCE.** *Information and Control* 1964, **7**(1):1-22.
3. Chaitin GJ: **To a mathematical definition of "life".** *ACM SICACT News* 1970, **4**:12-18.
4. Li M, Vitányi PMB: **An introduction to Kolmogorov complexity and its applications**, 2nd edn. New York: Springer; 1997.
5. Zuse K: **Rechnender Raum.** In: *English translation: "Calculating Space".* Cambridge, Mass.: Massachusetts Institute of Technology; 1969.
6. Schmidhuber J: **A Computer Scientist's View of Life, the Universe, and Everything.** In: *Foundations of Computer Science: Potential - Theory - Cognition.* Edited by Freksa C, Jantzen M, Valk R, vol. 1337. Berlin: Springer; 1997: 201-208.
7. Feigenbaum EA: **Some challenges and grand challenges for computational intelligence.** *Journal of the ACM (JACM)* 2003, **50**(1):32-40.

8. Blois MS: **Information and medicine: the nature of medical descriptions**. Berkeley: University of California Press; 1984.
9. Lenat DB, Guha RV: **Building large knowledge-based systems: representation and inference in the Cyc project**. Reading, Mass.: Addison-Wesley Pub. Co.; 1989.
10. Guha R, Lenat D: **Cyc: A Midterm Report**. *AI Magazine* 1990, **11**(3):32-59.
11. Lenat D: **CYC: A Large-scale Investment in Knowledge Infrastructure**. *Communications of the ACM* 1995, **38**(11):33-38.
12. Luger GF: **Artificial Intelligence: Structures and Strategies for Complex Problem Solving**, 4th edn: Addison-Wesley; 2002.
13. Winston PH: **Artificial intelligence**, 2nd edn. Reading, Mass.: Addison-Wesley; 1984.
14. Dennett D: **Cognitive Wheels: The Frame Problem in AI**. In: *Minds, Machines, and Evolution.* Edited by Hookway C: Cambridge University Press; 1984: 128-151.
15. Pylyshyn ZW: **The Robot's dilemma: the frame problem in artificial intelligence**. Norwood, N.J.: Ablex; 1987.
16. Janlert L-E: **Modeling Change - The Frame Problem**. In: *The Robot's dilemma: the frame problem in artificial intelligence.* Edited by Pylyshyn ZW. Norwood, N.J.: Ablex; 1987: xi, 156.
17. Kolodner J: **Case-Based Reasoning**. San Mateo, CA: Morgan Kaufmann Publishers; 1993.
18. Watson I, Marir F: **Case-Based Reasoning: A Review**. *The Knowledge Engineering Review* 1994, **9**(4):355-381.
19. Aamodt A, Plaza E: **Case-Based Reasoning: Foundational Issues, Methodological Variations, and System Approaches**. *AICom - Artificial Intelligence Communications* 1994, **7**(1):39-59.
20. Rumelhart DE, Hinton GE, Williams RJ: **Parallel Distributed Processing**, vol. 1-2: MIT Press; 1986.
21. Haykin SS: **Neural networks: a comprehensive foundation**. New York; Toronto: Macmillan; 1994.
22. Solomonoff RJ: **The Kolmogorov Lecture - The Universal Distribution and Machine Learning**. *The Computer Journal* 2003, **46**(6):598-601.
23. Wieland W: **Diagnose: Uberlegungen zur Medizintheorie**. Berlin, New York: de Gruyter; 1975.
24. Shortliffe EH, Blois MS: **The Computer Meets Medicine and Biology: Emergence of a Discipline**. In: *Medical Informatics: Computer Applications in Health Care and Biomedicine.* Edited by Shortliffe EH, Perreault LE, Wiederhold G, Buchanan BG: Springer Verlag; 2001.
25. Friedman CP, Owens DK, Wyatt JC: **Evaluation and Technology Assessment**. In: *Medical Informatics: Computer Applications in Health Care and Biomedicine.* Edited by Shortliffe EH, Perreault LE, Wiederhold G, Buchanan BG: Springer Verlag; 2001.

26. Musen MA: **Medical informatics: searching for underlying components**. *Methods Inf Med* 2002, **41**(1):12-19.
27. Patel VL, Arocha JF, Kaufman DR: **The Psychology of Learning and Motivation: Advances in Research and Theory**. 1994, **31**:187-252.
28. Kuncel NR, Hezlett SA, Ones DS: **A Comprehensive Meta-Analysis of the Predictive Validity of the Graduate Record Examination's Implications for Graduate Student Selection and Performance**. *Psychological Bulletin* 2001, **127**(1):162-181.
29. Klein GA: **A Recognition-Primed Decision (RPD) Model of Rapid Decision Making**. In: *Decision making in action: models and methods.* Norwood, N.J.: Ablex Pub.; 1993: 138-148.
30. Klein GA: **Decision making in action: models and methods**. Norwood, N.J.: Ablex Pub.; 1993.
31. Klein GA: **Sources of power: how people make decisions**, 1st MIT Press pbk. edn. Cambridge, Mass.; London: MIT Press; 1999.
32. Svenson O, Maule AJ: **Time pressure and stress in human judgment and decision making**. New York: Plenum Press; 1993.
33. Zakay D: **The impact of time perception processes on decision making under time stress**. In: *Time pressure and stress in human judgment and decision making.* New York: Plenum Press; 1993: 59-69.
34. Zsambok CE, Klein GA: **Naturalistic decision making**. Mahwah, N.J.: L. Erlbaum Associates; 1997.
35. Salas E, Klein GA: **Linking expertise and naturalistic decision making**. Mahwah, NJ: Lawrence Erlbaum Associates Publishers; 2001.
36. Fierz W: **Challenge of personalized health care:To what extent is medicine already individualized and what are the future trends?** *Med Sci Monit* 2004, **10**(5):111-123.
37. Kovac C: **Computing in the Age of the Genome**. *The Computer Journal* 2003, **46**(6):593-597.
38. Patel VL, Kaufman DR, Arocha JF: **Emerging paradigms of cognition in medical decision-making**. *Journal of Biomedical Informatics* 2002, **35**(1):52-75.
39. Sanford AJ, Sturt P: **Depth of processing in language comprehension: not noticing the evidence**. *Trends in Cognitive Sciences* 2002, **6**(9):382-386.
40. Baddeley A: **Working memory and language: an overview**. *Journal of Communication Disorders* 2003, **36**(3):189-208.
41. Johnson-Laird PN: **Human and machine thinking**. Hillsdale, N.J.: Lawrence Erlbaum Associates; 1993.
42. Bosch Avd, Daelemans W: **Do not Forget: Full Memory in Memory-Based Learning of Word Pronunciation**. In: *Proceeding of NeMLaP3/CoNLL98: New Methods in Language Processing and Computational Natural Language Learning: 1998; Sydney, Australia*: Association of Computational Linguistics; 1998: 195-204.
43. Riesbeck CK, Kolodner JL: **Experience, memory, and reasoning**. Hillsdale, N.J.: L. Erlbaum Associates; 1986.

44. Murdock B, Smith D, Bai J: **Judgments of Frequency and Recency in a Distributed Memory Model**. *Journal of Mathematical Psychology* 2001, **45**(4):564-602.
45. Saffran EM: **The Organization of Semantic Memory: In Support of a Distributed Model**. *Brain and Language* 2000, **71**(1):204-212.
46. Zipf GK: **Human behavior and the principle of least effort**. Cambridge, MA: Addison-Wesley; 1949.
47. Manning CD, Schütze H: **Foundations of Statistical Natural Language Processing**. Cambridge, Mass.: MIT Press; 1999.
48. Daelemans W: **Abstraction is Harmful in Language Learning**. In: *Proceedings of NeMLaP3/CoNLL98: New Methods in Language Processing and Computational Natural Language Learning: 1998; Sydney, Australia*: Association of Computational Linguistics; 1998: 1-1.
49. French RM: **The Computational Modeling of Analogy -Making**. *Trends in Cognitive Sciences* 2002, **6**(5):200-205.
50. Maher ML, Balachandran MB, Zhang DM: **Case-Based Reasoning in Design**: Lawrence Erlbaum Associates; 1995.
51. Keane MT: **Analogical problem solving**. Chichester, West Sussex, England New York: E. Horwood; Halsted Press; 1988.
52. Holyoak KJ, Thagard P: **Mental leaps: analogy in creative thought**. Cambridge, Mass.: MIT Press; 1995.
53. French RM, Labiouse C: **Four Problems with Extracting Human Semantics from Large Text Corpora**. In: *Proceedings of the 24th Annual Conference of the Cognitive Science Society: 2002; NJ*; 2002.
54. Cimino JJ: **Desiderata for controlled medical vocabularies for twenty-first century**. *Methods Inf Med* 1998, **37**:394-403.
55. Martin A, Chao LL: **Semantic memory and the brain: structure and processes**. *Current Opinion in Neurobiology* 2001, **11**:194–201.
56. Rector A, Rossi A, Consorti MF, Zanstra P: **Practical development of re-usable Terminologies: GALEN-IN-USE and the GALEN Organisation**. *Int J Med Inf* 1998, **48**(1-3):71-84.
57. Spackman K, Campbell K, Cote R: **SNOMED RT: A Reference Terminology for Health Care.** In: *Proceedings of the 1997 AMIA Annual Fall Symposium: 1997; Philadelphia*: Hanley & Belfus; 1997: 640-644.
58. Kintsch W: **Predication**. *Cognitive Science* 2001, **25**(2):173-202.
59. Kintsch W: **The potential of latent semantic analysis for machine grading of clinical case summaries**. *Journal of Biomedical Informatics* 2002, **35**(1):3-7.
60. Brants T, Chen F, Tsochantaridis I: **Topic-based document segmentation with probabilistic latent semantic analysis**. In: *Proceedings of the eleventh international conference on Information and knowledge management: 2002; McLean, Virginia, USA*: ACM Press; 2002: 211-218.
61. Hofmann T: **Unsupervised learning by probabilistic latent semantic analysis**. *MACHINE LEARNING* 2001, **42**:177-196.

62. Landauer T, Dumais S: **A Solution to Plato's Problem: The Latent Semantic Analysis Theory of Acquisition, Induction and Representation of Knowledge**. *Psychological Review* 1997, **104**(2):211-240.
63. Hadley RF, Rotaru-Varga A, Arnold DV, Cardei VC: **Syntactic systematicity arising from semantic predictions in a Hebbian-competitive network**. *Connection Science* 2001, **13**:73-94.
64. Miller G: **WordNet: A Lexical Database for English**. *Communications of the ACM* 1995, **38**(11):49-51.
65. Rector AL: **Clinical terminology: why is it so hard?** *Method Inf Med* 1999, **38**(4):239-252.
66. Kohonen T: **Self-Organizing Maps**, vol. 30, 3rd edn. Berlin Heidelberg New York: Springer-Verlag; 2001.
67. Schank RC, Abelson RP: **Scripts, Plans, Goals, and Understanding: An Inquiry into Human Knowledge Structures**. Hillsdale, N.J.: Erlbaum; 1977.
68. Miller RA: **Medical diagnostic decision support systems--past, present, and future: a threaded bibliography and brief commentary**. *J Am Med Inform Assoc* 1994, **1**(1):8-27.
69. Parker R, Miller R: **Creation of a Knowledge Base Adequate for Simulating Patient Cases: Adding Deep Knowledge to the INTERNIST-1/QMR Knowledge Base**. *Meth Inform Med* 1989, **28**:346-351.
70. Greene W, Hsu C-y, Gill JR, Saint S, Go AS, Tierney LM: **Case Records of the Massachusetts General Hospital: A Home-Court Advantage?** *N Engl J Med* 1996, **334**(3):197-198.
71. Macura RT, Macura K: **Case-based reasoning: opportunities and applications in health care (editorial)**. In: *Artificial Intelligence in Medicine.* vol. 9: Elsevier; 1997: 1-4.
72. Montani S, Bellazzi R, Portinale L, Fiocchi S, Stefanelli M: **A CBR System for Diabetic Patient Theraphy**. In: *Proc Intelligent Data Analysis in Medicine and Pharmacology (IDAMAP 98): 1998*: Wiley & Sons Publ.; 1998: 64-70.
73. Montani S, Bellazzi R: **Integrating Case Based and Rule Based Reasoning in a Decision Support System: Evaluation with Simulated Patients**. In: *JAMIA Symposium supplement: 1999*; 1999: 887-891.
74. Armengol E, Palaudàries A, Plaza E: **Individual Prognosis of Diabetes Long-Term Risks: A CBR Approach**. *Methods of Information in Medicine Journal* 2000, **5**:46-51.
75. Armengol E, Plaza E: **Relational Case-based Reasoning for Carcinogenic Activity Prediction**. *Artificial Intelligence Review* 2003, **20**(1-2):121.
76. Fritsche L, Schlaefer A, Budde K, Schroeter K, Neumayer H-H: **Recognition of Critical Situations from Time Series of Laboratory Results by Case-Based Reasoning**. *J Am Med Inform Assoc* 2002, **9**(5):520-528.
77. **UCI Repository of machine learning databases** [http://www.ics.uci.edu/~mlearn/MLRepository.html]

78. Pantazi S, Kagolovsky Y, Moehr JR: **Cluster Analysis of Wisconsin Breast Cancer Dataset Using Self-Organizing Maps**. In: *Medical Informatics in Europe: 2002; Budapest, Hungary*: IOS Press; 2002: 431-436.

79. Pantazi SV, Moehr JR: **Automated Knowledge Acquisition by Inductive Generalization**. In: *e-Health 2004*. Victoria, BC, Canada; 2004.

3. Analysis and Architecture of Clinical Workflow Systems using Agent-Oriented Lifecycle Models

James P. Davis[1], Raphael Blanco[2]

[1] Department of Computer Science and Engineering, University of South Carolina, Columbia, South Carolina, 29208 USA

[2] Florida Hospital Home Care Services, Adventist Health Systems, 1600 Tamiami Trail, 4th Floor, Murdock, Florida, 33938 USA

3.1 Introduction

Healthcare executives are grappling with a climate of great change in the healthcare industry. This is coming from a number of sources. First, there is increased activism among consumers and their employers who want a greater say in healthcare service delivery and reimbursement options; consumers want access to services, while employers and other payers want affordability. Second, in the clinical provider organizations, there is increased pressure to make operations more efficient in response to the need to hold down spiraling costs, to better manage utilization of health care resources among populations, and to more effectively compete in healthcare markets. (It should be noted that the market-oriented context for the application discussed in this paper is considered from the standpoint of the predominantly private healthcare sector, which is how the system is organized in the United States. However, the primary clinical application domain in which we focus our attention is one where the U.S. Government provides reimbursement for services under its Medicare program.) Finally, there is increased regulatory scrutiny across the spectrum of service providers, service payers and life science companies.

Through the adoption of advanced information technologies (IT), including the Internet, many organizations are seeking to transform the ways in which they do business. These technologies are making it possible for professionals and administrators in a number of different industries to leverage the power of greater automation, better workflow, and more effective deployment of IT across their organizations—to better manage their cost structure, improve their delivery of service, and be assured of regulatory compliance when required.

The Healthcare industry has been slower than most in the deployment of advanced IT systems, as has been cited in the literature. There are a number of root causes for this inability to bring the success of other industries in the application of IT to Healthcare. First, the practice of Healthcare involves people, populations, and their related health issues; thus, the primary "artifact" of work that drives activities in Healthcare is defined with respect to these people—patients, caregivers, clinicians, and the like. Given that the healthcare "system" has as its purpose to execute

J.P. Davis and R. Blanco: *Analysis and Architecture of Clinical Workflow Systems using Agent-Oriented Lifecycle Models*, StudFuzz **184**, 67–119 (2005)
www.springerlink.com

care-related activities in regards to these people, the information systems surrounding these activities take on a different significance than they do in other industries, for example, Manufacturing. Failure in carrying out manufacturing activities typically means a re-work of some production activity, or scrapping a resource and starting the line again. In Healthcare, a probable outcome of a failure in the system is the loss or diminished capacity of human life. Thus, the stakes are much higher in Healthcare than in most other industries (except, perhaps, in the Military/Aerospace industry).

Second, in many other industries, such as Manufacturing, practitioners started applying IT to the systemic problems of their industry earlier than in Healthcare. Companies, standards bodies and governments overcame difficulties in these industries, developing comprehensive standards, which has made possible the construction of application frameworks, systems development methodologies, and a rich set deployed IT systems. The impact is that, in an industry such as Manufacturing, practitioners have been able to increase productivity, lower cost structures, and improve product quality, whereas this is not the norm in the Healthcare industry.

Finally, the artifacts of a domain such as Manufacturing, although complex in their own right, are nowhere near the complexity of the human body, nor the human social institutions, that surround the practice of medicine. It is in this complexity that we find ourselves today—attempting to grapple with the plethora of terminology and standards of practice that differ across clinical domains, medical disciplines, and geography. There is still considerable lack of standardization in the ways we collect and share information in Healthcare, which is improving but still has a long way to go; and there is a growing desire to take stock in the lessons learned using information technology application across the board in the Healthcare industry.

One such application of IT in Healthcare involves the intelligent management of clinical processes associated with delivering care to a population of patients. In general, patients enter a healthcare system, they are subject to treatment by a loosely coordinated team of clinicians, and they subsequently leave the system. This basic pattern is reproduced in most clinical domains, and differs in terms of where the individual is in terms of a set of care guidelines. The set of activities that are taken on by the clinicians with regards to patients may differ, but the basic steps that occur with respect to a patient are very similar [2, 10, 34]. In many ways, it follows the pattern of work observed in any business enterprise: something enters our sphere of attention, we assess what we need to do in regards to this event, and we act, assessing the result once we are done. Business processes are built around taking this basic pattern, connecting its many instantiations together in sequences, and forming descriptions of the flow of work related to carrying out some activity or performing some useful function within the context of the organization [18].

In this chapter, we look at the application of an Agent-Oriented Method for effectively architecting complex workflow-driven healthcare applications for distribution across diverse healthcare enterprises. This method is based on the following components:

- Use of conceptual modeling methods to analyze business practices, identify conceptual structures, and, using "pattern finding", identify the patterns of organization in the healthcare enterprise that can be leveraged with information technology;
- Use of object-oriented and agent-oriented software engineering techniques in the detailing of the architecture of the clinical system; and,
- Use of a pattern of interaction between humans and computing systems, employing a number of mediating representations, which allow analysts and healthcare practitioners to reach agreement on the scope of coverage for a new system.

In this chapter, we discuss the clinical domain, as it exists in the US, and its regulatory backdrop, which forms the basis for understanding the need for a lifecycle-based, compliance-driven workflow model. Then, we discuss aspects of the lifecycle model itself, augmenting the management of artifact lifecycles through the deployment of software agents. We illustrate this activity using two different clinical domains by way of example, based on our experiences with two different applications: HealthCompass™ and CareCompass™. This discussion is carried out in reference to creating a *conceptual model* comprised of relevant artifacts, each with its own constituent state sequencing. The basic premise of this work is that these modeling techniques, and the abstract patterns of agent behavior that derive from them, form an effective methodology for creating flexible, customizable and extensible architectures for implementing agent-oriented, workflow-based clinical information systems across a diverse collection of clinical environments.

We discuss a set of methods for quickly analyzing and architecting complex clinical workflow applications for delivery across diverse healthcare enterprises. These methods are based on the following notions:

- Complex clinical management processes consist of a sequence of process steps, involving people playing many different *roles* that invariably involve the movement of information (in the form of defined clinical and financial documents) through the organization.
- There is a patient on which the organization's processes act. This action is represented in a computing system as a series of *activities* undertaken to change the status of the patient or agent as reflected by changes or additions to the organization's documents.
- This sequencing of activities around the patient and the corroborating documents forms a *workflow*, and the status of information in the document artifacts constitutes the current *state* of affairs pertaining to the patient under care. The joining together of these process *activities*, and the sequencing of these *states*, forms a *lifecycle*.
- Each clinical or financial document represents an *artifact* that is tracked by the system, and each patient under care has his/her own specifically defined lifecycle, each with its own set of clinical documents and allowable state sequences. Methodologically, a business analyst can

capture these state sequences beforehand, and can enter this sequence into a workflow system in order to explicitly represent the lifecycle activities to be supported by the system.

- The workflow for a particular patient, carried out according to a plan of care or treatment plan, is "shepherded" by a collection of autonomous software agents that act on objectives as stated in components of these plans.
- Such formulations are very flexible, extensible and customizable—all important attributes desired of clinical IT applications to allow systems to grow and evolve over time.

In this chapter, we present the conceptual model for a state-based lifecycle analysis pattern, followed by a discussion of the basic artifacts and processes associated with these healthcare enterprises. We then discuss the interesting aspects of the agent models and their relationships to the selected application architecture, and how that architecture is realized in a diverse health care enterprise.

We begin by providing some background on the underlying technologies and analysis methodologies that are part of this work. Next, we discuss the two healthcare domains of interest—namely, post-acute home-based care and disease management—in their regulatory and workflow context. We examine the healthcare workflow models in these domains using a collection of UML model views, discussing the creation of a robust enterprise model for supporting an extensible set of clinical transactions, whose compliance is monitored by collections of software agents. Finally, we discuss the results of the deployed systems built using the methods presented in this chapter.

3.2 Agent-Oriented Analysis Methods and Architecture Development

Before we delve into the clinical domains of interest, we'll look at the underlying methodology presented through the clinical system examples discussed here. Specifically, there are several methods we are using in our analysis, architecture and "operationalization" of clinical information systems. We refer to this amalgam of ideas as a singular Agent-Oriented methodology, as it involves the creation of workflow management functionality in the information system that is built around the operation of autonomous agents acting on behalf of stakeholders of the system. These agents—pieces of software operating with a specific, context-sensitive set of objectives—operate so as to fulfill their obligations with these stakeholders.

Our use of the term "agents" is consistent with much of the literature on software agents [14, 46, 60, 62, 64, 65, 70]; however, our interest is in defining a set of agents that operate in a narrowly-defined context of insuring that specific activities undertaken by human clinicians within the purview of the clinical system meets specific obligations. As such, our agents operate as "compliance monitors" [57]—insuring that tasks within the workflow complete in a timely manner, and complete such that time- and care-sensitive obligations are met with respect to guidelines.

3.2.1 Workflow-based modeling of a business

Workflow methods and workflow-based systems have been around for quite some time, having been used across many domains. Simply stated, workflow involves the completion of tasks in a business by the coordinated activities of the people involved in performing the work. The flow of work in a business enterprise is decomposed into a set of partially ordered tasks, which can be further decomposed and ordered. The end result is both a descriptive and prescriptive model of the business, one whose business functions can be supported by information systems. The automation of business processes is carried out using workflow-based information technology, specifically in the form of applications software that automate tasks, allowing information in the form of documents or other "artifacts" to be passed between work participants, according to some form of workflow description. There are a number of recent references that are good sources for detailed discussion of the state-of-the-art practices of workflow analysis, management and automation [3, 4, 5].

A recent trend in this field has been to link the definition and execution of workflow using the Internet. The Internet, specifically the World Wide Web, has been recognized as a platform for delivering services in loose collections of electronic commerce forums, and as a means to coordinate business functions through service-oriented architectures for the web [54]. Workflow systems are a natural extension to this point of view, as many business enterprises have embraced information systems delivered over the web [3, 5, 6, 14, 51]. Much of the work focused on the web involves mapping between terminology sets through the use of Ontologies, linking concepts together for indexing the massive amounts of web-based information and services, giving rise to a notion of a "semantic web" that has innate knowledge about itself—with the goal of transforming the web into a "organism" with highly distributed intelligence [3, 5, 6].

Formalizing workflow practices has been recognized in the Healthcare Informatics community as an essential aspect of building successful clinical systems [1, 2, 54]. As such, a consensus is forming around codification of clinical workflow. Our interest in this trend is relative to nursing disciplines—in terms of clinical standards of practice [27, 31, 32, 34, 37, 38], clinical concepts and terminology [27, 28, 29, 30], and clinical documentation (most importantly, the computer-based patient record [40, 41, 42]). Much of the Healthcare industry involves execution of workflow by clinical staff with nursing credentials; therefore, our studies to date, using IT to enhance workflow, have primarily focused on this set of process participants in the clinical domains.

3.2.2 Conceptual models and meta-models

Another key trend that plays into our work in clinical workflow is the use of conceptual modeling as a means to capture the essential semantics of underlying clinical domains, such that systems with greater robustness can be built. Conceptual modeling has been applied in the design of database systems for almost three decades, originally based on the Entity-relationship model [58, 59]. More recently, the Object-Oriented Software community has taken work done here and in the Artificial Intelligence community to devise a collection of modeling methods for use across the entire lifecycle of object-oriented software development—from business analysis through program deployment. This collection of standard graphical modeling notations is known as the Unified Modeling Language [16], and it is receiving wide usage in modeling dynamic workflow processes [4], for modeling the semantic hierarchy of healthcare concepts being encoded for the DICOM document model [23] and in the recently released HL-7 RIM [10, 34]. In addition, ongoing efforts to create conceptual models to organize clinical terminology and vocabulary across medical disciplines and clinical domains have involved ontological modeling with UMLS [53. 55] and LOINC schemata [31, 32, 33].

The use of conceptual modeling methods have different objectives, namely: (1) to observe and capture, in an "operationalizable" model, the structural semantics of a diverse set of clinical domains, where such models allow the translation of clinical vocabularies and application message sets [13, 20, 21, 23, 32, 55]; and, (2) to capture the essential structure of data relationships for creating widely applicable patient records and patient-oriented clinical documents, such that clinical data can be used more effectively in outcomes study and population health management [9, 24, 26, 34]. The mapping of these structural models is being made operational via conversion to the document markup language XML [22, 23, 24].

In addition to modeling the structural semantics of clinical domains, conceptual models are used to model the dynamic behavior of healthcare processes as a basis for architecting clinical systems [43]. Here, the UML modeling methods are used to model the collaboration and interaction of entities captured in structural views of models of the clinical enterprise [1, 2, 56]. Other modeling notations that have been examined in context of healthcare include Petri Nets [3] and the IDEF0 standard [7]; these modeling notations have been used in business process and workflow modeling in other domains. The notion of the internal "state" of an artifact or entity in the clinical domain is modeled using State diagrams [8, 15] or the UML Statechart notation [16]. Modeling the behavior of entity interactions, and the changing state of these entities during their lifetime, allow the modeling of a clinical workflow from different levels of abstraction.

Finally, in terms of systems development using conceptual modeling techniques, the cognitive aspects of computing are receiving greater attention in the analysis, planning and outcomes assessment of clinical systems in terms of user acceptance, effectiveness and performance [1, 12, 19, 24, 38, 39, 40, 43, 47, 48, 56]. In this perspective, the creation of clinical systems involves considering the broader issues of clinical user acceptance and the "organic" nature of the surrounding clinical environment. In relation to using the Internet, the dynamic nature of processes that are subject to change over time is being considered in other domains [3, 5, 6]. However, it is unclear whether the need to standardize clinical practice and terminology will mesh with the dynamic and changing nature of processes that occurs in other domains outside of healthcare [1, 2], as the need for follow-on outcomes studies generally requires healthcare systems to be static for longer time horizons.

The use of meta-models stems from an understanding that systems can be made more "intelligent" and, therefore, more robust by having an explicit internal representation of their own state [64, 68]. This ability of a piece of software to reflect on its own activity enables implementation of system functionality that is more adaptive to changes in the system environment. Often, this ability to change behavior is simply the ability to encode processing directives in an application by storing patterns of operation as data in system database tables, what is referred to as "declarative" representation of knowledge. Typically, such knowledge about patterns of operation are encoded in actual program code, implying that a human programmer has inflexibly represented some business rule or policy in the program in a manner that makes it necessary to change the code if the guideline or policy changes.

By identifying such patterns beforehand—and representing them in the systems architecture in a scheme that allows policies and guidelines to be inspected—means that the policies, rules and guidelines can be updated either manually by humans or by automated means using other programs, such as software agents. Meta-modeling is the practice of defining models of models, where the underlying domain model would characterize an "instance" of a meta-model. Therefore, multiple domains could be accommodated in a single system by having different domain model instances stored in some form enabling their query and use in application processing, thereby supporting the mapping between these domains. Meta-modeling is a fundamental supported property of the UML [16]. The use of meta-models is recognized in the healthcare research community as a means to achieve interoperability between clinical domains [34, 35, 47, 55].

3.2.3 Software-based compliance agents

Considerable work is also being done in the development of methods and architectures for systems employing autonomous software agents across different problem domains [14, 44, 45, 46, 51]. The literature for software agents, multi-agent systems, and agent-oriented software engineering techniques is extensive. However, we have not seen much work involving the use of agent-oriented methods or agent-based architectures applied in healthcare domains [57].

Software agents are small pieces of application code (sometimes implemented as Java "applets" executing on an application framework) that execute autonomously, their purpose and function focused on achieving specific goals and performing tasks on behalf of users. Agents have been applied to such tasks as information filtering, information retrieval, email sorting, meeting scheduling, resource management, and entertainment [60, 62]. There is much research and commercial product development being done using agents. In the commercial arena, most agent-related product efforts are focused on solving information explosion problems associated with using the Internet in general and the World Wide Web in particular [5, 6, 64]. The "intelligence" capabilities of these agents are only limited in terms of what tasks they can perform and what "understanding" they have about their environments. Work being done in university and commercial research labs is focused on the broader problems of applying agent-based software technology, harnessing techniques for knowledge representation and reasoning, problem solving, planning, and learning strategies.

There are a number of application domains that involve compliance (or adherence) monitoring, where the performance of activities must be monitored to insure that the impact or outcome of performing these tasks complies with guidelines set by a standards body. In a manufacturing enterprise, guidelines exist for tolerances on machined parts that must be checked. In healthcare enterprises, it is up to healthcare workers to insure that appropriate workplace practices minimize the risks of transmission of disease and other health risks, or that patient care meets guidelines of clinical practice. In all these instances, there is a general relationship that exists among the entity responsible for setting guidelines, the entity responsible for implementing specific procedures for adhering to guidelines, and the entity responsible for carrying out daily activities such that procedures defined for guideline compliance are followed.

Compliance agents work to insure compliance to a set of prescribed guidelines. The methodology uses object-oriented analysis techniques to determine the behaviors of the agents. The principal observation about identifying agent behaviors is that compliance agents track "artifacts" of compliance through a lifecycle, and that deviations from prescribed compliance indicate opportunities for compliance agents to take remedial action. Compliance can also be thought of as enforcing a "contract", in that activities that take place in context of some workflow must be completed within a certain time limit and according to certain standards. In a clinical setting, this is generally true with regards to completing clinical documents where reimbursement for services is involved, or managing patient behaviors according to treatment guidelines.

3.3 Agent-oriented Method and Architecture for Healthcare

In this section, we discuss the method for creating clinical workflow systems that use autonomous agents to track compliance in artifact lifecycles, and the general architecture for the two systems discussed in this paper that have been implemented to do this in two different clinical domains.

3.3.1 A methodology for agent-oriented analysis and design

During the course of creating systems to monitor compliance using software agents, we have abstracted the essential process steps into a specific methodology for creating compliance agents. The process steps are defined as follows:

- *Partition and decompose the problem space.* In the compliance domains we have examined, the process starts with the partitioning of the problem domain into *strategic*, *tactical*, and *operational* components. These flow in the manner shown later in Figures 3.3 and 3.13. We have found that a high-level stylized dataflow diagram (DFD) is useful for visualizing this partitioning, as we find that the *data stores* of DFDs [8] provide the linkage between these different organizational level processes.

- *Identify and create inventory of use cases.* A use case is a mechanism for identifying and describing the operational interactions between a system and the "actors" in its domain [16]. We use the notation for use cases defined in the UML standard. We augment the notation by adding an actor icon to those use cases that likely contain one or more agents acting on behalf of external users.

- *Identify and localize compliance monitoring activities.* Given the inventory of use-case interactions, we refine each of these so as to (1) highlight the essential functional transformations of the interaction, (2) define the order and direction of interactions, and (3) identify the important "artifacts" of interaction, namely, the data storage elements and knowledge sources required to process the interaction. We prefer to use the data flow diagram (DFD) notation for this purpose [8, 15]. At this time, we identify opportune locations in processes supporting the system interactions that might have autonomous agents associated with them.

- *Create an inventory of agents.* Once the agents are identified relative to the system processes, we create an inventory, indicating the agent category name, the actions that trigger the agent to take action, the data sources the agent uses in its reasoning activities, the basic nature of its output actions, and the destination "actors" who receive some notification of compliance information. We use a tabular form to present this information.

Figure 3.1. Iterative agent-oriented analysis and architecture definition process.

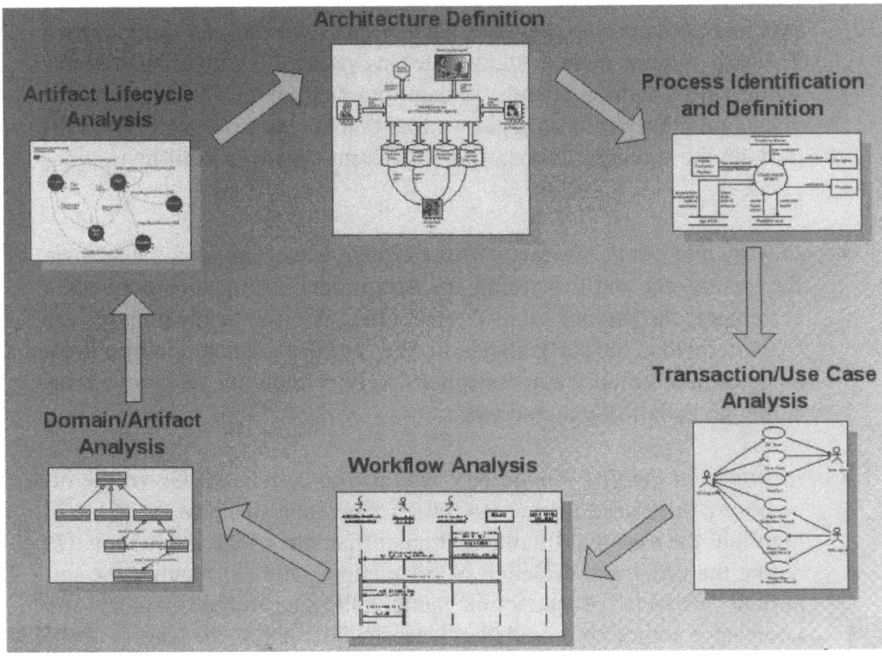

- *Identify and model the essential compliance lifecycles.* In our formulation of compliance problem solving, each compliance agent manages one or more "artifacts", each having a sequence of state transitions constituting a "lifecycle". Our treatment of lifecycle is based on that defined in the object-oriented analysis literature [15, 16]. Each specific category of compliance agent has its own lifecycle objects that it manages—which are document artifacts. We have had good success in using the state transition diagram (STD) notation [8, 15] as well as the UML Statechart [16] as an analysis and documentation medium for assessing the completeness of lifecycle depiction.

- *Map the abstract architecture onto the agent environment.* At this point, we need to map each compliance agent into the processing environment into which it will be delivered. In addition, we also need to indicate how the agents will interact with one another in that environment. It has been our experience that additional "helper" agents are needed in practice to facilitate distributed, coordinated agent behavior [65, 66]. To that end, we next model the sequences of interactions among the agents comprising the agent protocol. We use the UML sequence diagrams [16] for this modeling activity.

The sequence of steps is comparable to those described for other agent-based systems in the literature [44, 45, 46, 51, 64, 65, 66, 69]. Specifically, the subject of architecting agent-oriented systems has been discussed recently in the literature [44, 64, 65, 66, 67, 70], embodied in specific conference devoted to the subject. The work on agent architectures stems from earlier work in distributed artificial intelligence [67, 68], and is the confluence of ideas from this field and later work done in object-oriented systems architecture [6, 15, 44, 45, 46, 64].

3.3.2 An architecture for agent-based clinical workflow

The methodology steps described in the previous section, and the design artifacts created from their application, results in the creation of a conceptual architecture for a collection of applications that follow a compliance lifecycle model. In this section, we describe this architecture. In later sections, we discuss how the artifacts and agents for two clinical domains were developed using this architectural pattern [18].

In Figure 3.2, we organize the proposed workflow management infrastructure system around three principal functions, as shown by the boxes. To further refine this description, we indicate the key sources of information that would either be generated or required to carry out the functions of each component. Finally, we indicate the principal users of each component.

Note that the Protocol Management activity associated with clinical oversight is divided into two sub-parts in this figure, namely: Protocol Development and Treatment Plan Individualization. This reflects a natural delineation between features and functions to support the actual capture and management of the more general protocols (which would likely be prescribed for use in a given medical community by MCO, PSO or Provider organizations) and those to support selecting a protocol to formulate an individual treatment plan (as a physician or clinician would do for a particular patient). Overall, the system would function as follows.

Figure 3.2. Conceptual architecture of agent-oriented clinical workflow system for disease management.

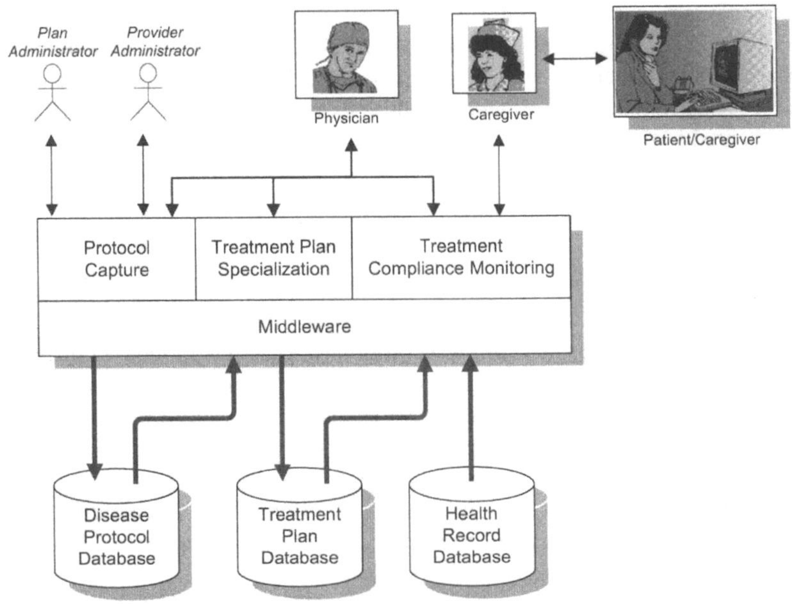

1. Protocol Development - Users of a Protocol Capture module specify treatment or compliance protocols for each artifact—which could be a document, disease under management, or other defined artifact for which the system will have protocols developed. These protocols are stored and indexed in a repository of protocols. The protocol descriptions could be modified and extended over time, in light of new clinical results or changes in compliance guidelines.

2. Plan Individualization - Users of this module (most likely, physicians or clinicians responsible for patient care) would select protocol(s) from the protocol database for purposes of constructing a specialized treatment plan. This might entail selecting a drug regimen, specifying target values or ranges for measures reflecting progress toward a desired patient outcome, or identifying specific treatments to be administered by the patient's care giver(s). Using the protocol as a guide, a treatment plan is specifically drawn up for the patient and stored in the treatment plan database; each clinical domain has its own set of forms and standards for this step. The treatment plans are also linked to the patient's record stored in a database, accessible by clinicians and the autonomous agents (subject to access control policies).

3. Compliance Monitoring - Users of this module are the practicing physician, clinician or caregivers for the patient, who would interact with software

agents in monitoring compliance activities. Software agents execute in the application environment on behalf of a patient under care. These agents perform highly specialized tasks associated with (1) monitoring for activities that show compliance with treatment plan (also referred to as a plan of care in some domains) prepared by clinician; (2) checking for certain trends in encounter data, stored in clinical documents or the patient record, which would place the patient outside of the care guideline as represented in the compliance plan; and, (3) notifying, reminding and/or alerting either the care giver, physician or clinician, or all parties when the agents detect non-compliance according to their internal rules.

Note that we do not consider the patient as a user of this system. We view the patient as a purely "passive" entity in this environment. In the context of self-administered care in a disease management setting, we consider the patient to play the role of "caregiver". We adopt this perspective in all further discussion in this document.

For the remainder of this chapter, we focus on discussing two example applications built using the architecture of the Compliance Monitoring functionality, which is where the autonomous agents execute. The Protocol Development and Plan Individualization components are not discussed in any further detail in this chapter, as they are the subject of further research and study. We will make mention of the interface between Plan Individualization and Compliance Monitoring modules in the discussion of the disease management application, as the compliance plans created in the former is how the agents get their directives for behaviors they exhibit while executing in the latter.

3.4 A Post-Acute Healthcare Domain Example

Before we can discuss the domain artifacts themselves, we need to discuss the environment (and typical structure) of a Post-acute healthcare business in the US. This business deals with the delivery of care to patients who are generally home-bound, as a result of age-related deterioration in health, or as a result of procedures of care requiring at-home convalescence. It should be noted that the basic sequence of activities—in fact, the very organization of the business—is built around strict adherence to a clinical methodology of care. In this case, the Home Health enterprise uses a basic nursing process [26, 27, 28], adapted for the needs of care delivery in the patient's home.

It should be noted that the authors have studied several such clinical domains, finding them to conform to the same basic workflow organization. This generic organization of processes around a set of document-based artifacts constitutes the architectural "pattern". Such enterprise-level business patterns are becoming recognized as being directly applicable to the identification and selection of appropriate system architectures [3, 17, 18].

In considering the functionality of the example, we partition the application space into a constituent set of functional components, laid out into an architecture that maximizes flexibility, customizability and extensibility. This partitioning is done along a natural basis, namely, that which is recognized in the healthcare enterprise itself. Traditionally, these functions have been carried out manually, and without much oversight between operations in the enterprise. This changed about five years ago, with the advent of stricter guidelines on reporting and oversight imposed by the agency in the US federal government responsible for reimbursement for services delivered under its Medicare program [71]. (This agency was known as the Health Care Financing Agency (HCFA), which was renamed in 2001 to the Centers for Medicare and Medicaid Services (CMS). This organization provides oversight on matters of quality of care and guidelines compliance, managed through its policies governing reimbursement for services to healthcare providers.) Because of requirements for increased data collection and reporting imposed by CMS, this home healthcare provider organization began an investigation of document-based workflow automation. The description that follows is a result of that initiative.

3.4.1 Characterizing the Enterprise Organization

As depicted in Figure 3.3, there is a primary flow of work indicated in this class of healthcare enterprise, starting with the "Referral" of a patient to the home health (or, post-acute care) agency. This figure takes the patient referral through the following process sequence. First, the referral passes through the Intake process. Next, the resulting program admission representing the patient passes into the Care Delivery process, where actual care is delivered, and care delivery documented, according to agency and regulatory guidelines for practice.

Finally, each clinical encounter with the patient culminates with passing documentation to those processes associated with the agency being paid for services rendered by the appropriate payers. The workflows associated with these business processes are those that are *operational* in nature, as they constitute the day-to-day execution of the business on a continuous basis.

Figure 3.3. Top-level workflow diagram for the Post-acute care enterprise.

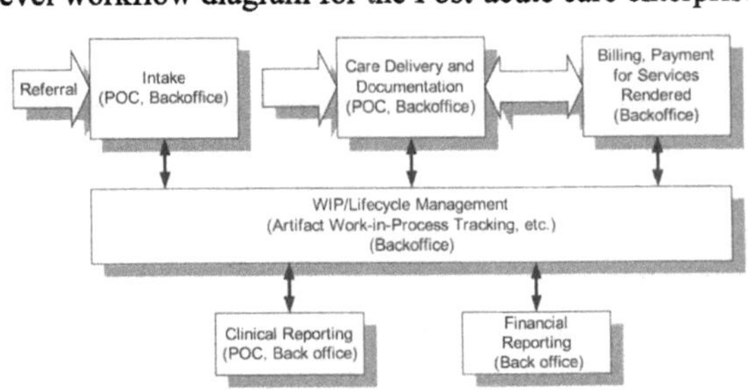

Also depicted in the figure is a box located at the *tactical* level of business operation, labeled "WIP/Lifecycle Management". This component encapsulates all system functionality of the application facilitating the back-office workflows for managing the flow of documentation and other information through the healthcare enterprise. We are following a practice employed in manufacturing domains for tracking the status of patient workload, defined as *work in process* or WIP [3].

In the US, a home health or post-acute care facility gets reimbursed for services based on some quantification of "work", where the billing is generally identified according to a procedure coding scheme. The components of this workflow need to be explicitly tracked and managed in order to represent the causal relationships between artifacts and activities leading to the coding presented to the payer entity (in this case, the US federal government's CMS agency). The Lifecycle management component provides a set of interfaces and services, allowing the end user—as well as other modules in the system itself—to act upon the artifacts representing the flow of work through the enterprise. Note that there may be many different end users, each representing an agency staff member playing different roles in the various point of care (POC) and back-office processes. The functionality and tasks encapsulated in this component are *tactical* in nature--they are associated with insuring effective and optimal operation of the business in satisfying the enterprise's specific business performance objectives.

Many aspects of running a healthcare facility require conformance to regulatory guidelines that are temporal in nature. Time-in-process becomes a critical concern—in the same way that time in process for product inventory would be critical for cost management for a factory. A business objective for such facilities is, thus, to minimize work-in-process, i.e., the amount of time an "artifact" stays active in the process by not completing its passage through its requisite sequence of lifecycle states. Furthermore, as a result of CMS guidelines, there are hard constraints on the amount of time a specific unit of work (such as an unsigned Assessment form) can be in the process. This component implements the set of functionality, using a set of artifact-specific autonomous agents, allowing monitoring and management of the artifacts, to insure that specific tactical business objectives are met.

Finally, as depicted in Figure 3.3, there are several components indicated to be *strategic* in nature—in that they are concerned with facilitating the healthcare enterprise's management with tools for meeting strategic business objectives. These objectives tend to be aligned with patient outcomes and financial performance of the agencies. The primary functionality in these components is involves reporting capabilities. The Clinical and Financial Reporting components are shown as separate boxes primarily because of the different objectives that each part of the business pursues.

3.4.2 Characterizing the post-acute care problem domain

The complex weave of clinical procedure in care delivery with changing business and regulatory realities has made home health and post-acute care a difficult problem domain in which to devise an effective computing solution to meet demands of the many stakeholders. This complexity comes from several basic characteristics of the home care enterprise and its general business model as practiced in the US.

- The delivery of quality health care to a homebound population encompasses a highly *distributed*—yet *synchronous*, *coordinated* and *tightly coupled*—range of activities. It involves collecting timely information and dispensing care services across an oftentimes-large geographical area. It also involves coordinating care for a patient among multiple clinicians (e.g., nurses and therapists) as well as physicians and other service providers.
- The deployment of agency clinical staff resources, management of materials and supplies, and coordination of patient care among multiple disciplines requires a sophistication of planning and schedule logistics management. As is quite the case, these activities must be performed in what is termed a *noisy*, *dynamic* and *non-monotonic* environment [64]. In other words, most information obtained from, and about, the patient under care can be suspect—and thus subject to revision, affecting the outcome of the delivery of care and payment for services. In addition, the plan and schedule of care for a patient is dynamic and is often subject to high volatility. A clinician may be scheduled to visit a patient in the home to deliver care, but the patient may not be home for a variety of reasons—thus forcing the clinician to adapt the care plan and reschedule the visit. Finally, a patient's medical condition may change significantly, causing the clinical team to re-evaluate and re-plan the treatment.
- The nature of many aspects of the clinical and financial workflows involves completing key tasks within pre-specified regulatory time windows. Missing these time windows—for example, in the submission of POC/485 forms—has a negative impact on the business. Furthermore, timing of events in the delivery and documentation of care, as well as in being paid for services rendered, can be interdependent across tasks and events. For instance, the time points for OASIS [73] events may be partially ordered but are sequentially time dependent.
- The execution of a home health enterprise's workflow involves all of these *interacting sub-problems* crossing the clinical space (in a multitude of clinical disciplines) as well as the financial space (covering the range of financial and administrative business functions). The results of clinical care, and its concomitant documentation, affect the financial transactions, and vise versa. With PPS, the nature of the regulatory constraints have become more restrictive in recent years on the business, in terms of the timing and payment amounts, for a large sector of the managed patient population. (PPS, or Prospective Payment System, is the claims processing and billing system for use with Medicare-based reimbursement of services provided by the CMS in the United States.)

In the deployment of IT solutions in many domains, acceptable solutions to these problems involve doing one of the following: (1) making simplifying assumptions to reduce the complexity of the application to be implemented; or, (2) identifying abstractions allowing the management of inherent complexity such that a flexible, extensible and conceptually simpler suite of applications can be devised. The application development discussed herein has sought to employ both strategies to obtain an aggressive solution—which is comprised of using agents to manage the compliance-driven lifecycle represented in the constituent lifecycles and connectivity between document artifacts moving through the domain.

Before doing so, however, we should make one additional statement about this application by way of example. We constructed a system for a set of workflows and business processes that did not yet exist. In other words, one of the requirements for this system at the outset of development was to not simply automate the existing paper-based procedures in use at the time the project started. Rather, the intent was to come up with new processes, supported by a well-founded clinical methodology, and build the system to support these new processes. This brings us to an important principle associated with the analysis methods and architecture patterns presented in this paper:

> **Principle #1:** A large part of the process of creating automated IT solutions involves doing the requisite business process definition such that there are appropriate manual procedures in place that the automated enterprise system can subsume and support. Furthermore, the creation and implementation of these processes must be carried out either before, or in parallel, with the systems development process.

As such, the focus of the IT systems development is on leveraging and magnifying the productivity and decision-making capacity of the various knowledge workers in the healthcare enterprise. Each of these workers plays a role in the completion of the various workflows required in operating the business, delivering the care, and getting payment for services. Therefore—in defining a conceptual model for the system—our task was to create an abstraction allowing the various users to effectively interact with the system to complete their designated workflow tasks. In addition, our objective was to find methods to assist these users, where possible, in managing the inherent complexity of their work environment. The system should, thus, address these concerns by providing the following services in the back-office:

- Facilitating coordination among workflow participants;
- Managing dependencies among workflow tasks;
- Tracking the critical time windows imposed by business and regulatory factors, and;
- Reporting timely information for steering the business.

At the outset, we wanted to have a means to measure healthcare worker productivity and the financial cost-reduction achieved through workflow automation.

This represents short-term, episodic data on the value of the methods presented. However, the longer-term effect, measured in terms of patient outcomes in a population of the elderly, for example, is outside the scope of the treatment given here.

3.4.3 Modeling domain workflow with agent-oriented lifecycles

As stated, the home health enterprise consists of a number of coordinated, interdependent workflows, which have traditionally been paper-based, but for which we automate using the system architecture developed in this chapter. In the short-term, we will not be able to eliminate the complete "paper trail" that exists and is still required by regulatory surveyors. However, we desire to support the effective management of these elements, or *artifacts*, of workflow in the back-office, and thus enable the healthcare knowledge workers to better manage the complexity of their work environment.

We now discuss a conceptual model defined to allow this objective to be met. We use the basic abstraction of the *artifact* and its *lifecycle*. In this, we recognize another important principle in the construction of enterprise applications:

> **Principle #2**: Interacting *artifacts*—and users interacting with artifacts through a browser-based user interface—can have the effect of chaining together a sequence of events and actions affecting the flow of real work through the enterprise. This flow can be affected in terms of what is stored in the system about the status, or *state*, of each corresponding real-world thing represented by the artifacts (such as documents, billings and the like). The flow can also be affected by the actions taken by a user to make changes to the underlying state of an artifact through the browser interface.

Here, we discuss the characteristics of the state-based lifecycle abstraction and its embodiment using software agents. We present how its use allows us to solve our problems (as stated in the previous section), and what descriptive elements we'll use to document this state-based behavior and the interactions between agents managing the artifacts, and between artifacts and end users. In the following sub-sections, we take a sampling of the identified domain artifacts, in turn, and develop the narrative of its underlying compliance-based lifecycle model.

3.4.3.1 Overview of artifacts and the state-based lifecycle

In the healthcare enterprise of interest, we are dealing with a number of things whose basic status changes over time. As a natural course of business, the statuses are of interest, but also the time sensitivity of the status changes. For example, a standard OASIS Assessment for a patient undergoes a series of ordered transformations over time, as clinicians and agency administrators act upon it. This series of ordered steps is referred to as a *lifecycle*, and the individual steps themselves are known as *states* in the lifecycle. Both are significant to healthcare knowledge workers, as they are used to track the movement of work through the enterprise, and are thus a very natural means of thinking about the elements, or "artifacts", of work.

More formally, a *state* is a stable, discrete state of existence for some artifact (such as an Assessment document) where certain policies, practices and activities apply to the artifact while it is in that state [8, 15, 16]. An example would be the "unsigned" state of an Assessment form, where certain rules apply to its handling that would differ from those that would apply once it has been "signed" by the authoring clinician. Here, we mean that a duly authorized clinician has either signed, or not signed, a document. When an authorized practitioner has signed a document, it is possible to move patient processing on to other activities in the process, which have their own stream of required documentation. A clinical document with a signature has special clinical significance, and is generally a requirement from a regulatory compliance standpoint.

It has been observed that a core set of artifacts in the enterprise have discrete states, through which they transition, from the time they are created until the point in the process where they are no longer referenced clinically. Furthermore, we observe that the ordering and sequencing of these states for a given artifact is *deterministic*. In other words, the set of possible state sequences for an artifact can be specified beforehand, as part of care planning, and can therefore be encoded and understood by agents acting in the system.

Finally, this state sequencing directly correlates to the workflow carried out on the artifact in the real world. For example, the real world activity of a patient clinical Assessment is reflected by an event indicating the activity has occurred, thus allowing those artifacts having this sensitivity to transition to new states. We build this sequencing into the system's underlying database structure, allowing agent-driven transactions to drive workflow through the enterprise as a result of state-changes among artifacts managed in the application. Agent-oriented document management has been investigated in a more general context in the literature [69].

There is a comprehensive set of artifacts having this behavioral characteristic of a state-based lifecycle in the healthcare enterprise. As shown in Figure 3.4, there are two broad categories of artifacts—those representing real world documents, *DocumentArtifacts*, and those representing other types of sequencing relations in the workflow, *RelationArtifacts*. The first category includes artifacts representing documents such as Assessments, Care Plans, and Visit Notes. The second category includes more abstract, "relational" notions in the clinical domain, such as Encounter (or Visit), Episode of Care, and Program Admission. The artifacts of both categories share the following basic characteristics:

- They are created by the system as a result of a specific creation event, either initiated by an end user through the browser interface or by actions taken by agents on behalf of other artifacts in the system. For example, when a back-office agent detects that a new Assessment form has been completed and signed for patient 'John Smith', the agent determines that a new Assessment artifact would need to be created by the system, being placed into the appropriate state.

- While cycling through their various states, agents carry out actions on behalf of artifacts, representing workflow in the enterprise. An action is an activity that must be performed, and either exists in the purview of the system or in the real world. If the specified action exists outside of the system, it implies that the action is some task to be performed by an end user playing a role in the workflow.
- In order to indicate to the system that the user has performed the action, the user must inform the agent managing the artifact instance through the user interface. For example, a valid action for a completed Assessment form is when an authorized clinician has signed it. If the clinician subsequently signs the hardcopy version of this document, the clinician or an administrator in the back-office makes note of this fact by an entry in a U/I dialogue box via a checkbox, for the given Assessment form, indicating that it has been signed. If status concerning the authorized review of this Assessment form isn't entered into the system within a prescribed time frame, the agent sends a reminder notice (in the form of a pop-up or email), followed by alerts to clinical supervisors.
- Specific actions are associated with specific states of an artifact agent's lifecycle. The user will be restricted from performing these actions in the system unless the artifact is in the appropriate state for such action to be taken. This notion of *state-based* access authorization is defined in addition to *role-based* access control, i.e., whether a user has sufficient privileges to carry out such actions on the type of artifact.
- Artifacts cycle through their various state sequences based on the occurrence of events to which they are sensitive while in a given state. Something can happen causing the artifact to change its state, referred to as an *event*. Lifecycle states are defined along with the events to which they are sensitive. The state behavior description indicates what the artifact is to do if the event is received. Generally, events cause state transitions. Once transitioned to a given state, other events would be generated to affect state transitions in agents for other types of artifacts.
- Most types of artifacts ultimately reach a "terminal" state, where further action on the artifact by the system is severely limited. In this terminal state, the system would generally limit access to the underlying stored document for viewing, reporting or archival purposes only. Often, regulatory guidelines dictate that documents cannot be destroyed once completed.
- Sometimes artifacts are forced into a state where they are replaced by a newly created artifact in the system. This is versioning, or "replay" of the artifact, where the original version is kept for historical purposes (usually required for regulatory reasons), although the new version is the one that is operated on in subsequent.

Artifacts are time-sensitive, in that they carry all information about timestamps as to when they entered a specific state in their lifecycle. It may be that only some entry dates of an artifact's states are significant in the lifecycle, in which case only those dates would be stored in the underlying database. The use of timestamps allows time point calculations to be performed. These are generally used in generating report *flow sheets* (such as those paper ones traditionally used in many healthcare agencies) and in calculating compliance timeout values.

The *DocumentArtifact* category of artifacts share many characteristics not held by *RelationArtifact* types, namely the following:

- All document instances in the system are created from a source template for that document category. Each source document template may have versions. Each template version may have its own lifecycle with a set of valid state transitions (such as "Active" and "Discontinued"). This state information associated with document templates might be used in the content distribution between the Back-office and an offline "point of care" (POC) device, such as a laptop or palmtop PC, used in the field—when such templates are cached locally.

Figure 3.4. Domain taxonomy of clinical lifecycle artifacts in the Post-acute care enterprise.

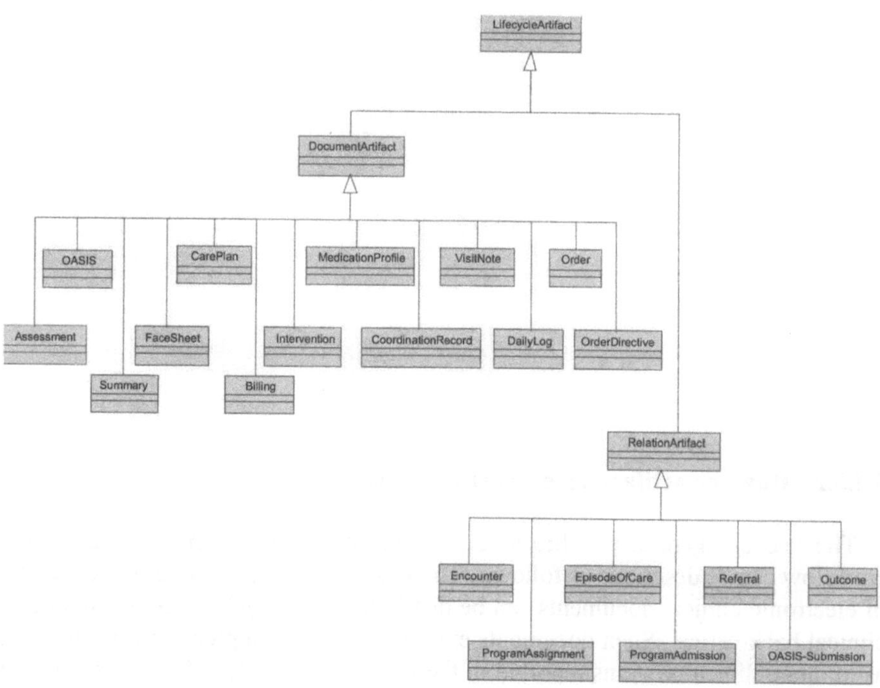

- All documents are of a given *category* and may also have a specific *type*. For example, Assessment document is the *category*, but SOC (start of care) Assessment would be the *type* of Assessment document.
- All documents have a *creator* (Author) as well as an *owner*. In addition, documents have *signatories*. Usually the author, a clinician, is a *signor*, whereas some document categories require additional signatures, such as from an agency supervisor and/or attending physician.
- Some document categories are defined such that they consist of document components, or *sub-documents*, which themselves may be treated as document *categories*. In other words, a document may be atomic, or it may be a compound artifact that can be decomposed into other compound or atomic document artifacts. Each component document category has its own state-based lifecycle, which may be implicitly embedded in the lifecycle of the compound document artifact.

Figure 3.5. UML Class diagram depicting the core semantic relations of the document artifact.

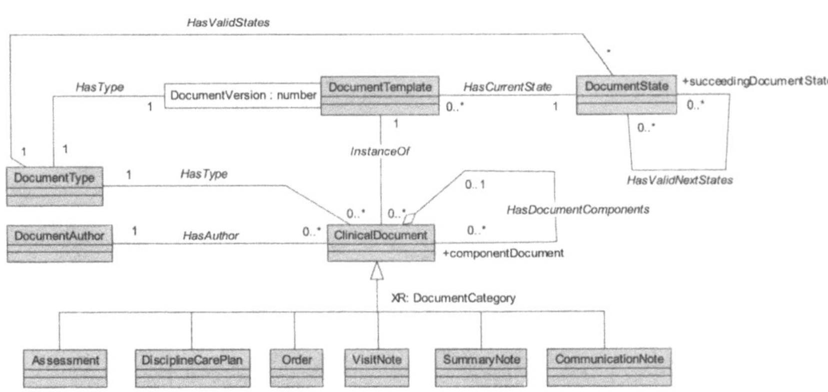

3.4.3.2 How the artifact agent works in practice

The use of agent-driven lifecycle artifacts in the management of document workflow can be described as follows. There is a means whereby actual renderings of electronic clinical documents can be distributed to a POC device or used in the clinical back-office. Such documents exist as templates, implemented using XML as in other clinical systems reported in the literature [21, 22, 23], and managed by other software components in the system. Our interest in this discussion is not what specific technologies are used or how the documents are rendered or stored but, rather, whether or not the system has a means to consistently manage document lifecycles regardless of form or location in the enterprise.

Each document *category* as depicted in Figure 3.4 has a collection of allowable state sequences constituting its lifecycle. The defined sequencing for a particular document is significant, in that it follows the workflow of the document—whether in electronic or paper form—as it moves through the enterprise. Each document created as a result of a clinician delivering and documenting patient care results in an instance of one of the document *artifacts* being created in the system. As the clinician and other healthcare staff act upon the real "hardcopy" document, the artifact instance's state information is updated to reflect the latest status of the real document. Sometimes the state transition can take place due to a triggering event, while other transitions may be initiated directly by an end user (either a clinician or data entry coordinator).

As the state of the document artifact is updated to reflect the current status of the real document, agents tied to the artifact are able to perform meaningful tasks on behalf of the users. For instance, the agent for the affected artifact may perform specific actions upon entering the new state, such as sending messages to instances of other artifact agents appropriately linked.

In addition, the artifact agent provides information indicating which User Interface functions are valid for a set of screens given the state of the current document. This allows the "graying out" (i.e., invalidating certain buttons in the browser interface from accepting input) of functions, so that invalid functions are not available to users when the artifact is in a particular state.

3.4.4 A state-based lifecycle example

In this section, we present an example of the agent lifecycle for artifacts in the home health domain discussed earlier. We present a subset of important artifacts and their respective lifecycles, discussing specific rules and constraints for each that are embodied in software using agents. We start in the order in which the document artifact instances are likely created as a result of a patient entering the sphere of care of the healthcare agency, flowing into the clinical care process. This order is shown in the business process model depicted in Figure 3.6. We present an overview of this clinical process, to set the stage for describing the example document artifacts, their state-based lifecycles, and how this state-based information is used to carry out workflow management using a set of agents.

3.4.4.1 Modeling detailed clinical workflow

As we saw in Figure 3.3, there is a component of the system associated with the *Intake* process. During *Intake*, a referral for a patient is received by the agency. A set of activities ensues to collect information on the patient regarding the referral, so that a decision can be made as whether to accept the referral or not. Factors such as insurance eligibility, geographical location, and homebound status are considered when making this decision.

If a patient referral is accepted by the agency, the patient still must be evaluated in order for staff to decide whether s/he will be admitted for care. The decision to admit a patient is based on additional factors not considered during evaluation of whether to accept or reject the referral. This invariably requires a visit be made by a duly certified clinician to the patient's home to assess the patient's status and the patient's propensity to benefit from a regimen of care provided by the agency.

Upon assessing the patient, the attending clinician decides whether the patient will be admitted for care in one or more of the Agency's programs of care. The clinician may decide that the patient could benefit from receiving care under multiple programs offered by the agency simultaneously. At this point, the patient is admitted for care, and care commences usually on this initial visit. By accepting the patient, the clinician responsible for assessing the patient sets in motion a number of required actions that must be responded to by different entities in the agency. Each of these actions is tracked by agents executing in the system according to specific state-based lifecycles—which we develop in this section for several artifacts. It is at this point that the "episode of care" with the patient begins.

One of the preconditions for delivering care to the patient is the authorization by the attending physician for care to be given. This authorization is provided as a set of orders for a plan of care, and may initially be given verbally as part of the referral. Once the clinician has made an initial assessment of the patient, s/he drafts a set of Orders, consisting of a number of directives, which must be signed by the physician in a manner consistent with the literature [19, 36]. There are several Order-related document types allowing this to be done, depending on when during the episode of care the clinician requests a signing of orders. Outstanding orders for a patient have a time horizon over which they are valid. Once this period expires, the patient must have new orders for care drafted, and s/he must be "recertified" for care in the programs to which s/he was admitted. Otherwise, the patient is discharged from the agency's care.

While the patient is actively receiving care, the clinician makes scheduled visits to the patient's home. As part of a clinical care delivery methodology [31, 34, 37], the clinician documents the care on a number of different document artifacts. Various types of *Assessment* documents are used to capture the status of the patient and his/her environment, depending on when during the episode of care the visit is being made and the assessment performed. The clinician prepares a *Care Plan* for the patient, which is updated frequently during the episode of care [34]. This care plan establishes the set of expected outcomes (or Goals) for the patient and the set of Interventions to be performed, along with their frequency and duration, during delivery of care.

Once care is delivered in accordance with a Care Plan previously drawn up for the patient, the specific care-related activities are duly documented on a *Visit Note*. The Visit Note's contents are generated from data garnered from the Assessment and the Care Plan. In addition, any procedures not covered under an existing physician's order must have an Order (such as a 485 or Supplemental Order) form completed. Finally, the attending clinician documents the visit on a Daily Log time sheet, which is used downstream for agency payroll and billing.

As mentioned, care is delivered for the course of the episode of care. For Medicare-related services in the US, this is 60 calendar days. After this time, the patient may be "recertified" for another "certification period" or discharged from the programs of care. Recertification consists of performing a comprehensive re-assessment of the patient, developing a new Care Plan, and obtaining a new set of signed Orders for the proposed plan of care. The delivery of patient care could also be interrupted by one of the following events: (1) transfer of the patient to an In-patient facility; (2) suspension of care because the patient is otherwise unavailable for care; or, (3) death of the patient. Each of these events affects the status of the program admission and its corresponding episode of care.

3.4.4.2 Artifacts of the Intake process

Figure 3.7 depicts the conceptual model for the key concepts and relations associated with managing lifecycles for artifacts in the Intake workflow. The principal hierarchy of relations exists between a Patient and one or more Referrals of the patient to the agency. A patient can be referred on many occasions, each of which may not be disjoint in time (in other words, one or more referrals may overlap in time).

Figure 3.6. IDEF0 dataflow model of the clinical process in the Home Health clinical domain.

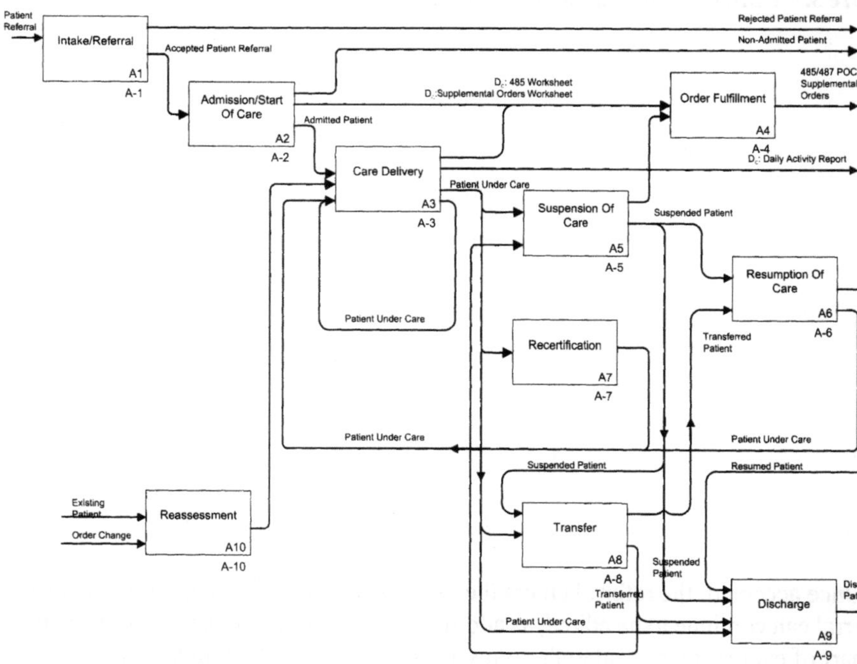

A given Referral, if accepted by the agency, results in one or more Program Assignments. As part of the same referral, a patient could be assigned for evaluation by clinicians in different programs of care. Each such program assignment may result in an Admission to that program, depending on the results of the clinical evaluation. Once admitted to one or more programs of care, a new Episode of Care is established for each Admission.

3.4.4.3 The Referral artifact lifecycle

A Referral artifact would be created at the time a new referral is entered into the system by an end user via an Intake screen. The specific browser screen sequence is not relevant to the development of this discussion. Suffice to say that, the user creates a new referral, resulting in one or more records being written to the database for the referral. A new Referral artifact should also be created, being initialized to the "*Incomplete*" state. The state transition diagram in Figure 3.8 shows the sequencing of states.

While the Referral artifact is in the "*Incomplete*" state, the referral information associated with the patient can be edited. The Intake process has a significant amount of patient information that must be collected as part of evaluating whether to accept the referral. Availability of the editing capability is exposed to the end user as an enabled button on a U/I screen. In addition, while in this state, the user can update the status of the patient referral to indicate that it is either accepted or rejected. Updating this status results in the Referral artifact transitioning from the Incomplete state to either the "*RejectedReferral*" or "*AcceptedReferral*" state.

Figure 3.7. UML Class diagram for the Intake process artifacts.

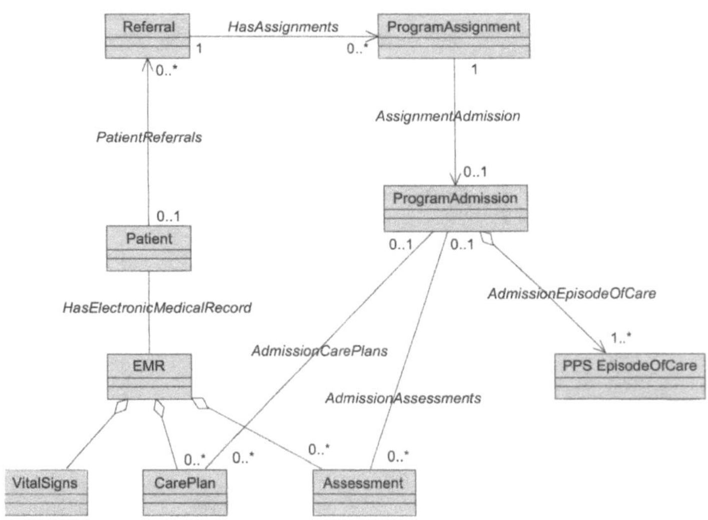

Once accepted, the referral enters the "*AcceptedReferral*" state. In this state, the referral can continue to be edited, as additional data must be collected for the patient as part of evaluating the patient's admissions status. Note that, in this state, the subsequently created *ProgramAssignment* artifact may also be "replayed" through the U/I (as discussed in the next paragraph). Alternately, if a referral is rejected, placing it in the *RejectedReferral* state, the referral cannot be operated on by the user other than for read-only viewing or reporting.

Figure 3.8. UML Statechart diagram for the Referral artifact lifecycle.

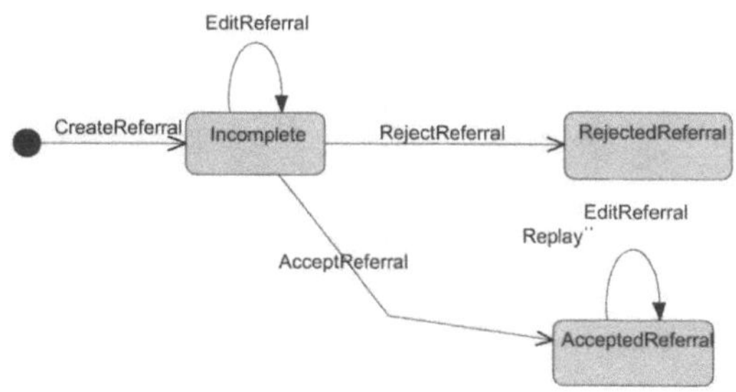

3.4.4.4 The Program Assignment artifact lifecycle

Once a patient referral is accepted into one or more of the agency's programs of care, new instances of *ProgramAssignment* artifacts are created—one for each program assignment made on behalf of the patient. When the Referral artifact enters its *"AcceptedReferral"* state, a message is sent by its agent, signaling the creation of the *ProgramAssignment* artifacts.

Note that we are not dictating how the program assignment process is performed or how it is exposed through the browser interface. However, the user must perform two actions in order for a *ProgramAssignment* artifact to be properly initialized. First, the user must indicate that a particular patient referral has been accepted (by clicking a check box in the U/I). Second, the user must indicate the specific program of care.

The lifecycle diagram is depicted in Figure 3.9 for the *ProgramAssignment* artifact. The event labeled as "*Link Referral to Program*" initiates creation of the artifact instance, placing it into the "*Undecided*" state. This indicates that it is not yet known whether the patient is to be admitted into the assigned program of care. While in this state, data can continue to be entered into the patient's medical record. In addition, the Referral artifact is automatically linked to the *ProgramAssignment* artifact.

Figure 3.9. UML Statechart diagram for the Program Assignment artifact lifecycle.

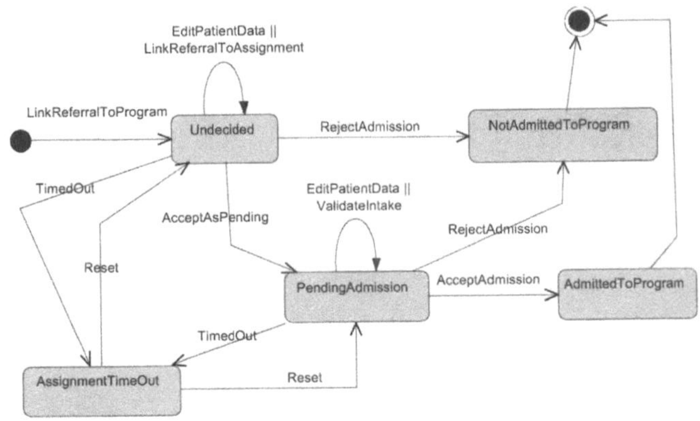

Finally, on entering the *"Undecided"* state, the responsible agent sets a "watchdog" timer for the given *ProgramAssignment* artifact. The timer is set up around the length of time that the assignment artifact can exist, not being either admitted or rejected for admission into the program. This time frame is significant, in that an assignment can't be held in either the *"Undecided"* or *"PendingAdmission"* states indefinitely. In fact, agencies have specific time limits on this length of time.

By supporting the setting of timers, the agents keep track of the bookkeeping associated with these time frames, alerting an Administrator when the time is about to be exceeded for a set of assigned referrals. Presumably, the agency staff would have some procedure to insure that appropriate action is taken—for example, making sure an Admissions visit is scheduled and Assessment of the patient's condition is performed. To facilitate this, the responsible agent sends a reminder to an assigned clinical staff member, such as the Intake Supervisor, indicating that the referral assignment is tardy in closure.

During the valid time window, before the timer is exceeded, the end user may change the status of the assignment to a "*PendingAdmission*" status, indicating the agency has scheduled a clinician to visit the patient's home to make an evaluation for admission. The user makes a status change through the browser, causing the associated *ProgramAssignment* artifact for the patient's referral to transition to its *"PendingAdmission"* state. Alternately, a decision could be made to reject the patient's admission into the program outright, without making an evaluation visit. In this case, the user would set the status through the browser to cause a transition to the *"NotAdmittedToProgram"* state.

While in the *"PendingAdmission"* state, patient data can continue to be entered and modified in the patient's medical record. Once the assignment has been "pended" and all patient data has been collected, the system validates the Intake data set. As long as the agent's timer doesn't expire, the user can indicate through the U/I that the admission has been either accepted or rejected for the program referral. If the user indicates that the admission is rejected, the corresponding artifact transitions to the *"NotAdmittedToProgram"* state. Conversely, if the user indicates that the patient has been admitted to care, it transitions to the *"AdmittedToProgram"* state. On entry to this state, the agent sends a message to create an instance of a *ProgramAdmission* artifact for the newly admitted patient.

3.4.4.5 The Program Admission artifact lifecycle

Figure 3.10 depicts the lifecycle model for the *ProgramAdmission* artifact. An instance is created on accepting the patient into the specified program of care. We have not stated how this information is communicated to the system, only that there is a U/I element communicating this information to the associated agent. It could be indirectly conveyed by the creation of a SOC Assessment for the current episode of care, but this treats program admission as a side effect of assessment, which is not the case. We opt to explicitly represent this by the interaction of multiple agents, given the workflow specification that is declaratively stored in the Plan database.

On creation of a *ProgramAdmission* artifact, the agent sets its state to "*Active*". In this state, the patient's record can be edited (which, by this point in the clinical process, the record has been downloaded to the offline POC device); a patient can be recertified to the same program of care; or, the patient can be transferred to another agency facility (such as when the patient changes location of residence).

If the patient is transferred to an Inpatient facility, such as occurs when the patient enters the hospital, the associated *ProgramAdmission* artifact must transition to the "*Hold*" state through some status update via the U/I. The artifact should remain in this state until one of the following events occurs:

- Patient is discharged from the hospital, such that the agency can resume the delivery of care, in which case the artifact transitions back the "*Active*" state.
- The program certification period expires while the patient is in *"Hold"* status, resulting in the automatic discharge of the patient from the current program admission ("*Discharged*" state).
- The patient moves away, or is otherwise transferred out of the service area for the agency, resulting in a discharge of the patient (the *"Discharged"* state).
- The patient dies while under the current admission to care, causing the transition to the *"Death"* state for the *ProgramAdmission*.
- The agent's timer around the *ProgramAdmission* expires, meaning that the time frame for which the Process Plan sets a tolerance for action has been exceeded. In this situation, the agent sends a *reminder* to the Case Manager or Supervisor indicating that the patient's Recertification date is approaching. If a subsequent timer expires, the agent escalates the *reminder* to an *alert* to the agency Supervisor.

Figure 3.10. UML Statechart diagram for the Program Admission artifact lifecycle.

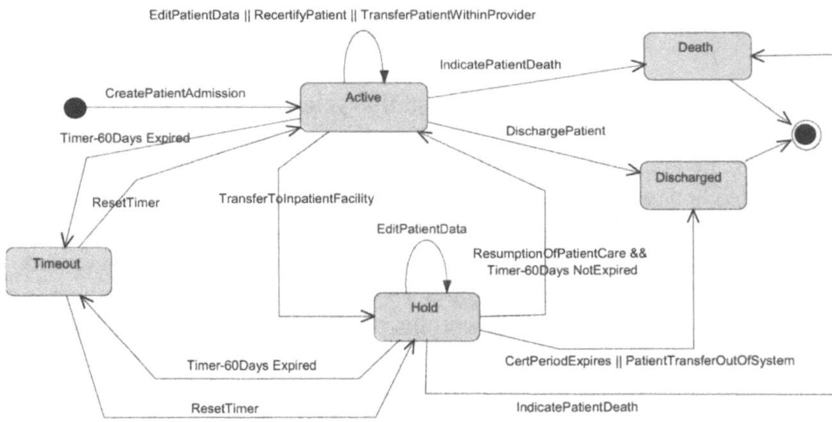

Note that the lifecycle allows for "cycling" through different sequences of states, as long as the patient has a valid admission status. The agent places the artifact in a terminal state when the patient either has died or is discharged. As before, if one of the process timeouts is exceeded, the agent resets timer and continues with its process directives.

3.4.4.6 The Episode of Care artifact lifecycle

There is an Episode of Care associated with the admission of a patient into a program of care. It used to be that these two concepts were the same. However, under the terms of Medicare's PPS payment scheme [71], the differing characteristics of the episode of care necessitate tracking it in the workflow with a separate lifecycle. As we mentioned, a given *ProgramAdmission* can have one or more *EpisodeOfCare* artifacts associated with it. Although we won't attempt to enumerate the reasons for this distinction in PPS, we simply present the required state behavior.

Figure 3.11 depicts the lifecycle for the *EpisodeOfCare* artifact. It has a similar set of state sequences as the *ProgramAdmission* artifact, with some differences. An instance of this artifact is created at the same time as the associated *ProgramAdmission* artifact--when the patient was admitted to the program of care. The *EpisodeOfCare* artifact is initialized into the *"ActiveEpisode"* state. While in this state, users may edit patient data, create new patient encounters (i.e., document visits to the patient's home) or transfer the patient to another agency. Note that, up until this point, new *PatientEncounter* artifact instances cannot be created; the end user would experience this in the U/I, as the browser buttons associated with a "New Encounter" would be disabled.

Figure 3.11. UML lifecycle diagram for the Episode of Care artifact.

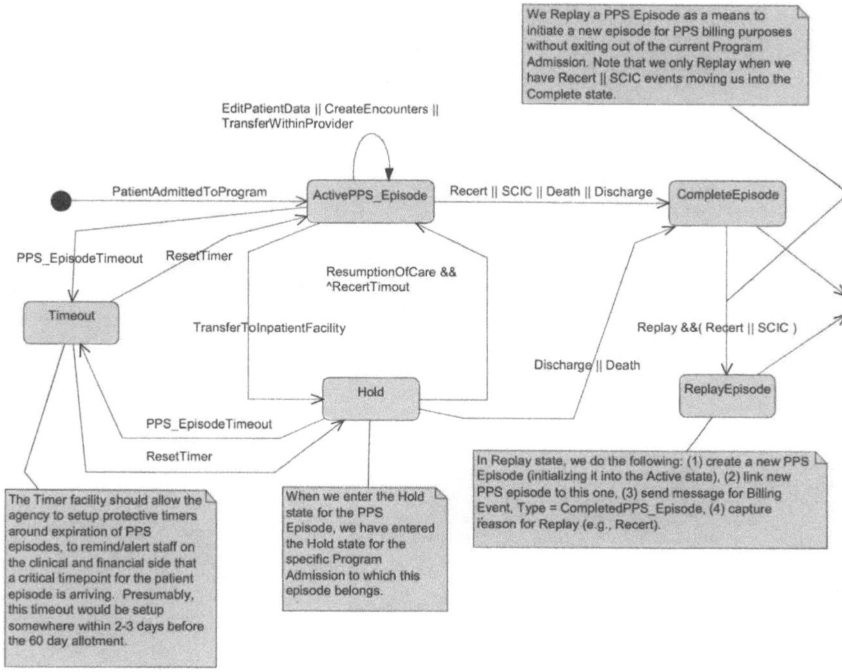

The artifact can transition between *"ActiveEpisode"* and *"CompleteEpisode"* states, based on the user indicating that the patient has been discharged, has died, has been recertified, or has had a significant change in his/her condition. These latter two conditions are what define the difference between a *ProgramAdmission* and an *EposideOfCare*. Specifically, if a patient is recertified after the initial duration for an episode of care (for example, for Medicare PPS in the US, this is 60 days), the episode is complete. In addition, if the clinician deems that the patient's condition has changed considerably from that which was originally assessed—which formed the basis for the plan of care—then the episode is prematurely terminated (i.e., set as being "complete"). In both cases, an additional transition would be made from the *"CompleteEpisode"* to *"ReplayEpisode"* state for the associated instance of this artifact type, indicating that the current episode of care is to be linked to a new one for the patient's current *ProgramAdmission*.

As is the case for the bracketing *ProgramAdmission* artifact instance, the *EpisodeOfCare* artifact can transition to the *"Hold"* state, indicating through the U/I that the patient has transferred to an Inpatient facility. While in this state, the artifact waits until an event indicating that the patient has been discharged or has died, the patient has resumed receiving care from this organization, or the timer has expired. Indicating the patient has died or been discharged is signaled by the bracketing *ProgramAdmission* artifact instance and its controlling agent, since it has more sensitivity to events concerning these conditions, and is within its area of responsibility.

Figure 3.12. UML Sequence diagram modeling interactions and lifecycle management among Intake agents.

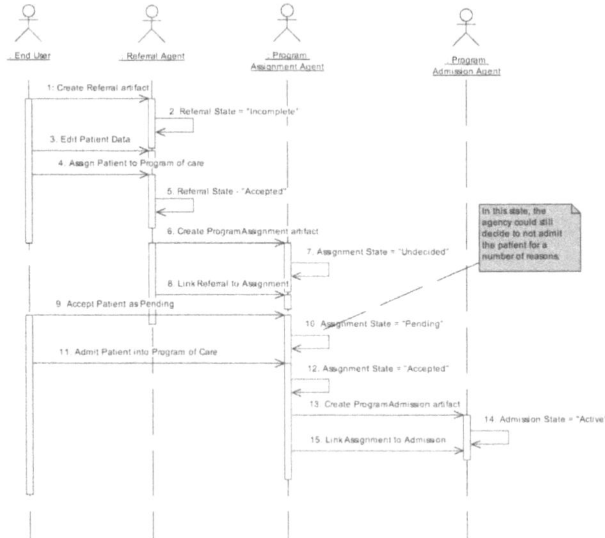

3.4.5 Managing system complexity using agent-oriented protocols

Figure 3.12 depicts the sequencing of the various agent types associated with the artifacts stored in the backend database. We should note that there are several different ways in which to realize this sequencing of workflow: (1) use transaction and triggering capabilities of a relational DBMS; or, (2) use capabilities of standard object frameworks. Having looked at both of these alternatives, we opted for an architecture that allowed the pieces of software to be loosely coupled to the underlying document and other "artifact" data in the database, yet more tightly bound in the execution of workflow protocols that were themselves stored in the database. The architecture relies heavily on the workflow specifications that are captured by an administrator to drive the behavior of the agents. The agents collaborate relative to artifacts based on the linkages defined in the protocol data.

Given the example of linking all the artifacts of the Intake process (cf. process boxes for Intake in Figures 3.3 and 3.6), we see that a number of software agents work together to "shepherd" the workflow in support of the clinical process. The agents in this application carry out the following functions: (1) insure the connectivity among artifacts that are related according to their workflow specification (stored as "meta-data" in the backend database); (2) insure that compliance constraints involving the completion of clinical documentation are met (to the degree that the agent can remind the clinical staff and alert the clinical supervisor when the process flow for a given patient is in danger of being non-compliant with guidelines).

What is important to note in the sequencing and coordination of Intake agent behaviors in Figure 3.12 is the coordination of state transitions of the various agents, and how they are causally linked between agents managing their associated lifecycle artifacts. The messaging that transpires between agents for the different artifacts is defined such that the workflow sequencing is mapped directly onto this interaction pattern. Instead of viewing the system behavior as a monolithic execution of different application modules, we developed an application model that conceptualizes the system as a collection of document agents that manage the lifecycles of many types of artifacts, and that these artifacts represent the "imprint" of the patient onto the higher-level clinical care lifecycle. The lifecycle of document artifacts in the system are monitored by agent instances, whose responsibility it is to insure that the various compliance guidelines specified in the protocol portion of the system are monitored. At the higher-layer of process execution, there are also instances of Process Agents that insure that the operation of the artifact lifecycles comply with broader functioning within the whole enterprise. We will leave the discussion of this type of agent for the next application we discuss.

3.5 A Disease Management Domain Example

In this section, we present a high-level overview of the problem space for using an agent-oriented clinical architecture as the basis for creating a disease management application, once again using compliance protocol-driven autonomous software agents [56]. As in the previous example, we discuss the architecture using UML diagrams of the principal elements of the architecture. These serve as an aid to succinctly capture the essential aspects of the system.

The concept embodied in this application of agents to healthcare is as follows: an appropriately designed lifelong summary, consumer-oriented, electronic health record can be augmented with intelligent agents to provide "active" and "collaborative" support to assist the consumer in maintaining their health, and in helping their physician to monitor their progress along a treatment plan. This objective is embodied in the HealthCompass™ e-Health portal, an application that remained on the web as a distinct entity from 1996 until 2001.

The specific tasks that comprise this system were: (1) create a suite of software agents that interact and collaborate among themselves to provide health advocacy functions on behalf of users, whose collective purpose is to promote desired changes in healthcare related behavior so as to enhance health and reduce the rate of negative outcomes in selected disease states; (2) develop an appropriate psychologically-based model of patient/consumer behavior, so that this model could be effectively represented as a set of goals and plan actions for the automated agents; and, (3) study the correlation between automated, personal health advocates for our service study population and their health outcomes, comparing against a control population of users that don't have benefit of agent-based health advocates and electronic health record at their disposal. We discuss the results of the first task in this chapter, namely, the agent-oriented architecture of the disease management component for HealthCompass.

3.5.1 Managed care and disease management infrastructure

In the universe of managed healthcare in the US, a constant tension exists between care providers and healthcare payers about the appropriate balance between quality of care and cost of care. This tension becomes acute when considering the subject of disease management. Managed Care Organizations (MCOs) have the objective of controlling costs through efficient allocation of healthcare resources by applying some "appropriate" kind and amount of resources to a disease process so that the best patient outcomes can be achieved. By maximizing outcomes through controlled interdiction, they wish to better manage spiraling costs. The care providers, on the other hand, have the objective of dispensing the highest quality care to their patients within the constraints imposed by current payer models.

However, both parties understand the relationship existing between patient behavior, outcomes and cost in the healthcare system, as borne out by various studies [73, 74, 75, 76, 77]. As patient outcomes for a particular disease (such as hypertension, diabetes or ischemia) worsen, the cost of care for the patient escalates. One recognized factor affecting medical outcomes for a large segment of the population with ambulatory diseases is the lack of patient compliance (or adherence) to medical treatment guidelines. Lack of adherence to treatment comes in many forms, such as (1) patients not taking medication properly; and, (2) patients not following prescribed guidelines for diet, exercise, weight control, and/or other habitual behaviors. Lack of adherence may also due to the patient not understanding the purpose and goals of therapy.

A central premise to our work is that outcomes need to improve in order to lower the cost of healthcare in our target population—namely, sponsored subscribers to the HealthCompass™ system. In order for outcomes to improve, patient treatment adherence rates need to improve. To improve compliance levels in the population, we created a "workflow" product set that ties together the development of treatment protocols by MCOs, the individualization of protocols into treatment plans for specific patients by care providers, and the monitoring of compliance to prescribed treatment by intelligent software agents in the HealthCompass environment. Compliance and outcomes data could presumably be collected and provided to MCOs for subsequent analysis in order to refine the protocols for increased effectiveness.

There are two points in the health care process ripe for exploration as places for mitigating spiraling health care costs, characteristic of the nature of healthcare in the US. These are at the boundaries of the healthcare system: (1) before the consumer enters the health care system or interacts with a care provider in that system; and, (2) after the consumer leaves the healthcare system, having had an "encounter" with a care provider. An "encounter" with the healthcare system includes any interaction that a consumer may have with some care provider, such as a physician (in private practice or public clinic), a hospital, an in-home nurse, a pharmacist, etc. Such encounters usually result in billing claims made by care providers to MCO health plans for which the consumer has policy coverage.

Figure 3.13. A view of a partitioned healthcare space into clinical management domains.

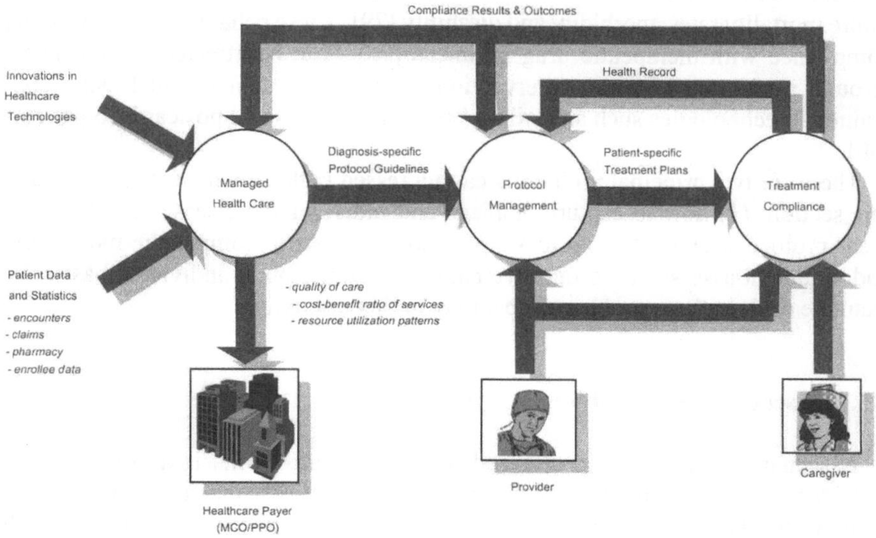

It has been reported that consumers make 70-80% of all decisions about their choices in healthcare before they enter the healthcare system [72]. This includes decisions about whether to seek care, what type of care to seek, which care provider to visit, and even whether to modify their "at-risk" behaviors in the face of chronic disease. When uninformed decisions are made by consumers about when and how to seek medical care, or about personal behavior towards health risks, inappropriate utilization of healthcare system resources—and thus, increased costs—often are the result.

Once a consumer leaves the health care system (i.e., is no longer under the watchful eye of a care provider), there is often a low rate of compliance with prescribed treatment [73]. Consumers who don't follow prescribed therapy (including not taking prescription medication, or not taking it through full term of prescription) evidence this lack of compliance. When uninformed decisions are made in regards to care follow-up, the ultimate impact can be higher costs—manifested through greater consumption of healthcare resources "downstream" during later stages of a disease state.

This increased consumer-side cost of healthcare is borne directly by Managed Care Organizations. This cost is indirectly passed on to employers (who often provide health coverage as part of non-wage compensation to their employees), to employees themselves (as co-payments, deductibles and reduced direct wage compensation due to increased cost of insurance coverage) and to consumers of goods and services (because goods and service providers employing workers covered under the managed care health plans pass along these costs in the form of higher prices to the economy at large). This is a logical and common sense relationship, easily comprehended by the general public: if you can limit inappropriate consumption--and thus the cost--of healthcare, individual consumers and the whole economy will benefit.

It has been reported in literature that certain consumer health behaviors predict future mortality rates, morbidity and disability [79]. These behaviors—for example, compliance with therapeutic drug regimens [73]—can be affected in consumers through a program of active intervention, having been demonstrated using conventional technologies such as mailing "reminder" letters and postcards to patients [80].

There are two principal problem areas addressed in the architecture presented in this section: (1) how to capture, manage and individualize disease-specific treatment protocols; and, (2) how to support disease-specific compliance monitoring and treatment assessment to improve patient outcomes on an individual basis. We examine each of these problems separately in this discussion.

3.5.2 A scenario with multi-agent systems

A scenario of how an agent-based health advocate works is as follows: We consider a care guideline for hypertension, a chronic disease that affects millions of Americans. The agent reads data in the healthcare consumer's longitudinal health record, locating his/her status on the care guideline. If there are nodes in the care guideline that have not been completed, an agent will email a notice to the user reminding them to complete the care node, based on a compliance timeline stored for the care guidelines protocol in the system.

A specific example of an "unvisited" care node occurs when a patient with hypertension, being treated with a diuretic, has not had a potassium level taken during the time frame specified in the care guideline. On expiration of a timer, without a notice by the user otherwise, the agent would email a reminder to the user, requesting confirmation that the user read the email reminder and has complied with the request for a potassium value. If there is no confirmation, the frequency of email reminders increases. If confirmation is still not received, the agent then sends a regular mail reminder, finally alerting the physician responsible for the patient.

Figure 3.14 depicts the architecture of the Treatment Compliance Monitoring component of the HealthCompass infrastructure, which is similar in scope and function to that developed for CareCompass, described earlier. The four sets of numbered actions show the flow of activity in the process of monitoring compliance for a prescribed medication. A clinician or physician would create a Treatment Plan through a tool set in the Plan Individualization module. Once the treatment plan is specified, a compliance agent would have the necessary direction needed to monitor compliance of various elements of the plan. There are specific types of agent for each type of compliance objectives contained in the Treatment Plan. The agents use the plan's elements to define its compliance monitoring activities. Most activities follow the pattern of checking for data in their patient's health record against the contents of the plan.

Over time, it is likely that a subset of consumers with hypertension, who are using the system, will go on to have a negative outcome (e.g., a stroke). Studying the correlation of specified agent characteristics with negative and positive outcomes in hypertension to further develop and strengthen the agent characteristics most correlated with positive outcomes (i.e., the lack of stroke, in hypertension) is outside of the scope of the methodology and architecture discussed in this chapter. This is the subject of ongoing research.

Figure 3.14. Depiction of the disease management system and its principal user roles.

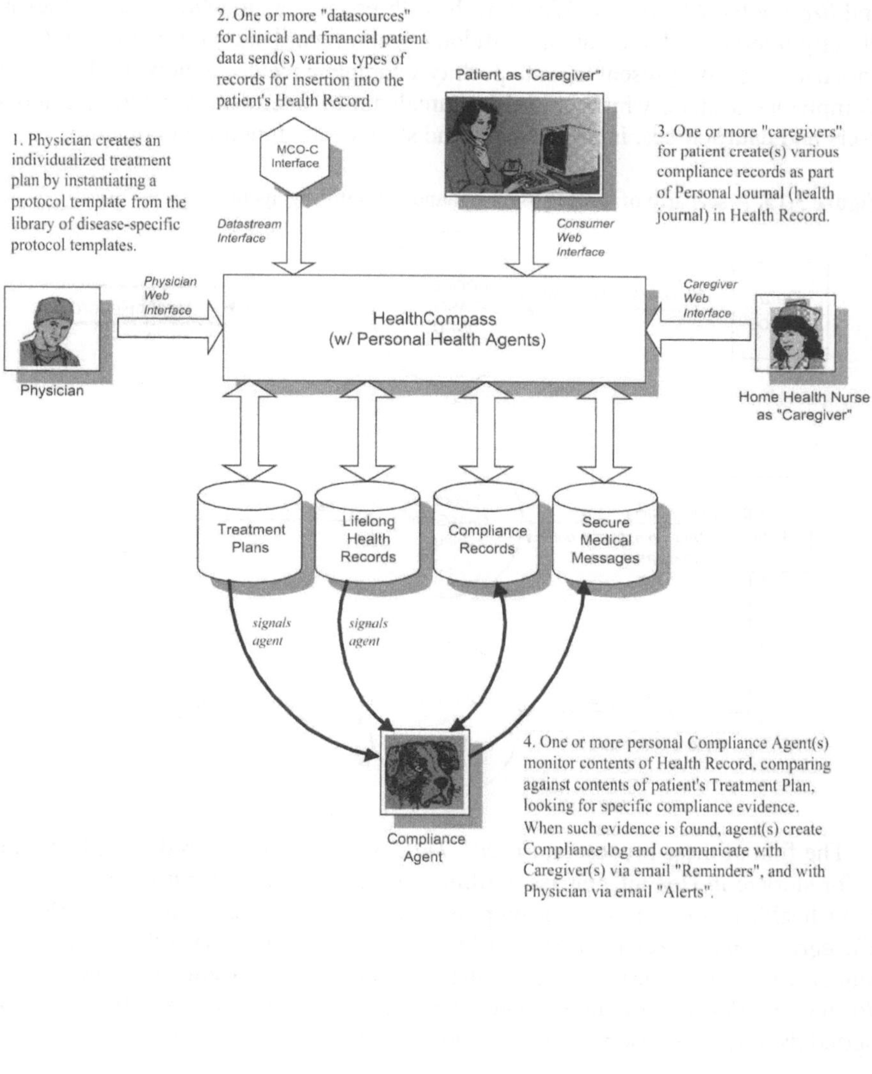

3.5.3 Transaction analysis for identifying agent responsibilities

Up to this point in our analysis, we have not made any statement about where the intelligent agents are located, or what specific tasks they perform. We now begin thinking about this part of the system's functionality. As we "peel" the layers of the system apart, working from outside to inside, the presence or absence of needed agent functionality for each transaction process will become clear. We walk through this process for one specific type of agent in the disease management system.

In Figure 3.15, we see three transactions (or "processes", in the parlance of the Data Flow method [8, 15]): *Process Data Source Input, Process Caregiver Input* and *Browse Health Record.* We show these three grouped together because they all directly interact with the patient's lifelong health record stored in the HealthCompass database. We present them to portray a complete picture of how the Treatment Compliance system, which is itself an amalgam of interactions between external users and data sources, internal agents and stored data, functions in practice.

Figure 3.15. A scenario of the use of compliance monitoring agents.

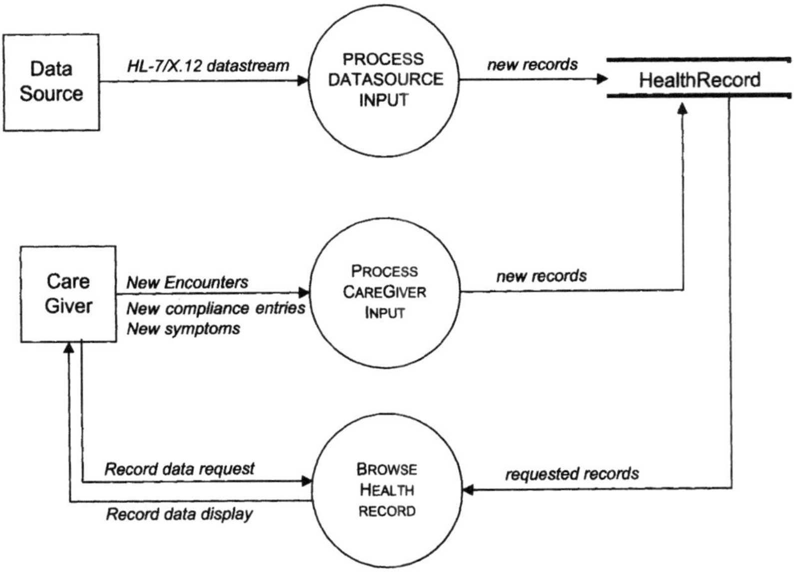

The first of these processes, *Process Data Source Input,* takes data and prepares it for storage in HealthCompass, writing new record entries for insertion into lifelong health records of HealthCompass subscriber members. Similarly, *Process Caregiver Input* takes data entered by a subscriber via the HealthCompass consumer web page interface and creates new health record entries. The process *Browse Health Record* simply notes that there is a means to view this newly inserted data by those users who have appropriate access privileges.

What is relevant to our consideration of these HealthCompass-defined processes is how they are augmented in the Treatment Compliance Monitoring module. For both *Process Data Source Input* and *Process Caregiver Input*, agents notice that new health record entries of particular types being placed into a specific consumer-patient's health record. In other words, the fact that new records are present must cause certain other transactions to take place. This implies some means to "wake up" agents to look at new data when that data becomes available. The second thing to note, regarding the *Process Caregiver Input* process, is that we are focusing on those HealthCompass subscribers playing the role of "caregiver" in the context of post-visit treatment compliance.

The figure below shows the principal transaction associated with each type of compliance monitoring agent. Each category of monitoring agent uses its own unique information sources in the *Compliance Record* and *Compliance Plan* data structures for the healthcare worker. However, all agent categories share the same general pattern of behavior, described as follows.

Figure 3.16. Essential data flow diagram for general form of a compliance agent.

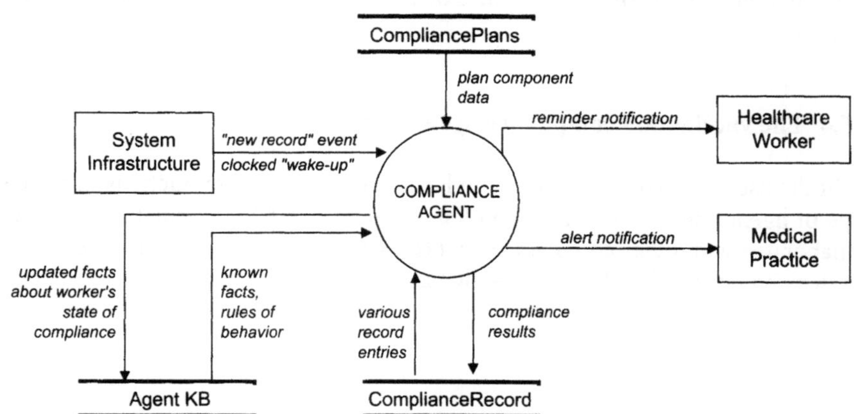

The system provides some event triggering mechanism, indicating that new data has been placed into the *Compliance Record* or into the *Compliance Plan* for a specific healthcare consumer. The type of record entry and content of the entry must be examined to determine whether the event is a type recognized and claimed by any of the agents currently attached to the worker. A special service-oriented agent, known as the *Activity Monitoring Agent* (AMA) performs this checking activity. The AMA agent will send a message to "start" or "wake up" the appropriate compliance agent that might be interested in the new compliance record or compliance plan entry for its healthcare worker.

Once activated, the specific monitoring agent would evaluate the information for itself to see if it is of interest. The agent determines whether new data is of interest based on the type of compliance record or compliance plan entry. For example, a given patient's vaccination compliance agent (VCA) would be interested in entries in the *Compliance Plan* related to vaccination requirements, created by the physician through a browser interface. It also evaluates where the subject currently resides on the vaccination guideline, as defined by their specific *Compliance Plan* record. Once relevance is established, the agent would evaluate the data and compare it to target information contained in the plan.

The agent retrieves its instructions, evaluates its possible actions, and selects its decision criteria from its own database of facts and rules. The facts component of an agent's knowledge base represents its current understanding of its sphere of interest and responsibility (generally, the state of the "subject" and his/her whereabouts on the particular "node" of the compliance plan). Its rules define the limits of what the agent can conclude from the data sources, and provide direction for its actions based on new information it derives as a result of "ruminating" over the facts it has stored.

As a result of the agent's actions, one of the following will happen: (1) new information is written into its internal facts base; (2) new information is written into the *Compliance Record* database; or (3) notification messages are initiated through an appropriate "mediating" interface (such as through a pager or email), or through corollary data generated for display on a dynamic page, whose URL is to be passed to a managing physician or compliance officer for the disease management medical practice.

3.5.4 The vaccination compliance agent example

In the use case shown below, we indicate the individual transactions in which a type of agent, the Vaccination Compliance Agent (VCA), participates. The VCA collaborates with other compliance agents, as well as agents that provide specific services, in performing these transactions.

Figure 3.17. Use-case diagram for compliance agents.

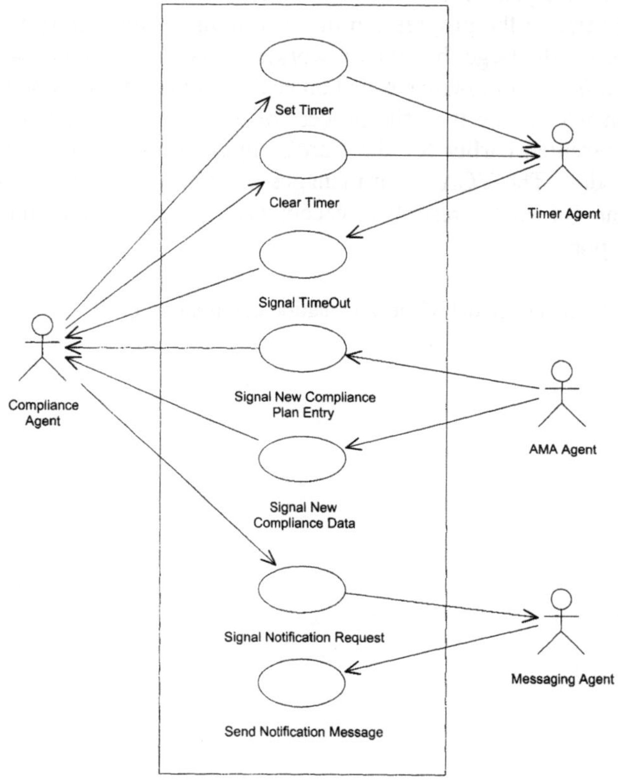

The first three Use cases (the "ovals" in the figure) involve interactions between the VCA agent and a Timer agent. The Timer agent uses system timers to control the length of time that the VCA agent spends waiting for compliance input from the healthcare consumer, caregiver or clinician. This mechanism allows the VCA agent to take specific actions when anticipated data fails to arrive within prescribed time limits. This time limit is to be specified by the managing physician or compliance officer for the medical practice, and would be input into the healthcare worker's individualized compliance plan for each prescribed vaccination. Each of the following transactions—*SetTimer*, *ClearTimer*, and *TimeOut*—requires a "handshaking" protocol between the VCA and Timer agents, the details of which are not presented here. The next three use-case transactions involve interaction between the VCA agent and the AMA agent. The AMA agent is alerted to events occurring in the system environment by other application processes, and has responsibility of determining which agents have interest in these events, and forwarding appropriate information to them.

3.5.4.1 A state-based model for prescribed vaccination

During our analysis of the VCA agent, it was observed that the agent's actions were closely tied to the progression of a given vaccination entry within the Compliance Plan for the target healthcare worker or patient. In other words, the agent follows a *Subject's* compliance based on each vaccination that s/he is prescribed to take, and on where s/he is in the process of having it administered. As with the examples presented earlier for the CareCompass system, we define this using a lifecycle model. The VCA agent manages a collection of *PrescribedVaccination* artifacts, one for each prescribed vaccination record written into the subject's compliance plan.

Figure 3.18. Lifecycle model of the vaccination compliance agent.

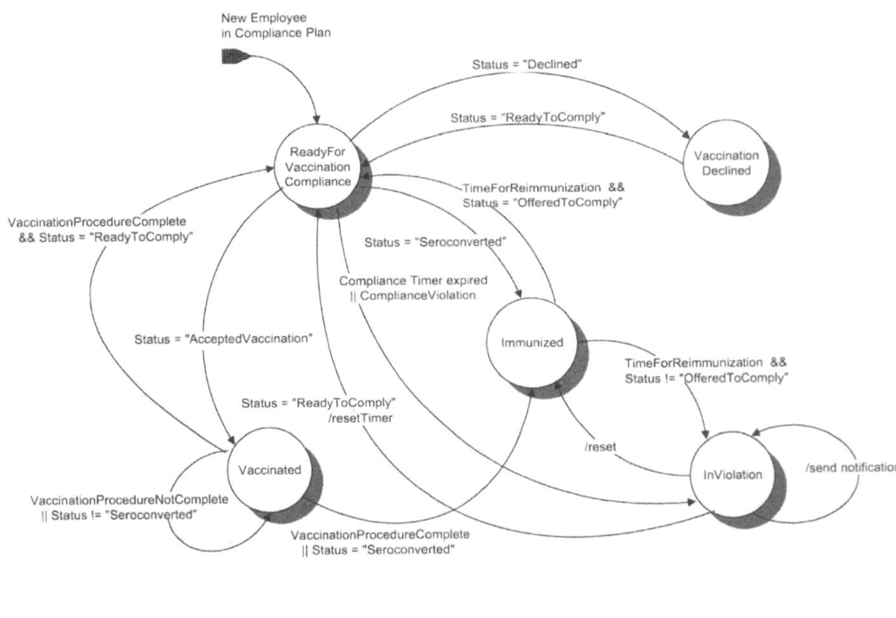

Note that, for this particular compliance management task, we could be carrying out monitoring on behalf of a patient or a clinical worker in a healthcare enterprise; the general structure of compliance monitoring follows the same pattern, regardless of who is playing the role of compliance *Subject*. The lifecycle for the *PrescribedVaccination* object used by the VCA agent is shown in the Figure 3.18, depicted as a state transition diagram [8, 15]. When the managing physician or compliance officer for the medical practice prescribes a vaccination for each new employee or patient, and enters it as a record in the subject's *Compliance Plan*, the event causes the AMA agent to signal the worker's VCA agent. The VCA agent creates a new *PrescribedVaccination* artifact for this new *Compliance Plan* entry, placing the artifact in the initial "*Ready*" state. While in this state, the agent sets a timer to "remember" the vaccination timeout period specified in the *Compliance Plan* entry while it waits for a new entry in the subject's *Compliance Record* indicating the vaccination has been performed.

3.5.4.2 Interaction scenario for the vaccination compliance agent

The vaccination compliance agent performs several different activities to check the patient's compliance to prescribed regimen defined according to compliance guidelines. Here, we examine one of these scenarios in detail and illustrate the agent protocol using a sequence diagram.

Figure 3.19. High-level sequence diagram for the vaccination compliance protocol.

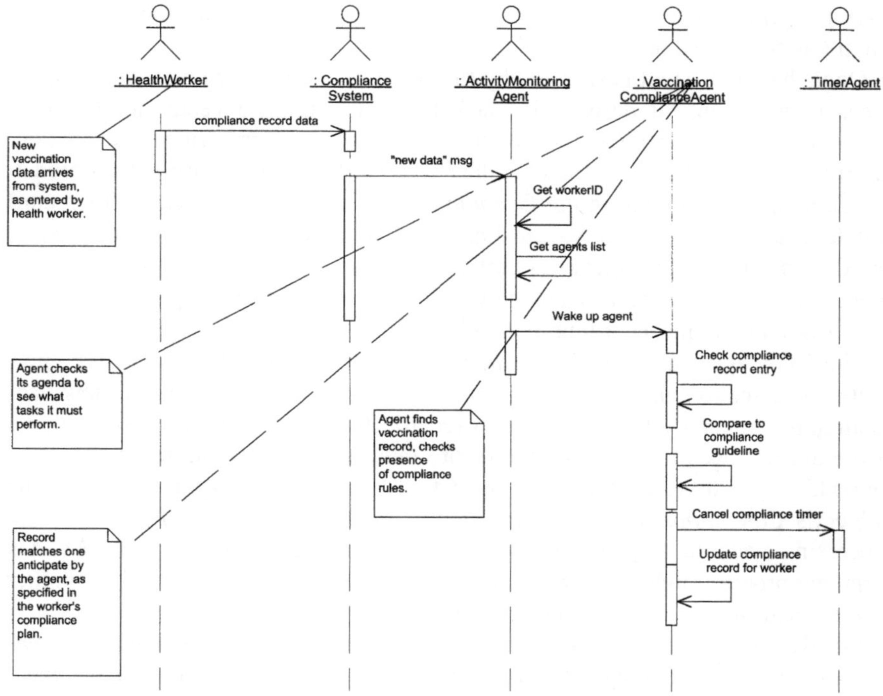

The sequence diagram graphically depicts the ordered sequence of activities transpiring between the agents in the system and the *Subject*. Along the top of these diagrams are listed the entities involved in the scenario. This usually includes one or more categories of intelligent agents. Time flows along the vertical lines dropping from the box representing each entity. The action on these vertical lines may involve a single entity or may involve one entity interacting with one or more other entities in the system. These interactions are depicted in the figure by the use of horizontal lines, with an arrow and text label indicating the nature of the communication.

3.5.4.3 Vaccination compliance checking

One of the key responsibilities of the VCA is to monitor vaccination compliance, in that the *Subject* has the appropriate vaccinations (such as for Hepatitis B or the latest strain of Influenza). For compliance checking, a vaccination entry is written into the worker's *Compliance Record* in the database, which would also signal the activity monitoring agent (AMA) that new record data has been written. The diagram shows that the data source provides a data record for the *Subject* to the system, which writes the data and signals AMA. The AMA agent gets the *Subject's* ID and determines the record type of new data, and uses this information to select the appropriate agents to wake up. For new vaccination records, the AMA will select the patient's VCA to be activated. The VCA agent then attempts to match the new vaccination record with any of its currently active vaccinations for the patient. If it finds a match, it notes this in the *Compliance Record*, then signaling the AMA agent that it has completed its current task.

Once the VCA agent is signaled by the AMA agent, it determines what tasks it needs to work on. It derives this task list from the state vector for the *PrescribedVaccination* artifact associated with the current prescribed vaccination. Information about the current state of the *PrescribedVaccination* artifact is stored in the *Compliance Plan* and in the *Compliance Record* for the *Subject.* The record maintains a persistent log of vaccination compliance actions that have been noted, based on prior tasks the agent has performed. In the current discussion, the VCA agent is interested in whether any new vaccination records correspond to specific ones it is anticipating according to the plan.

The VCA agent uses the *PrescribedVaccination* artifact of each "active" prescribed vaccination entry in the *Compliance Plan* for matching against new vaccination records placed in the *Subject's* record. In this scenario, we assume that a new entry has been inserted into the record indicating a vaccination has been performed. Using its rules, the VCA agent finds a match and logs the event in the Subject's *Compliance Record.* This completes the VCA's tasks for the current processing cycle, so it signals the AMA that it is finished. At this point, the MCA's computer process might either be put to sleep until reawakened by arrival of another external data stream of health record entries.

Finally, in the event of a match, the VCA agent writes an entry into the *Compliance Record*, containing the following: (1) that a vaccination compliance event has occurred, (2) the identity of the vaccination (given either by its batch number and NDC drug code) and, (3) the compliance date.

3.5.4.4 Timer setting and timeout checking

At certain points, the AMA awakens the VCA to process one of the "timeout" events specified for the given vaccination in the *Compliance Plan*. A "timeout" is simply another type of event anticipated by the agent, set up around actions defined in the plan, to allow it to take its own default actions when something it expects doesn't occur within a prescribed amount of time.

A separate timer agent carries out timer management. This agent handles initializing and resetting the timers. When a timer expires, the timer agent signals the AMA agent, which determines the appropriate agent to wake up. The AMA wakes up the VCA agent for a timeout event when no vaccination record has been written into the worker's *Compliance Record* within the allotted time frame that matches the anticipated vaccination from the *Compliance Plan* entry.

Given either scenario, the VCA agent responds by sending either a *reminder* or *alert* message indicating a compliance violation. For example, in the event of a vaccination timeout, a reminder message is first sent to the *Subject*, instructing him/her to complete the vaccination within a certain time frame. On the other hand, if a specified *Reminder Count* threshold in the plan is exceeded, the VCA agent sends an *alert* message to the physician (or the assigned compliance officer in the medical practice) indicating that it has not received information on the vaccination. The physician or compliance officer may choose to take action by making a more direct inquiry into the *Subject's* follow-up actions.

3.6 Discussion of the Architecture and its Performance

In previous sections, we have presented two example applications of this approach to modeling and analysis of complex workflow applications in healthcare using compliance agents managing artifact lifecycles. The first system, the CareCompass™ clinical application, has been deployed since 1999, and has been operating in over 300 home health agencies across the United States. The HealthCompass application was an e-Health portal operating on the Internet from 1996 until 2001.

One of the principal tenets of the approach discussed in this chapter is the separation of the analysis and architectural formulation of the system solution from any consideration of its implementation. It should be noted that the HealthCompass and CareCompass systems have been implemented using a combination of Microsoft technologies, according to methods for using Microsoft tools, platforms and technologies. However, later releases of the HealthCompass system have been implemented using Java and other commercially available middleware and web development platforms.

The CareCompass system is implemented as a multi-tiered, web-enabled client-server Intranet system. There are different tiers of the system, corresponding to resources at the level of the enterprise (a collection of post-acute care facilities), the business unit (a specific care facility), the front office of a care facility, and the point of care (POC) terminals used by clinicians during patient encounters. The terminals employed include desktop PCs used in the facility, laptops used by the clinicians in the field, and palmtop computers being prototyped in the field.

For most encounter and intervention activities, the clinicians may be using the document entry portions of the application in an off-line mode, capturing data that is stored locally to their POC device. Once they return to the office, they are able to connect to the servers and upload the new/modified documents in a set of transactions. It is against these centrally stored documents that the lifecycle compliance agents execute. Implemented as a set of Java servlets, the agents are enabled using database triggers that are fired on insertion or update to the clinical document database. Some transactions are carried out against the document store, while others are carried out against the patient record.

Figure 3.20. Distributed multi-tiered architecture for the CareCompass clinical system.

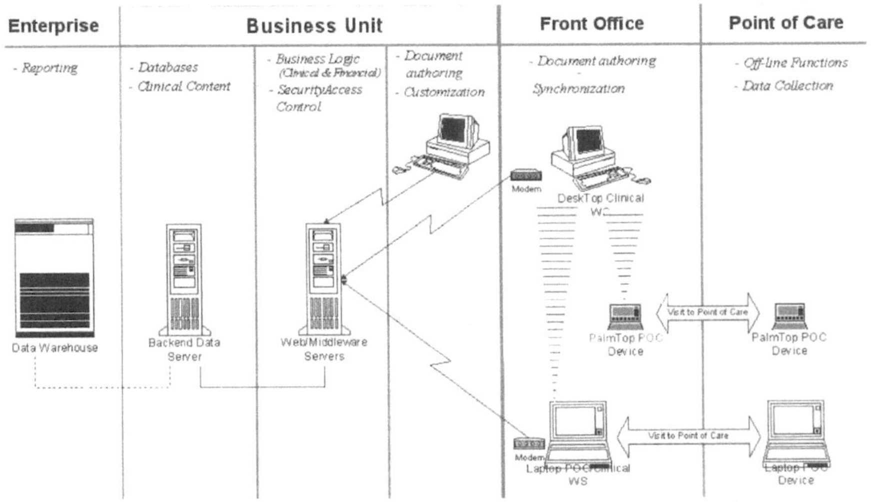

Figure 3.21. Screen for the assesment module in the CareCompass system.

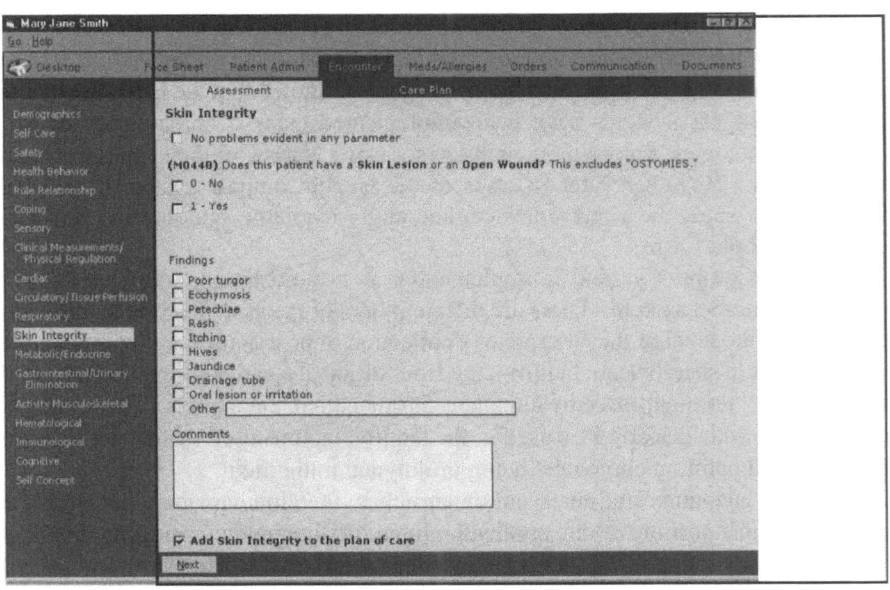

A sample browser screen shot shows the type of interface available to a clinician creating a new artifact instance of an Assessment document. The agents were not programmed to react to specific data within a document artifact, as the target population of clinicians was not comfortable with giving this level of capability to the agents. However, they do follow the lifecycles of document artifacts as a whole, issuing reminders and alerts to Clinicians and Administrators alike. The agents are interested in specific compliance behaviors in regards to completion time frames on various activities within the care processes, as dictated by regulatory agencies that are charged with oversight and payment for services.

The basic structure and flow of document lifecycles are the principal means of organizing agents in the CareCompass system, whereas the set of specific compliance events defined according to a treatment plan is the means for agent organization in HealthCompass. The performance assessment of the systems involved using basic measurements of application load, transaction throughput, and application response time for a number of different operation scenarios. This is conventional practice for client-server systems. However, an additional element in this analysis had to do with the impact of a large number of agent-oriented servlets executing on the servers, accessing the various databases to obtain document information, and accessing patient data and compliance plan data for determining their operation behavior at any given time. Here is where the architecture required the leverage of the particular technology being used in order to provide runtime optimization.

The JAT (Java Agent Toolkit) and other tools used to construct the agents had to be tuned to work with the JDBC programming interface due to the structure of transactions imposed by the database designers. We consider the effective integration of lightweight agents with relational DBMS environments as an ongoing area of study. It was observed that tighter coupling of the agents to the database, through the use of stored procedures and triggers (thus partitioning some agent functionality into the DBMS) improved performance considerably. However, there are limits to the number of agents that can effectively be executed, as the DBMS transaction processing capability becomes the limiting bottleneck. Care was needed when considering the workload for a given server, and caching of data records in the underlying object system became a means of dealing with the bottleneck.

It should be noted that these extensions to the CareCompass and HealthCompass applications were not run in a day-to-day production environment. Agent-oriented techniques require more study in order for that to happen in a live healthcare environment in the ways in which we seek to employ them. The critical question is whether the use of agents has any effect on quality of care and, by implication, the subsequent outcomes in a patient population. It is known that, for the home health environment, compliance on meeting the process guidelines for turning in paperwork to payers with regulatory oversight improves significantly. Further study is needed to correlate the system performance with care guidelines and outcomes. Given the nature of clinical data processing, such studies will likely be required before healthcare organizations will accept the perceived risk of using agent-based applications.

3.7 Chapter Summary

In this chapter, we have presented a method for the analysis and architecture of clinical systems based on the principle of agent-oriented design using state-based compliance lifecycles. We presented the method in terms of modeling two different clinical domain applications, illustrating the procedure by discussing design models of portions of these applications. We also discussed this type of system in terms of an architectural pattern for use in the construction of enterprise-wide workflow applications, using the two examples of this workflow pattern—clinical document-based workflow in a post-acute care facility and treatment record-based workflow in a disease management environment. Although the direct application of our approach has been in predominately nursing-driven workflow domains, we believe the method and its accompanying architecture is applicable in any clinical care domain where the characteristics of the problem fit the method and architecture pattern. The work presented in this chapter was carried out over a five-year period, covering two different product development life cycles for the applications.

One of the principal benefits of the approach presented in this chapter is that it is possible to reuse this approach—the analytical methods and architecture pattern—to solve problems in a wide variety of problem domains, where the underlying business processes for the enterprise follow this model. The model was originally created for the disease management application, was extended for the post-acute care application, and then re-applied to an extended version of the original application.

It turns out that there are many such problem domains—both within and outside of healthcare—that can benefit from this agent-based, compliance-driven workflow model. As we demonstrated, this basic architecture for organizing workflow compliance was done in terms of software agents that managed some collection of domain artifacts. We are currently examining the use of this approach in other clinical domains, and will be evaluating the benefits of reuse across enterprise applications at a much high-level of abstraction. Furthermore, we will also be examining the logical independence of the architecture from its implementation, to measure how such decoupling allows for the faster construction of enterprise-wide business applications addressing this type of lifecycle-based workflow problem.

3.8 Acknowledgements

We gratefully acknowledge the cooperation and support of Florida Hospital, Sunbelt Home Health Care, and the Adventist Healthcare System of Orlando, Florida, HealthMagic, Inc., and the Center for Information Systems, University of South Carolina, in the research and reporting during the five years in which the projects reported in this chapter were active, without which this work could not have been carried out. The following individuals are acknowledged for their contributions to the work reported in this chapter: Nelson Hazeltine, Calvin Wiese, Fred Druseikis, PhD, Ken Armstrong, MD, Ronald Lankford, MD, Michael Huhns,

PhD, Prof. Ronald D. Bonnell, John Morrell, PhD, Lynne Stogner, RN, Lisa Cook, RN, Donna Murphy, RN, Caroline Murphy, RN, Patrice A. Cruise, RN, Ruth Irwin, RN, Don Dinkel, Mark Mauldin, Joel Johnston, Joe Duty, Mike Williamson, Jon Harley, Dave Kythe, Gail McFaddin, MPH, and Sonya D. Rankin, RN.

Literature

1. Pratt, W., Reddy, M.C. , McDonald, D.W., Tarczy-Hornoch, P., and Gennari, J.H.: Incorporating ideas from computer-supported cooperative work. J Biomed Inform 37 (2004) 128-137.
2. Lenz, R., Elstner, T., Siegele, H., and Kuhn, K.: A practical approach to process support in health information systems. J Am Inform Assoc. 9 (2002) 571-585.
3. vander Aalst, W., and van Hee, K.: Workflow management: models, methods, and systems. Cambridge, MA, MIT Press, 2004.
4. Sharp, A., and McDermott, P.: Workflow modeling: tools for process improvement and application development. Artech House Publishers, 2001.
5. Marinescu, D.: Internet-based workflow management: toward a semantic web. New York, John Wiley and Sons, 2002.
6. Cardoso, J. and Sheth, A.: Semantic e-workflow composition. Journal of Intelligent Information Systems. 21,3 (2003) 191-225.
7. Marca, D., and McGowan, C.: IDEF0/SADT business process and enterprise modeling. Eclectic Solutions Corp. 1993.
8. Edwards, K.:Real-time structured methods–system analysis. John Wiley and Sons (1993).
9. Malet, G., Munoz, F., Appleyard, R., and Hersh, W.: A model for enhancing Internet document retrieval with "medical core metadata". J Am Inform Assoc. 6 (1999) 163-172.
10. Dolin, R., Alschuler, L., Beebe, C., Biron, P., Boyer, S., Essin, D., Kimber, E., and Mattison, J.: The HL-7 clinical document architecture. J Am Inform Assoc. 8 (2001) 552-569
11. Patel, V., and Kaufman, D.: Medical informatics and the science of cognition. J Am Inform Assoc. 5 (1998) 493-502.
12. Kushniruk, A., and Patel, V.: Cognitive and usability engineering methods for the evaluation of clinical information systems. Jour Biomed Infor. 37 (2004) 56-76.
13. van der Maas, A., ter Hofstede, H., and ten Hoopen, A.: Requirements for medical modeling languages. J Am Inform Assoc. 8 (2001) 146-162.
14. Buhler, P., and Vidal, J.: Multiagent systems with workflow. IEEE Internet Computing Jan-Feb 8(1)2004 76-82.
15. Shlaer, S., and Mellor, S.: Object lifecycles: modeling the world in states. Englewood Cliffs, NJ, Prentice Hall, 1992.
16. Booch, G., Rumbaugh, J., and Jacobson, I.: The unified modeling language user guide. Reading, MA, Addison Wesley Longman, Inc., 1999.
17. Gardner, K., Rush, A., Crist, M., Konitzer, R., and Teegarden, B. Cognitive patterns: problem-solving frameworks for object technology. Cambridge, UK. Cambridge University Press, 1998.
18. Gabriel, R. Patterns of Software. Oxford, UK. Oxford University Press, 1996.

19. Staggers, N., and Kobus, D.: Comparing response time, errors, and satisfaction between text-based and graphical user interfaces during nursing order tasks. J Am Inform Assoc. 7 (2000) 164-176.
20. Moorman, P., Branger, P., van der Kam, W., and van der Lei, J.: Electronic messaging between primary and secondary care: a four year case report. J Am Inform Assoc. 8 (2000) 372-378.
21. Shiffman, R., Karras, B., Agrawal, A., Chen, R., Marenco, L., and Nath, S.: GEM: a proposal for a more comprehensive guideline document model using XML. J Am Inform Assoc. 7 (2000) 488-498.
22. Schweiger, R., Hoelzer, S., Altmann, U., Rieger, J., and Dudeck, J.: Plug-and-play XML: a health care perspective. J Am Inform Assoc. 9 (2002) 37-48.
23. Tirado-Ramos, A., Hu, J., and Lee, K.: Information object definition-based unified modeling language representation of DICOM structured reporting: a case study of transcoding DICOM to XML. J Am Inform Assoc. 9 (2002) 63-71.
24. Laerum, H., Karlsen, T., and Faxvaac, A.: Effects of scanning and eliminating paper-based medical records on hospital physicians' clinical work practice. J Am Inform Assoc. 10 (2003) 588-595.
25. Poon, A., Fagin, L., Shortliffe, E.: The PEN-Ivory project: exploring user interface design for the selection of items from large controlled vocabularies of medicine. J Am Inform Assoc. 3 (1996) 168-183.
26. Bakken, S., Cashen, M., Mendonca, E., O'Brien, A., and Zieniewicz, J.: Representing nursing activities within a concept-oriented terminological system: evaluation of a type definition. J Am Inform Assoc. 7 (2000) 81-90.
27. Hwang, J., Cimino, J., Bakken, S.: Integrating nursing diagnostic concepts into the medical entities dictionary using the ISO reference terminology mode for nursing diagnosis. J Am Inform Assoc. 10 (2003) 382-388.
28. Staggers, N., and Thompson, C.: The evolution of definitions for nursing informatics: a critical analysis and revised definition. J Am Inform Assoc. 9 (2002) 255-261.
29. Hardiker, N., and Rector, A.: Structural validation of nursing terminologies. J Am Inform Assoc. 8 (2001) 212-221.
30. Henry, S., Warren, J., and Lange, L.: A review of major nursing vocabularies and the extent to which they have the characteristics required for implementation in computer-based systems. J Am Inform Assoc. 5 (1998) 321-328.
31. Matney, S., Bakken, S., and Huff, S.: Representing nursing assessments in clinical information systems using the logical observation identifiers, names, and codes database. Jour Biomed Inform 36 (2003) 287-293.
32. White, T., and Hauan, M.: Extending the LOINC conceptual schema to support standardized assessment instruments. J Am Inform Assoc. 9 (2002) 586-599.
33. Bakken, S., Cimino, J., Haskell, R., Kukafka, R., Matsumoto, C., Chan, G., and Huff, S.: Evaluation of Clinical LOINC (logical observation identifiers, names, and codes) semantic structure as a terminology model for standardized assessment measures. J Am Inform Assoc. 7 (2000) 529-538.
34. Danko, A., Kennedy, R., Haskell, R., Androwich, I., Button, P., Correia, C., Grobe, S., Harris, M., Matney, S., and Russler, D.: Modeling nursing interventions in the act class of HL-7 RIM version 3. Jour Biomed Inform 36 (2003) 294-303.
35. Harris, M., Graves, J., Solbrig, H., Elkin, P., and Chute, C.: Embedded structures and representation of nursing knowledge. J Am Inform Assoc. 7 (2000) 539-549.

36. Payne, T., Hoey, P., Nichol, P., and Lovis, C.: Preparation and use of preconstructed orders, order sets, and order menus in a computerized provider order entry system. J Am Inform Assoc. 10 (2003) 322-329.
37. Ruland, C.: Decision support for patient preference-based care planning: effects on nursing care and outcomes. J Am Inform Assoc. 6 (1999) 304-312.
38. Sintchenko, V., Coiera, E., Iredel, J., and Gilbert, G.: Comparative impact of guidelines, clinical data, and decision support on prescribing decisions: an interactive web experiment with simulated cases. J Am Inform Assoc. 11 (2004) 71-77.
39. Bell, D., Cretin, S., Marken, R., and Landman, A.: A conceptual framework for evaluating outpatient electronic prescribing systems based on their functional capabilities. J Am Inform Assoc. 11 (2004) 60-70.
40. Ammenwerth, E., Mansmann, U., Iller, C., Eichstadter, R.: Factors affecting and affected by user acceptance of computer-based nursing documentation: results from a two-year study. J Am Inform Assoc. 10 (2003) 69-84.
41. McHugh, M.: Nurses' needs for computer-based patient records. Ball, M, and Collen, M. (eds.) Aspects of the computer-based patient record. New York, NY, Springer-Verlag, Inc., 1992.
42. Amatayakul, M., and Wogan, M.: Record administrators' needs for computer-based patient records. Ball, M, and Collen, M. (eds.) Aspects of the computer-based patient record. New York, NY, Springer-Verlag, Inc., 1992.
43. Bourke. M. Strategy and architecture of health care information systems. New York, NY, Springer-Verlag, Inc., 1994.
44. Wooldridge, M., and Jennings, N. R.: Pitfalls of agent-oriented development, Proceedings AGENTS-98, 1998.
45. Kendall, E.A., Malkoun, M.T., and Jiang, C.: The application of object-oriented analysis to agent-based systems," JOOP. 2 (1997) 56-65.
46. Kautz, H., et al.: An experiment in the design of software agents. Huhns, M.N., and Singh, M.P. (eds.) Readings in Agents. Morgan Kaufmann Publ. (1997) 125-130.
47. Patel, V., Kushniruk, A., Tang, S., and Yale, J-F.: Impact of a computer-based patient record system on data collection, knowledge organization, and reasoning. J Am Inform Assoc. 7 (2000) 569-585.
48. Menon, A., Moffett, S., Enriquez, M., Martinez, M., Dev, P., and Grappone, T.: Audience response made easy: using personal digital assistants as a classroom polling tool. J Am Inform Assoc. 11 (2004) 217-220.
49. von Fuchs, T.: More than just networking. Mobile Enterprise 6 (2004) 11-12.
50. Westfall, R.: Does telecommuting really increase productivity? Comm ACM 47,8 (2004) 93-96.
51. Huhns, M., and Stephens, L.: Automating supply chains. IEEE Internet Comp. July-Aug (2001) 90-93.
52. Chen, E., Mendonca, E., McKnight, L., Stetson, P., Lei, J., and Cimino, J.: PalmCIS: a wireless handheld application for satisfying clinician information needs. J Am Inform Assoc. 11 (2004) 19-28.
53. Zeng, Q., Cimino, J., and Zou, K.: Providing concept-oriented views for clinical data using a knowledge-based system. J Am Inform Assoc. 9 (2002) 294-305.
54. Anyanwu, K., Sheth, A., Cardoso, J., Miller, J., and Kochut, K.: Healthcare enterprise process development and integration. Jour Res Prac Info Tech. 35:2 (2003) 83-98.

55. Zhang, L., Perl, Y., Halper, M., Geller, J., and Cimino, J.: An enriched unified medical language system semantic network with multiple subsumption hierarchy. J Am Inform Assoc. 11 (204) 195-206.
56. Aarts, J., Doorewaard, H., and Berg, M.: Understanding implementation: the case of a Dutch university medical center. J Am Inform Assoc. 11 (2004) 207-216.
57. Armstrong, K., and Davis, J.: Increasing treatment adherence using the Internet and intelligent agents. Proc AMIA-98, Philadelphia, PA, 1998.
58. Chen, P.: The entity-relationship model: towards a unified view of data. ACM Trans Database Sys 1,1 (1976) 9-36.
59. Teorey, T., Yang, D., and Fry, J.: A logical design methodology for relational databases using the extended entity-relationship model. ACM Comp Surv. 18,2 (1986) 197-222.
60. Maes, P.: Agents that reduce work and information overload", Comm ACM. 37,7 (1994) 31-40.
61. Silverman, B.: Computer reminders and alerts. IEEE Computer. Jan (1997) 42-49.
62. Genesereth, M., and Ketchpel, S.: Software agents. Comm ACM. 37,7 (1994) 48-53.
63. McKie, S.: Software agents: application intelligence goes undercover, DBMS. Apr (1995) 56-60.
64. Huhns, M.: Interaction-oriented programming. Cianciarni, P., and Wooldridge, M. (eds.) Agent-oriented software engineering. Berlin, Springer-Verlag (2001) 29-44.
65. Lind, J.: Issues in agent-oriented software engineering. Cianciarni, P., and Wooldridge, M. (eds.) Agent-oriented software engineering. Berlin, Springer-Verlag (2001) 45-58.
66. Shehory, O.: Software architecture attributes of multi-agent systems. Cianciarni, P., and Wooldridge, M. (eds.) Agent-oriented software engineering. Berlin, Springer-Verlag (2001) 78-80.
67. Bauer, B., Muller, J., and Odell, J.: Agent UML: a formalism for specifying multiagent software systems. Cianciarni, P., and Wooldridge, M. (eds.) Agent-oriented software engineering. Berlin, Springer-Verlag (2001) 91-103.
68. Pattison, H., Corkill, D., and Lesser, V.: Instantiating descriptions of organizational structure. Huhns, M. (ed.) Distributed artificial intelligence. London, Pittman Publishing (1987) 59-96.
69. Huhns, M., Mukhopadhyay, U., Stephens, L., and Bonnell, R.: DAI for document retrieval: the MINDS project. Huhns, M. (ed.) Distributed artificial intelligence. London, Pittman Publishing (1987) 59-96249-283.
70. Lind, J.: Patterns in agent-oriented software engineering. Giunchiglia, F., Odell, J., and Weiss, G.: Agent-oriented software engineering III, LNCS 2585. Berlin, Springer-Verlag (2003) 47-58.
71. Center for Medicare and Medicaid Services, Home health prospective payment system (HH PPS), A3-3639 (2001).
72. Fazzi, R., Harlow, L., and Wright, K.: 3M national OASIS integrity project: Recommended questions and techniques for OASIS M0 questions. Final Report. 3M Home Health Systems. http://www.3m.com/us/healthcare/his/products/home_health/
73. Sobel, D.S.: Self-care in health: information to empower people. Levy, A.H., and Williams, B. (eds.), Proceedings of the American Association for Medical Systems and Informatics, Congress 87, San Francisco, CA, American Association for Medical Systems and Information (1987) 12-125.
74. Buckalew, L.W., and Buckalew, N.M.: Survey of the nature and prevalence of patients' non-compliance and implications for intervention. Psychological Report. 76:1 (1995) 513-321.

75. Sclar, D.A., Tartaglione, T.A., and Fine, M.J.:Overview of issues related to medical compliance with implications for the outpatient management of infectious diseases. Infect Agents Dis, 3:5 (1994) 266-273.
76. Britten, N.: Patients' ideas about medicine: a qualitative study in a general practice population. British Journal of General Practice, 44:387 (1994) 465-468.
77. Kruse, W., Rampmaier, J., Ullrich, G., and Weber, E.: Patterns of drug compliance with medications to be taken once and twice daily assessed by continuous electronic monitoring in primary care", International Journal of Clinical Pharmacology Therapy. 32:9 (1994) 452-457.
78. Lowe, C.J., Raynor, D.K., Curtney, E.A., Purvis, J.. and Teale, C. : Effects of self medication programme on knowledge of drugs and compliance with treatment in elderly patients", British Medical Journal. 310:6989 (1995) 1229-1231.
79. White, J. E.: Telescript technology: mobile agents". Bradshaw, J. (ed), Software Agents. Cambridge, MA, AAAI Press (1996).
80. Donaldson, S.I., and Blanchard, A.L.: The seven health practices, well-being, and performance at work: evidence for the value of reaching small and underserved worksites. Preventive Medicine. 24:3 (1995) 270-277.
81. McCarthy, B., Baker, A., Yood, M. U., Winters, M., Scarsella, F., and Gurley, V.: Evaluation of the flu vaccine reminder trial. Center for Clinical Effectiveness (1997). http://www.hths-cce.org/whatsnew/cce_flu.html.

4. Virtual Communities in Health Care

George Demiris PhD

Department of Health Management and Informatics, University of Missouri-Columbia, 324 Clark Hall, Columbia Missouri 65201, USA

4.1 Introduction

A virtual community is a social entity involving several individuals who relate to one another by the use of a specific communication technology that bridges geographic distance. Traditional communities are determined by factors such as geographic proximity, organizational structures or activities shared by the members of the community. The concept "virtual" implies properties that unlike these of a traditional community are based on the utilization of advanced technologies enabling interactions and exchange of information between members who may not physically meet at any point in time.

A report resulting from the workshop held at the ACM CHI (Association for Computing Machinery-Computer Human Interaction) conference on the theory and practice of physical and network communities identified several core attributes of virtual communities [1]:

- Members have a shared goal, interest, need, or activity that provides the primary reason for being part of the community.
- Members engage in repeated, active participation and they have access to shared resources. Defined policies determine the type and frequency of access to those resources.
- Reciprocity of information, support, and services among members play an essential role. In this context there is a shared context of social conventions, language, and protocols.

A virtual community in health care refers to a group of people (and the social structure that they collectively create) that is founded on telecommunication with the purposes of providing support, discussing issues and problems, share documents, consult with experts and sustain relationships beyond face-to-face events. Such communities include peer-to-peer networks and virtual health care teams. Advanced telecommunications enable health care providers to interact and work on cases as members of so-called virtual teams. Such teams can ensure continuity of care as they utilize a common platform for exchange of messages, opinions and resources. Home care patients or patients with chronic conditions utilize different types of health care services at different points in time. Advanced technology enables physicians, nurses, social workers, nutrition and rehabilitation experts to interact and conduct team meetings in a virtual mode, namely bridging geographic distance and time constraints. Virtual teams are considered essential to

G. Demiris: *Virtual Communities in Health Care*, StudFuzz **184**, 121–122 (2005)
www.springerlink.com

successful disease management and to providing continuity of care for the patients.

Many applications of virtual communities function as self-help groups of individuals diagnosed with the same medical condition or undergoing the same treatment. One study [2] found that virtual self-help groups can provide many of the processes used in face-to-face self-help and mutual aid groups. The emphasis in such virtual communities is on mutual problem solving, information sharing, expression of feelings, mutual support and empathy.

Technologies for virtual communities include, among others, online message boards and automatic mailing list servers for asynchronous communication, or video conferencing, Internet relay chat, group and private chat rooms for synchronous communication. Some of the discussion groups are not "moderated"; that is, there is no individual or group responsible for reviewing and filtering posts that are thought to be provocative, inappropriate or in violation of any of the rules of the virtual community. Anybody may post any message they wish. In such non-moderated groups, the community relies largely on the normative processes of their own internal social norms "to define and enforce the acceptable behavior of the community members [3]."

This chapter providers an overview and discussion of virtual communities and specifically, patient and caregiver-centric support groups, peer-to-peer networks and virtual teams. Ethical and legal considerations as well as privacy and security issues associated with virtual communities will be discussed. The concept of patient empowerment in this context and issues of identity and deception in a virtual health care community will be defined and analyzed.

4.2 Virtual teams in health care delivery

Chronic illnesses require specialized and complex treatment protocols that involve a team of healthcare professionals and disciplines to address the multiple dimensions of care and social, psychosocial and clinical needs of patients. Such teams are essential to effective care provided to ensure continuity and to improve the patient's quality of life. However, there are often practical constraints such as time conflicts, geographic distances, other coordination challenges and lack of resources that limit the type and frequency of interactions among health care professionals. The use of advanced telecommunication technologies provides an opportunity to bridge geographic distance and create "virtual" health care teams.

Is there really such a concept of a "virtual team"? Lorimer [4] defines a team as a "small number of consistent people committed to a relevant shared purpose, with common performance goals, complementary and overlapping skills, and a common approach to their work." The physical presence of team members at the same location and same time is not inherent as a requirement for the creation of a team. Rather, it is the nature of the interactions, namely the interdisciplinary character of the information exchange, that becomes essential to an effective team. Health care providers of different disciplines (such as physicians, nurses, social workers, physical therapists, etc.) can create a team in which they combine their knowledge and expertise to provide a comprehensive plan of care. It is essential to include patients in virtual health care teams. Patients must be well informed about their conditions, treatment options and how to access them and be actively involved in their treatment [5].

Heineman [6] describes four domains of team function that can guide interdisciplinary team development: 1) structure (composition of team members and representation of disciplines); 2) context (relationship to the larger institution); 3) process (of team functioning, hierarchy and communication) and 4) productivity. In this context, the third domain referring to the process is the one that would be defined differently for virtual teams. The communication in this case could be web-based synchronous interaction or video-mediated (via videoconferencing) or in an asynchronous manner using message boards and discussion forums. Some would argue that this mode of communication could lead to increased overall productivity of the team as professionals contribute at their own discretion and convenience, having the opportunity to review the files, notes and records carefully before communicating a message to the rest of the team.

Pitsillides et al [7] developed a system to support the "dynamic creation, management and coordination of virtual medical teams for the continuous treatment" of home care patients. This system was designed using a patient centric philosophy and focused on care delivered at the patient's home and not a health care facility. Some of the goals were to create a virtual team that will be accessible to patients and families at all times, to improve communication among the team members and to improve the collection of monitoring data and enhance decision making. The team in this project includes oncologists, family physicians, home care nurses, physiotherapists, psychologists, social workers and the patient. The system architecture utilized the Internet and included a centralized electronic medical record system and mobile agents and devices distributed to members of the team to ensure accessibility and timely dissemination of up-to-date information.

Another example of virtual interdisciplinary teams is implemented within the Telehospice Project at the University of Missouri. The goal of hospice care is to improve the quality of dying patients' last days by offering comfort and dignity, focusing on palliation and the relief of suffering, individual control and autonomy. Good pain and symptom management for patients at the end of life requires the intervention of all disciplines in a holistic approach [8]. The philosophy underlying hospice care is supported by four principles that recognize the critical nature of interdisciplinary teamwork and patient/family participation: 1) wholistic care - the patient and his/her family are the unit of care [9]; 2) self determination – care that is governed by the patient and his/her family's values culture, beliefs and lifestyle [10]; 3) comfort -- focus on one's quality of life, assuring a patient "lives until he dies", rather than on prolonging futile medical treatment [11]; 4) development continuum – death is viewed as the final stage of development, filled with great opportunity for growth on many dimensions [12, 13]. These principles mandate an interdisciplinary approach to managing care at the end-of-life.

In most cases, hospice patients/families are not able to participate actively in the IDT discussions during which a care plan is agreed upon, a plan which patients/families, paradoxically, are advocated to control. Because hospice focuses on the family, patient/family inclusion is conceptually very appropriate [14]. While the hospice team meets at least every other week to review care plans and coordinate service provision [15], the patient/family is currently absent from the discussion. Numerous barriers prevent patients/ families from attending interdisciplinary team (IDT) meetings in which they would represent their experiences, values, and concerns. The symptoms and stresses associated with dying and caregiving are barriers to traveling to attend IDT care plan meetings. Physical limitations prevent the patient from traveling and require the family to remain in the home and attend to the patient's physical needs. Additionally, the team meetings usually are held at the hospice office location, requiring patient/family to travel many miles, especially in rural areas, to participate in person. Moreover, should these hurdles be overcome, usually only a few minutes are spent on any single case, making the journey to join the team meeting even less efficient. Hospice patients/families, therefore are not able to participate in the discussions developing the plan of care they are advocated to control, and participation is not a routine practice.

The Telehospice Project at the University of Missouri utilizes commercially available videophones that operate over regular phone lines to enable patients at home and their caregivers to interact with hospice providers at the clinical site [16]. This interaction enables the "virtual" participation of patients in interdisciplinary team meetings and allows for them and their caregivers to interact with hospice providers, even ones who they would not normally meet at their home (i.e., hospice medical director) [17].

4.3 Virtual communities and patient empowerment

Patient empowerment is a concept that has emerged in the health care literature in the last few years. It is based on the principle that patients are entitled to access health information and determine their own care choices. Feste argues that the empowerment model introduces "self-awareness, personal responsibility, informed choices and quality of life.[18]" Empowerment can be perceived as an enabling process through which individuals or groups take control over their lives and managing disease. Advances in telecommunication technologies have introduced new ways to enhance and supplement communication between health care professionals and patients. The implication is a shift of focus for system designers who had primarily focused on designing information technology applications that addressed the needs of health care providers and institutions only. As a result, the data models included episodic patient encounters as one group of health care related transactions, but did not aim to evolve around the life course of the individual patient or ensure continuity of care. New technologies and advancements in informatics research call for the development of informatics tools that will support patients as active consumers in the health care delivery system. Virtual communities are one of the tools that enable a shift from institution-centric to patient-centric information systems.

4.3.1 Virtual Disease management

The concept of disease management refers to "...a set of coordinated healthcare interventions and communications for populations with conditions in which patient self-care efforts are significant. [19]" These interventions aim to enhance the care plan and the provider-patient relationship while emphasizing prevention of deterioration and complications using evidence-based practice guidelines. In addition, further goals include the improvement of outcomes, decrease of costs, patient education and monitoring.

The concept of "virtual disease management" is defined by the utilization of information technologies such as the Internet to allow patients suffering from chronic conditions to stay at home and be involved in the care delivery process. Such technologies can link home care with hospital and ambulatory care, and facilitate information exchange and communication between patients, family members, and care providers. Patient education is an essential component of disease management and can be supported by the transmission of tailored health information or automated reminders to patients or their caregivers. The integration of commercially available household items such as television sets, mobile phones, videophones, medication dispensing machines, and handheld computers introduces new communication modes and patient empowering tools.

The Internet has been used as a platform for several disease management applications and in different clinical areas. Disease management for asthma patients, for example, has the potential of early detection and timely intervention as demonstrated by the home asthma telemonitoring (HAT) system [20] which assists patients in the daily routine of asthma care with personalized interventions and alerts health care providers in cases that require immediate attention. Diabetes is also a clinical area where web-based disease management could enhance care delivery due to the requirement for long-term prevention and intervention approaches. The Center for Health Services Research, Henry Ford Health System in Detroit, Michigan, developed a web-based Diabetes Care Management Support System (DCMSS) to support care delivery to diabetic patients [21]. The system was evaluated within a non-randomized, longitudinal study and findings suggested that web-based systems integrating clinical practice guidelines, patient registries, and performance feedback have the potential to improve the rate of routine testing among patients with diabetes. A distributed computer-based system for the management of insulin-dependent diabetes was developed and evaluated within the Telematic Management of Insulin-Dependent Diabetes Mellitus (T-IDDM) project funded by the European Union. The objective was to utilize Internet technology and monitoring devices to support the normal activities of the physicians and diabetic patients by providing a set of automated services enabling data collection, transmission, analysis and decision support [22].

Virtual disease management applications can be also developed for post transplant care. Regular spirometry monitoring of lung transplant recipients, for example, is essential to early detection of acute infection and rejection of the allograft. A web-based telemonitoring system providing direct transmission of home spirometry to the hospital was developed and evaluated demonstrating that home monitoring of pulmonary function in lung transplant recipients via the Internet is feasible and accurate [23]. Another application utilizing low-cost commercially available monitoring devices and the Internet was developed within the TeleHomeCare Project at the University of Minnesota aiming to enable patients at home, who were diagnosed with congestive heart failure, chronic obstructive pulmonary disease or required wound care, to interact with health care providers at the agency. Personalized web pages allowed patients to interact with their providers and fill out daily questionnaires including questions about vital signs (such as weight, blood pressure or temperature), symptoms, and overall well-being and nutrition. Alerts were triggered and providers were notified when a patient's entry required immediate medical attention based on predefined personalized rules [24].

4.3.2 Peer-to-Peer Applications

A peer-to peer system enables any unit within a network to communicate with and provide services to another unit within the network. All peers are of the same importance to the system; no single peer is critical to the functionality of the system and the application functions without the control or authorization of an external entity. Peers can be assumed to be of variable connectivity and can join and leave the system at their own discretion.

While peer-to-peer applications such as Kazaa or Napster that enabled users to exchange and download files gained increased media attention, there are similar applications that follow the peer-to-peer design in the health care field.

One such application is PeerLink [25] designed for people with disabilities. Persons with disabilities have high need for timely and complex information coordination and resource sharing. Most of the existing web-based structures and applications rely heavily on third parties to maintain and update information, resulting in high maintenance costs and limited direct control by users with disabilities. PeerLink is an information management system that allows users to share information instantaneously with others, and to selectively share personal and local community resource information according to their own specifications. Knowledgeable community members with disabilities have been recruited to provide local resource information and to make vetted information more broadly available to other community members.

Sharf [26] studied the communication taking place at Breast Cancer List, an online discussion group which continues to grow in membership and activity.

Three major dimensions of communication were identified: exchange of information, social support, and personal empowerment. The study concluded that this application fulfills the functions of a community, with future concerns about information control and the potential to enhance patient-provider understanding.

Hoybye et al [27] used ethnographics case-study methodology to explore how support groups on the Internet can break the social isolation that follows cancer and chronic pain. They studied the Scandinavian Breast Cancer List and using participant observation and interviews, followed 15 women who chose the Internet to battle social isolation. Study findings indicate that these women were empowered by the exchanges of knowledge and sharing experiences within the support group.

The widespread diffusion of the Internet has enabled the creation of electronic peer to peer communities, namely structures that allow for people with common interests, clinical conditions or health care needs to gather "virtually" to ask questions, provide support and exchange experiences. Such applications enable both synchronous and asynchronous communication and can serve as social support interventions. In July 2004 Yahoo!Groups (www.yahoo.com) listed 67450 electronic support groups in the health and wellness section.

Randomized controlled trials are required to measure the impact of peer-to-peer systems or virtual communities on clinical outcomes. Tate et al [28] conducted a randomized trial to compare the effects of an Internet weight loss program alone vs this program with the addition of behavioral counseling via e-mail provided for 1 year to individuals at risk of type 2 diabetes. The behavioral e-counseling group lost more mean (SD) weight at 12 months than the basic Internet group and had greater decreases in percentage of initial body weight. The authors concluded that adding e-mail counseling to a basic web-based weight loss intervention program significantly improved weight loss in adults at risk of diabetes.

Another study by Houston et al [29] focused on the characteristics of users of Internet-based depression support groups and assessed whether use predicts change in depression symptoms and social support. One hundred and three users of these groups were recruited into the study cohort and followed prospectively. They had high depression severity scores, and were socially isolated at baseline. They perceived considerable benefit from the web based support group indicating a potential of web-based support groups to play a positive role in the treatment of depression.

In a recent study [30], researchers compiled and evaluated the evidence on the effects on health and social outcomes of computer based peer-to-peer communities and electronic self support groups that are used by people to discuss health related issues remotely. The study conclusions were that no robust evidence exists, as of yet, of consumer led peer-to-peer communities, partly because most of these communities have been evaluated only in conjunction with more complex interventions or involvement with health professionals. However, given the great amount of non-moderated web based peer-to-peer groups, further research is needed to assess when and how electronic support groups can be effective.

4.4 Communication and information exchange in virtual communities

In the context of virtual communities it is important to address the actual process of communication that occurs between members and the type and frequency of information exchange that takes place.

In a content analysis of an online cancer support group, Klemm et al [31] identified a typology of information exchange which includes information giving and seeking, statements of encouragement and support, statements of personal opinion, and statements of personal experience.

Rafaeli and Sudweeks [32] argued that studying threads or chains of interrelated and interdependent messages can provide a representative snapshot of communication in virtual communities. They placed emphasis on examining threads instead of individual messages. Using this approach they determined that the content of communication in virtual communities is less confrontational than often anticipated. Specifically, they found conversations to be helpful and social rather than competitive. Interactive messages were identified as friendly and in many cases contained self-disclosure statements.

Burnett [33] presented a typology for information exchange in virtual communities. According to this classification, behaviors within virtual communities may be divided into two broad categories: non-interactive behaviors and interactive behaviors. The primary non-interactive behavior in virtual communities is referred to as "lurking", which is the act of limiting one's participation to the passive role of observing rather than also contributing to the discussion. Interactive behavior, on the other hand, based on the typology by Burnett, includes collaborative or positive interactive behavior, hostile behavior or behavior not specifically oriented toward information. Positive interactive behavior includes announcements, queries or specific requests and group projects. Hostile interactive behavior includes "trolling", "flaming", and "spamming." Trolling refers to deliberately posting a message aiming to elicit an angered response. Flaming is argumentation with the sole purpose of insulting one or several community members. Spamming refers to any unsolicited information or even any unwanted and extensive verbiage unrelated to the defined boundaries of the community. Finally, behaviors not related to information include smalltalk, pleasantries, jokes.

The study of the communication content and frequency between members of virtual health care communities where health care providers actively participate, can reveal the impact of the virtual community on the patient-provider communication and relationship.

4.5 Identity and deception in a virtual community

Identity is an essential component of members of virtual communities. Being aware of the identity of those with whom one interacts is essential for understanding and evaluating the interactions. Determining one's identity in the "disembodied" world of a virtual community becomes a challenge as many of the basic cues about personality and social role one is accustomed to in the physical world, are absent [34].

Members of virtual communities become attuned to the nuances of communication styles. Members are being distinguished by their own "voice" and language. There are specific identity clues that refer to the location or the hardware of the member (such as the IP address, domain name, browser type) and more general clues that refer to the writing style, tone and language used by the member.

However, these identity cues are not always reliable [34]. Members of a virtual community who have the intention to deceive the community about their identity could deliberately misuse such clues. A term that is often used in online communities is "trolling" which refers to an individual who attempts to falsely convince members of a community that he/she shares the group's common interest or concern with the intention to ultimately damage the feeling of trust in the community or disseminate inaccurate information, bad advice or anger participants.

Another dimension of identity deception is impersonation, namely, a case where one user pretends to be another member of the virtual community providing false identity cues that lead other members of the community to believe that he/she is the member the impersonator is portraying to be.

While the issue of identity deception has been often studied in online communities where members share common hobbies or cultural interests, the impact of this behavioral pattern has not been studied extensively in the context of health care related virtual communities. In such cases, the impact of deception can go beyond impacting the trust among members of the community and lead to a damaging effect on members' health care status.

Numerous cases of deception in virtual communities have been reported in the media and scientific literature. One of the earlier cases of deception that received great attention was that of the disabled "Joan" [35, 36], a young disabled and disfigured woman who chose not to meet people face to face due to her disability but formed relationships within an online community. When it was revealed that Joan did not really exist and was a persona created by an impersonator, a male psychiatrist in his fifties, members of the online community expressed that they felt outrage and betrayal, while several members stated they were mourning the loss of "Joan" [36]."

Feldman [37] reports several cases where people in on-line support groups falsely claim to suffer from specific medical conditions. In one case, Barbara became a member of a cystic fybrosis support group claiming she was approaching the end of her life at home receiving palliative care by her sister

Amy. Members of the support group exchanged messages with this individual over a long period of time and expressed their support and offered help. They all expressed distress when Amy announced to the community that Barbara had passed away. Members of the community, however, identified spelling errors and other identity clues in the communication with Amy and questioned the story. Amy admitted to being an impersonator pretending to be both the patient at the end of life and the caregiver.

The identity issue of virtual community members becomes obviously essential in the context of virtual medical teams, online communities that aim to enhance continuity of care or peer-to-peer communities where members exchange experiences and advice for a specific clinical condition.

Virtual Communities: A Case Study

Deborah was recently diagnosed with breast cancer. Her physician discussed with her the treatment options and enrolled her in a treatment protocol. He also informed her of a web-based virtual community for breast cancer patients. The web platform provides information about the diagnosis, treatment options and answers to patients' questions. The site identifies community support groups, alternative medicine centers and other facilities for different geographic regions across the country. It also includes a message board and chat room for interaction among the members of the community. Deborah can access her own medical history, scientific databases, consumer ratings, a personalized calendar with an email reminder service for medical appointments or virtual group discussions. She can fill out questionnaires assessing her overall well-being and symptoms on a daily basis or at a frequency of her choice. Copies of her responses are being automatically sent to her physician who keeps track of the overall health status and trends.

Furthermore, the site enables users to email specific questions related to the patient's personal history to be answered by medical experts or their own health care provider. These messages are being handled by Green Valley, which operates health-related call centers. Their employees are geographically dispersed. Green Valley utilizes an instant messaging platform and a web based messaging center for patients. Based on a network of medical contact centers and nurses, Green Valley offers medical messaging support for numerous clients such as health insurance companies, hospitals, physician group practices such as the one where Deborah's doctor is at, and other clinical settings. Based on the nature of the message and the patient's preference, Green Valley distributes the message securely to the intended recipient and ensures its appropriate and timely process. Web platforms and instant messaging have helped Green Valley create a distributed community for its employees and clients that supports the operation of the virtual community for breast cancer patients. Green Valley processes patient calls in a similar way to the handling of email messages from the members of the virtual community.

The challenges for the sustainability of this virtual community for breast cancer patients are the creation of a virtual environment that will facilitate communication using appropriate interaction channels and addressing breast cancer patients' needs, and the establishment of accessibility and authentication structures that enhance the sense of trust among the members of the virtual community.

4.6 Virtual research communities

The Internet and other advanced technologies enable health care researchers to communicate and exchange information. One such pioneering initiative is create a virtual community of cancer researchers with access to a vast array of previously unavailable scientific data [38]. This international initiative labeled the Strategic Framework, aims to revolutionize medical science by fostering a new context of information exchange and creating a large virtual research community. The UK's National Cancer Research Institute (NCRI) outlined its plans with the support of the US National Cancer Institute and other global leading cancer organizations.

Recent advances in cancer research due to developments in the fields of genomics, proteomics, and innovative clinical trials have led to a wealth of new datasets. While researchers are generating more data than ever before, the great majority remains unpublished and/or not analyzed. The UK NCRI (National Cancer Research Institute) identified the need for faster, more efficient and accurate ways of accessing, analyzing and disseminating research datasets and findings in order to achieve state of the art and continuously improved cancer treatments. Within the proposed virtual community, scientists in different fields of cancer research will agree on how best to record data in areas as different as genomics, medical imaging and epidemiology that will be made available to the entire research community using the web and other advanced technologies. Such an infrastructure will take advantage of existing resources and expertise and will foster communication and collaboration among members of the international scientific community of cancer research.

The Comprehensive Health Enhancement Support System (CHESS) developed by the University of Wisconsin is a platform that provides services designed to help individuals cope with a health crisis or medical concern, but also invites researchers to utilize resources and share knowledge and findings [39]. The system provides timely access to resources such as information, social support, decision-making and problem-solving tools when needed most. The CHESS Health Education Consortium (CHEC) brings together research and health care organizations known for excellence and innovation in health promotion and patient self-management. The CHESS application and its modules and consortia are good examples of a virtual community that serves individual patients' and caregiver needs while also providing an active laboratory for researchers and organizations.

4.7 Privacy and Confidentiality

The healthcare sector is facing many challenges in regard to the privacy and confidentiality of individual health information in the information age. Information Privacy is the patient's right to control the use and dissemination of information that relates to them. Confidentiality is a tool for protecting the patients' privacy. In 1998 the Notice of the Proposed Rule from the Department of Health and Human Services concerning Security and Electronic Signature Standards was introduced (U.S. Department of Health and Human Services 1999) as part of the Health Insurance Portability and Accountability Act (HIPAA) that was passed in 1996. This Proposed Rule became law in 2000 in the United States and proposes standards for the security of individual health information and electronic signature use for health care providers, systems and agencies. These standards refer to the security of all electronic health information and have a great impact on the design and operation of e-health applications.

Recent events that have attracted media attention include the case of the pharmaceutical company that violated its own privacy policy by inadvertently publicizing the e-mail addresses of more than 600 patients who took an antidepressant drug [40], and the case of the health care organization that mistakenly revealed confidential medical information in hundreds of e-mail messages to individuals for whom they were not intended [41].

The publicity surrounding such incidents creates confusion and can lead to patients' mistrust of this mode of communication.

When discussing privacy, issues related to the video- and/or audio-recording and maintenance of tapes, the storage and transmission of still images, and other patient record data have to be examined, and efforts have to be undertaken to address them to the fullest extent possible. The transmission of information over communication lines such as phone lines, satellite or other channels, is associated with concerns of possible privacy violations. An additional concern in some cases is the presence of technical staff assisting with the transmission procedure at the clinical site (or even at both ends) that could be perceived as a loss of privacy by the patients. Patients often are unfamiliar with the technical infrastructure and operation of the equipment which can lead to misperceptions of the possibilities of privacy violation during a videoconferencing session or online communication.

For disease management applications that are web-based, ownership of and access to the data have to be addressed. In many web-based applications in home care, patients record monitoring data and transmit them daily to a web server owned and maintained by a private third party that allows providers to log in and access their patients' data. This type of application calls for discussion and definition of the issue of data ownership and patients' access rights to parts or all of their records. The implications are not only possible threats to data privacy but extend to ethical debates about the restructuring of the care delivery process and introduction of new key players.

4.8 Sociability and Usability

Preece [42] introduces the terms sociability and usability in the context of virtual communities as two concepts that link knowledge about human behavior with appropriate planning and design of online communities. Sociability refers to the collective purpose of a community, the goals and roles of its members, and policies and rules defined to foster social interaction. There are numerous online communities and their members participate for different reasons, whether to share information, find friends, get advice, or coordinate services. The members' information needs can be addressed within the online community according to the social framework and the defined polices. Each virtual community is unique and its growth or development can be unpredictable. Developers and designers can influence the development trend by clearly communicating the purpose and policies of the community.

Usability in general refers to the accessibility of the design and the specifics of an interface that lead to rapid learning, increased skill retention and minimizing error rates. The implication for virtual communities, according to Preece [42], is that a usable virtual community is one where members are able to communicate with each other, find information, and navigate the community software with ease.

Usability and sociability are closely related, but not identical. This becomes more clear when considering an example, namely a virtual community for caregivers of diabetic patients. The designers of the community are faced with the question whether they should enforce a registration policy and how to define requirements for membership. These items constitute a sociability decision, as they will definitely impact the number and type of memberships of the community and the social interactions that will occur. The design specifications for the registration procedures (e.g., forms, buttons etc.) are related to the software issues and constitute usability decisions. Both usability and sociability will determine the feasibility and overall success of the virtual community and can be the object of both a formative and summative evaluation.

4.9 Ethical considerations

The administration of virtual communities faces challenges as such communities often include members from countries around the world. The first challenge relates to participation of health care providers and the issue of licensing. In the United States, for example, medicine is practiced at the location where the patient is. This issue has often been encountered with telemedicine applications that utilize videoconferencing systems. In these cases, physicians have to be licensed to practice medicine in the state where the patient is at, during the teleconsultation. Another challenge is to determine the extent to which rules on regulation of speech defined by existing geographical jurisdiction can be applied to a virtual community.

A further concern is the so-called "progressive dehumanization" of interpersonal relationships, namely the conduct of not only professional but also personal interactions online or via communication technologies with a decreasing number of face-to-face interactions. Virtual support groups while having the potential to bring people together from all over the world and allow for anonymity that might be desired for a specific medical condition, might be lacking the sense of touch and inter-human close contact that occurs in face-to-face meetings. Virtual communities represent a physically disembodied social order. While this virtual order exists in parallel with social structures in physical space, some argue [43] that it will eventually compete with a structure or network of entities which occupy spatial locations. It is often stated that "the fabric of human relationships and communities rests on real presences, real physical meetings and relationships [44]." It remains to be investigated whether the conventional notions of a social contract, personal rights, justice and freedom survive in a virtual world.

The concept of virtual health care communities is relatively new and there are no specific guidelines or regulations addressing some of these ethical considerations. The American Medical Informatics Association (AMIA) has provided guidelines for the electronic communication of patients with health care providers [45]. Based on these guidelines, a turnaround time for messages should be established, patients should be informed about privacy issues, and messages should be printed out and included in the patients' charts. Patients must be warned not to use the online mode of interaction in an emergency and should be aware of all recipients of their messages as well as general privacy issues.

For the conduct of virtual visits using videoconferencing technologies in home care, the American Telemedicine Association [46] has produced a set of clinical guidelines for the development and deployment of such applications. These guidelines refer to patient, technology and provider criteria. Patient criteria involved a set of recommendations such as the need for informed written consent obtained from patients, selection of patients able to handle the equipment, and training. Technology criteria refer to the operation and maintenance of equipment, establishment of clear procedures and safety codes and protection of patient privacy and record security. Health provider criteria refer to training issues and after hours support.

Such guidelines by professional organizations address some important concerns and provide an appropriate framework for the integration of virtual health care communities in the care delivery process. However, many issues such as licensing, accreditation, concerns of identity deception and dependency have not been fully addressed yet by legislative or professional entities.

4.10 Conclusion

Virtual communities are emerging in many health care related domains. Such communities aim to support patients, caregivers, families and health care providers and facilitate information exchange, provide support and enhance communication among people who do not have to be physically present at the same time at one location. Whether such communities are based on moderated or non-moderated discussions, it is important to have a clear, published and easily accessible set of rules and regulations or code of conduct for the members of the virtual community. Members of such a community need to claim ownership of the community so that they can be encouraged to provide constructive critiques and improve overall performance.

Powerful technologies and trends are emerging in the health care field. Advanced technologies that enable people to communicate and form virtual teams and communities can revolutionize the health care field and support a paradigm shift, namely the shift from institution-centric to patient-centric or consumer-centric systems. Policy, ethical and legal issues associated with virtual health care communities will have to be addressed. Furthermore, extensive research initiatives are needed that will determine the impact of virtual health care communities on clinical outcomes, the overall process and quality of and access to care. Such initiatives should go beyond pilot-testing an innovative application and employ experimental design methods to investigate the utility of virtual health care communities and the extent to which they empower patients and their caregivers. As advanced web-based applications continue to emerge and grow, system designers, health care settings, organizations and policy makers need to be prepared to properly adopt these technologies and develop the capacity to evaluate and make informed decisions about their appropriate use.

References

1. Whittaker, S., Issacs, E., & O'Day, V. (1997). Widening the net. Workshop report on the theory and practice of physical and network communities. *SIGCHI Bulletin, 29*(3), 27-30.
2. Finn J. An exploration of helping processes in an online self-help group focusing on issues of disability. Health Social Work 1999; 24(3): 220-231.
3. Burnett G, Besant M, Chatman EA. Small Worlds: Normative behavior in virtual communities and feminist bookselling. Journal of the American Society for Information Science and Technology 2001; 52(7): 571-535.
4. Lorimer W, Manion J. Team-based organizations: leading the essential transformation. PFCA Rev 1996 Spring:15-19.
5. Davis RM, Wagner EG, Groves T. Advances in managing chronic disease. Research, performance measurement, and quality improvement are key. BMJ 2000 Feb 26;320(7234):525-526.
6. Heinemann GZA. Team performance in health care—assessment and development. In: Stricker G, editor. Issues in the Practice of Psychology. New York: Kluwer Academic/Plenum Publishers; 2002. p. 400.
7. Pitsillides A, Pitsillides B, Samaras G et al. DITIS: A collaborative virtual medical team for home healthcare of cancer patients. In *M-Health: Emerging Mobile Health Systems*, Robert H. Istepanian, Swamy Laxminarayan and Constantinos S. Pattichis (Ed.), Kluwer Academic/Plenum Publishers 2004

8. Mazanec P, Bartel J, Buras D, et al. Transdisciplinary pain management: a holistic approach. Journal of Hospice & Palliative Nursing 2002; 4:228-34.
9. Jaffe C, Ehrlich C. All Kinds of Love: Experiencing Hospice. Amityville, NY: Baywood Publishing Co, 1997:346.
10. Eagan KA. Patient-family value based end of life care model. Largo: Hospice Institute of the Florida Suncoast, 1998.
11. Torrens PR. More than Semantics: What is a Hospice? In: Torrens P, ed. Hospice Programs and Public Policy: American Hospital Publishing, 1985:31-43.
12. Byock I. Dying well: Peace and possibilities at the end of life: (1997). xv, 299pp., 1997.
13. Reese DJ. Addressing spirituality in hospice: current practices and a proposed role for transpersonal social work. Social Thought 2001; 20:135-61.
14. Connor SR, Egan KA, Kwilosz DM, Larson DG, Reese DJ. Interdisciplinary approaches to assisting with end-of-life care and decision making. American Behavioral Scientist 2002; 46:340-356.
15. HCFA. Federal Register: Health Care Financing Administration, Agency for Health Policy Research, 1983.
16. Demiris G, Parker Oliver D, Porock D, Courtney KL. The Missouri telehospice project: background and next steps. Home Health Care Technology Report 2004; 1:49-55.
17. Demiris G, Parker Oliver D, Fleming D, Edison K. Hospice Staff Attitudes towards "Telehospice." American Journal of Hospice and Palliative Care 2004; 21(5): 343-348.
18. Feste C., and Anderson R. M. 1995. "Empowerment: from philosophy to practice." Patient Education and Counseling 26:139-144.
19. Disease Management Association of America. 2002. "Definition of Disease Management." [Online article or information; retrieved 9/20/2004.] http://www.dmaa.org/definition.html.
20. Finkelstein J., O'Connor G., and Friedmann R. H. 2001. "Development and implementation of the home asthma telemonitoring (HAT) system to facilitate asthma self-care." In MedInfo 2001, edited by V. Patel, R. Rogers and R. Haux, 810-4. Amsterdam, Washington, DC: IOS Press.
21. Baker A. M., Lafata J. E., Ward R. E., Whitehouse F., and Divine G. 2001. "A Web-based diabetes care management support system." Jt Comm J Qual Improv 27(4):179-90.
22. Riva A., Bellazzi R., and Stefanelli M. 1997. "A Web-based system for the intelligent management of diabetic patients." MD Computing 14(5):360-4.
23. Morlion B., Knoop C., Paiva M., and Estenne M. 2002. "Internet-based home monitoring of pulmonary function after lung transplantation." Am J Respir Crit Care Med 165(5):694-7.
24. Demiris G., Finkelstein S. M., and Speedie S. M. 2001b. "Considerations for the design of a Web-based clinical monitoring and educational system for elderly patients." JAMIA 8(5):468-72.
25. Schopp LH, Hales JW et al. Design of a Peer-to-Peer Telerehabilitation Model. Telemedicine Journal and e-Health Jun 2004, 10(2): 243-251
26. Sharf BF. Communicating breast cancer on-line: support and empowerment on the Internet. Women Health. 1997;26(1):65-84.
27. Hoybye MT, Johansen C, Tjornhoj-Thomsen T. Online interaction. Effects of storytelling in an Internet breast cancer support group. Psychooncology. 2004 Jul 15
28. Tate DF, Jackvony EH, Wing RR. Effects of Internet behavioral counseling on weight loss in adults at risk for type 2 diabetes: a randomized trial. JAMA. 2003 Apr 9;289(14):1833-6.
29. Houston TK, Cooper LA, Ford DE Internet support groups for depression: a 1-year prospective cohort study. Am J Psychiatry. 2002;159(12):2062-8.

30. Eysenbach G, Powell J, Englesakis M, Rizo C, Stern A. Health related virtual communities and electronic support groups: systematic review of the effects of online peer to peer interactions. BMJ. 2004 May 15;328(7449):1166.
31. Klemm P, Hurst M, Dearholt SL, Trone SR. Gender differences on Internet cancer support groups. Computer Nursing 1999; 17(2): 65-72.
32. Rafaeli S, Sudweeks F. Interactivity on the nets. In Sudweeks F, McLaughlin M, Rafaeli S. (Eds.) Network and netplay: Virtual groups on the Internet (pp. 173-189) Mento Park, CA: AAAI Press/ The MIT Press
33. Burnett, Gary (2000) "Information exchange in virtual communities: a typology" *Information Research*, **5**(4) Available at: http://informationr.net/ir/5-4/paper82.html
34. Donath JS. Identity and deception in the virtual community in Kollock, P and Smith, M (Eds.) Communities in Cyberspace. London: Routledge 1998.
35. Van Gelder, L. (1991). The strange case of the electronic lover. In C. Dunlop and R. Kling (Eds), Computerization and controversy: Value conflicts and social choice. Boston MA: Academic Press.
36. O'Brien, J. (1999). Writing in the body: gender (re)production in online interaction. In M. A. Smith and P. Kollock (Eds.). Communities in cyberspace (pp. 76-106). London: Routledge.
37. Feldman, M.D. (2000). Munchausen by Internet: Detecting factitious illness and crisis on the Internet. Southern Medical Journal, 93, 669-672.
38. Statement of Intent published in the British Medical Journal and Nature in March 2004
39. Gustafson DH, Bosworth K, Hawkins RP, Boberg EW, Bricker E. CHESS: A computer-based system for providing information referrals, decision support and social support to people facing medical and other health-related crises. Proc 16th Ann Symp Comput Appl Med Care. 1993;161-165.
40. Federal Trade Commission: *Eli Lilly Settles FTC Charges Concerning Security Breach*, Jan. 18, 2002. http://www.ftc.gov/opa/2002/01/elililly.htm (last access*ed Jun. 18, 2004).*
41. Rodsjo S.: *Hack Attack. Healthc Inform* 18:37-40, 42, 44, Jan. 2001.
42. Preece J. Online Communities: Designing Usability and Supporting Sociability. John Wiley & Sons 20000
43. Winner L. Living in electronic space. IN: Casey T, Embree L (eds.) Lifeworld and technology, Lonham MD: Center for Advanced Research on Phenomenology and University Press of America 1990; 1-14.
44. Sanford Horner D. The moral status of virtual action. Horner, D.S. (2001), The moral status of virtual action. In: T.W. Bynum et al eds. Proceedings of the Fifth International Conference on the Social and Ethical Impacts of Information and Communication Technologies: Ethicomp. Vol. 2.
45. Kane B, Sans D. Guidelines for the clinical use of electronicmail with patients. J Am Med Inform Assoc. 1998;5(1):104–11.
46. American Telemedicine Association (2003) 'ATA adopts Telehomecare Clinical Guidelines', 10 October 2004, http://www.americantelemed.org/icot/hometelehealthguidelines.htm

5. Evidence Based Telemedicine

George Anogianakis[1], Anelia Klisarova[2], Vassilios Papaliagkas[1], Antonia Anogeianaki[1,2]

1. Dept. of Physiology, Faculty of Medicine, Aristotle University of Thessaloniki, Greece
2. Dept. of Imaging Diagnostics and Nuclear Medicine, Medical University of Varna, Bulgaria

Summary

This chapter focuses on evidence based telemedicine and its various applications. Evidence based medicine is the integration of best research evidence with clinical expertise and patient values, for the best possible patient management. It is the explicit and judicious use of current best evidence in making decisions about the treatment and care of individual patients. In practice, it means integrating the individual clinical skills of the doctor with the best available clinical evidence from systematic research.

Telemedicine, on the other hand, is a process for delivering health services via telecommunication technologies to underserved regions (whether the poor in the metropolitan areas of the western world or the populations of the Sub-Saharan countries in Africa) or to special social groups around the world (e.g., merchant mariners, prisoners, the elderly etc). Its defining feature is that, in most cases, it does not rely on physical examination but mainly on patient history and that it normally utilizes a limited number of easily available pharmaceuticals. However, except for the case of emergency medicine, a great deal of the teleconsultant's time is devoted in routine items such as every-day consultations, test interpretation, chronic disease management, hospital or surgical follow-up and specialist visits.

Evidence based telemedicine differs from telemedicine, as we presently use this term, in that:

1. It requires the combination of highly honed medical history-taking skills with current best evidence on the prevalence of the different diseases at the point of health service delivery;
2. It uses best evidence to design treatments that take into account the state of the locally available resources (e.g., drug availability);
3. It actively seeks best evidence (even non-medical) regarding local customs in order to design treatments that do not contradict local beliefs and practices and are easily accepted and implemented by the recipients.

Evidence based telemedicine can be extremely useful in delivering emergency care, general practice and pre-hospital as well as home care telemedicine services in the case of cardiology, dermatology, ENT, general surgery, gynecology,

G. Anogianakis, et al.: *Evidence Based Telemedicine*, StudFuzz **184**, 139–172 (2005)
www.springerlink.com

hematology, nephrology, oncology, ophthalmology, pediatrics, psychiatry, respiratory medicine and urology. Finally, in a very transparent way, it is already a part of the modern practice of radiology (through outsourcing) and pathology.

Introductory Note

Evidence Based Telemedicine (EBT) is a field of telemedicine (TM) that combines the practice of Evidence Based Medicine (EBM) with the modern technological advances in Information Technology (IT) and telecommunications that gave rise to modern TM over the last 15 years. It is, therefore, the purpose of this paper to explain how this combination of techniques for health care delivery is taking place and to acquaint the reader with the concepts required to understand this synthesis. As a result, the emphasis was placed on presenting the basis for EBM, to the extent that it applies in TM, and to explore the contributions and potential applicability of TM in modern health care services. Finally, given the authors' conviction that the Internet will eventually be the basic, transparent, medium over which TM is going to be practiced, only a very small effort was expended in presenting other technologies that presently underlie the delivery of TM services

5.1 Introduction

What is TM?

TM derives from the combination of the Greek root "tele-" (τηλε-) which means "far" or "at a distance" and the root of the Latin verb "medere" which means "to heal". Literally, therefore, TM means "to heal at a distance". However simple this may sound, a good look at modern literature on the subject yields more than 30 different definitions of TM, depending on what the author (in most cases an academician, but quite often an administrator) is attempting to describe. Among the definitions the following seven, randomly selected, "typical" examples (Table 1) serve to demonstrate this point:

Table 1: Typical examples of the definition of TM encountered in the relevant literature

Origin	No.	Definition
European Commission: DG XIII (1993)	1	Rapid access to shared and remote medical expertise by means of telecommunications and IT, no matter where the patient or relevant information is located
WHO (1997)	2	The practice of medical care using interactive audiovisual and data communications. This includes medical care delivery, diagnosis,

		consultation and treatment, as well as education and the transfer of medical data
Preston J, Brown FW and Hartley B (1992)	3	The use of telecommunication technology to assist in the delivery of health care
	4	A system of health care delivery in which physicians examine distant patients through the use of telecommunications technology
Brauer GW (1992)	5	Patient-care oriented tele-health
Goldberg MA, Sharif HS, Rosenthal DI, Black-Schaffer S, Flotte TJ, Colvin RB and Thrall JH (1994)	6	The interactive transmission of medical images and data to provide patients in remote locales with better care
	7	The delivery of medical care to patients anywhere in the world by combining telecommunications and medical expertise

On the face of it, there are as many definitions of TM as there are writers on the subject. A quick look however at the examples presented, allows us to group them together and classify them on the basis of the particular characteristic of TM each definition intends to emphasize (Table 2). For example, definition "1," in contrast to all other definitions presented, subtly but definitely, identifies TM with emergency medicine. On the other hand, all definitions stress the distance between teleconsultant and patient as the characteristic that adds the prefix "tele" to "medicine". However, definitions "1," "6" and "7" explicitly state the distance between teleconsultant and patient as the important characteristic of TM, while definitions "2," "3" and "5" only indirectly mention distance as the important characteristic of TM. Interactivity does not seem to be a defining characteristic of TM since only two definitions ("2" and "6") explicitly refer to it, nor is the recruitment of IT or multimedia (definitions "1," "2" and "6") to the delivery of medical care . Finally, a number of definitions (definitions "3," "4," "5" and "7") view TM as the natural evolution of medicine in the age of telecommunications.

Table 2: Number of defining Characteristics included in the definitions of TM mentioned in Table 1

Defining Characteristic	Emergency Medicine	Separation of doctor from patient	Interactivity of process	IT and Multimedia content	Natural evolution of Medicine
Definitions	1 out of 7	6 out of 7	2 out of 7	3 out of 7	4 out of 7

If we take into account the circumstances under which these definitions were conceived, we will notice that definitions that are broad and generic rather than narrow and specific (with respect to the technology used or the medical discipline served) are most prevalent and/or useful. Along this line of thought, "the use of telecommunications to deliver clinically effective healthcare services to individuals, organizations and communities, where and when needed, in a cost effective manner" might presently (ca. 2004) be a more relevant definition of TM. European bureaucracies and academia uses the term "health telematics" to refer to the combined use of informatics and telecommunications in the delivery of healthcare. "Telehealth" or "e-health" is a synonymous term referring to the delivery of health services and products that is enabled by communication technology.

The advent of the information society concept in the early 1990's implied a substantive role of IT in medicine. Within this context the ministers responsible for the promotion and development of a global information society in the G-7 countries met in Brussels in February 1995 and, among other tasks, they established Global Healthcare Applications Project (GHAP) whose objective was to improve quality and cost-efficiency of healthcare delivery through IT tools. Within GHAP, "Subproject (SP)-4" was focused on TM [22, also http://mi.med.u-tokai.ac.jp/g7sp4/final.htm cited Dec 29, 2004]. Its objective was to lead the way towards a "24-hour multilingual and multidisciplinary TM surveillance and emergency service around the world". The scope of the effort was later extended to include all TM interventions rather than just emergency TM, including inter-operability of means, cost-efficiency of applications, legal aspects, and healthcare management. A number of challenges were identified and resolved at five separate meetings. In the Melbourne, Australia meeting (http://www.atmeda.org/news/2001_presentations/International/Lacroix.ppt cited Dec 29, 2004]) on Feb 19-20, 1999, it was suggested that: "TM is the delivery of health services through the transfer of information, via telecommunication technologies," irrespective of whether these services are clinical, educational or administrative in nature; "information," in the context of the "Melbourne definition", includes video, graphics and audio as well as text or data items. The key implication is that TM, by applying computing and IT in the practice of medicine, breaks the nexus between service delivery, on one hand, and time and place, on the other. Thus, lifting this inherent limitation of face-to-face medicine emerges as the only way to swiftly and massively improve health care in rural areas, in the home or in other places where medical personnel are not readily available. It is for this reason that advocates of TM insist that TM services must be covered by health insurance. However, as of today, TM benefits and actual TM costs continue to remain poorly defined (http://www.ingbiomedica.unina.it/teleplans_doc/wp5_d051_4.htm cited Dec 29, 2004).

No definition of TM would be complete without questioning the reasons for which, despite the, sometimes poor definition of its benefits or costs, TM is becoming a part of our lives; or why it emerges as a field of international collaboration, despite the fact that its economic and social benefits are of regional or, at most, of national importance. The answers should be sought in the rapid sharing of knowledge and expertise, which are no longer constrained by geographical and political barriers, and to the fact that industrialized nations openly declare their responsibility to develop and evaluate new technologies, which have the potential to improve the quality of life in the less developed countries.

Through TM, academic centres can offer their services to ever wider regions and they can help distant physicians and allied health workers to get involved in the delivery of highly specialized services to their locales. They also provide them with the means to discuss their difficult cases or share knowledge and experiences with distantly located world experts and to participate in healthcare training programs without necessarily attending traditional international conferences which are widely dispersed and have a low cost-to-benefit ratio.

Finally, the advent of Internet has resulted in better educated patients, with higher expectations for their physicians, which demand a high-standard, quality care. At the same time, the increase in travel and population migrations, that characterize the beginnings of the 21st century, require local healthcare providers to be more knowledgeable of diseases from distant geographical areas.

What is EBM?

As in the case of TM or any other still developing field of medicine, there are many definitions of EBM. Each of them underlines some specific aspects of EBM practice (Table 3) and it reflects the reasons for which the user is practicing EBM.

For our present purposes we will define EBM as "the integration of best research evidence with clinical expertise and patient values, so as to achieve the best possible patient management". Since in clinical practice physicians make decisions, one can argue that EBM represents an attempt to make better decisions by improving the quality of information on which those decisions are based. Furthermore, the information that is relevant to EBM is empirical evidence about what works and what does not work when treating a disease; it has nothing to do with the pathophysiology of the disease.

Table 3

Origin	Definition/quote
Sackett DL, Rosenberg WM, Gray JA, Haynes RB, Richardson WS (1996)	EBM is the conscientious, explicit, and judicious use of current best evidence in making decisions about the care of individual patients. The practice of EBM means integrating individual clinical expertise with the best available external clinical evidence from systematic research. By individual clinical expertise we mean the proficiency and judgment that individual clinicians acquire through clinical experience and clinical practice. Increased expertise is reflected in many ways, but especially in more effective and efficient diagnosis and in the more thoughtful identification and compassionate use of individual patients' predicaments, rights, and preferences in making clinical decisions about their

	care. By best available external clinical evidence we mean clinically relevant research, often from the basic sciences of medicine, but especially from patient centered clinical research into the accuracy and precision of diagnostic tests (including the clinical examination), the power of prognostic markers, and the efficacy and safety of therapeutic, rehabilitative, and preventive regimens. External clinical evidence both invalidates previously accepted diagnostic tests and treatments and replaces them with new ones that are more powerful, more accurate, more efficacious, and safer.
McKibbon KA, Wilczynski N, Hayward RS, Walker-Dilks CJ, Haynes RB (1995)	EBM is an approach to health care that promotes the collection, interpretation, and integration of valid, important and applicable patient-reported, clinician-observed, and research-derived evidence. The best available evidence, moderated by patient circumstances and preferences, is applied to improve the quality of clinical judgments.
Appleby J, Walshe K, Ham C (1995).	EBM involves evaluating rigorously the effectiveness of healthcare interventions, disseminating the results of evaluation and using those findings to influence clinical practice. It can be a complex task, in which the production of evidence, its dissemination to the right audiences, and the implementation of change can all present problems
Rosenberg W, Donald A (1995)	EBM is the process of systematically finding, appraising, and using contemporaneous research findings as the basis for clinical decisions. EBM asks questions, finds and appraises the relevant data, and harnesses that information for everyday clinical practice. EBM follows four steps: formulate a clear clinical question from a patient's problem; search the literature for relevant clinical articles; evaluate (critically appraise) the evidence for its validity and usefulness; implement useful findings in clinical practice. The term "evidence based medicine" (no hyphen) was coined at McMaster Medical School in Canada in the 1980's to label this clinical learning strategy, which people at the school had been developing for over a decade
Cook DJ, Levy MM. (1998)	EBM involves caring for patients by explicitly integrating clinical research evidence with pathophysiologic reasoning, caregiver

	experience, and patient preferences...EBM is a style of practice and teaching which may also help plan future research
Geddes JR, Harrison PJ (1997)	EBM is also a way of ensuring that clinical practice is based on the best available evidence through the use of strategies derived from clinical epidemiology and medical informatics
Muir Gray JA (1997)	Evidence based clinical practice is an approach to decision making in which the clinician uses the best evidence available, in consultation with the patient, to decide upon the option which suits that patient best
First Annual Nordic Work-shop on how to critically appraise and use evidence in decisions about healthcare, National Institute of Public Health, Oslo, Norway (1996)	Evidence-based healthcare is the conscientious use of current best evidence in making decisions about the care of individual patients or the delivery of health services. Current best evidence is up-to-date information from relevant, valid research about the effects of different forms of health care, the potential for harm from exposure to particular agents, the accuracy of diagnostic tests, and the predictive power of prognostic factors
Hicks N (1997)	Evidence-based healthcare takes place when decisions that affect the care of patients are taken with due weight accorded to all valid, relevant information
Marwick C (1997)	Evidence-based healthcare is a conscientious, explicit, and judicious use of the current best evidence to make a decision about the care of patients
Centre for Evidence Based Medicine Glossary http://www.cebm.net cited Dec 29, 2004	Evidence-Based Health Care extends the application of the principles of Evidence-Based Medicine (see above) to all professions associated with health care, including purchasing and management

This point is amply illustrated by the story of flecainide [16]. Flecainide was used in the 80's to treat heart attacks. The idea was that since a heart attack, many times, leads to ventricular fibrillation and results in death, the administration of "a safe and long-acting antiarrhythmic drug that protects against ventricular fibrillation" to people at risk should save millions of lives. This "pathophysiologically sound" suggestion led to the widespread use of flecainide, which was an antiarrhythmic agent. Indeed, patients on flecainide had fewer preventricular contractions than patients on placebo. Since arrhythmias were the cause of death from heart attack, researchers concluded that people who had survived a heart attack should be given flecainide. Within 18 months of flecainade's introduction, however, it was clear that the death rate in the group of patients who were treated by flecainide was double than that in the placebo group. Eventually, the treatment had to be abandoned.

The moral of the flecainide story is twofold:

1. Despite our knowledge of the underlying mechanisms, other factors, not important in terms of pathophysiology but clearly important in terms of the intended outcome (i.e. patient survival and better quality of life), are at play. In the case of flecainide these factors made the drug toxic/dangerous.
2. More than information on the pathophysiology of the disease they treat; practicing physicians need information on the effectiveness of the treatment they prescribe, both in terms of patient survival and in terms of the possible improvements in the quality of their patients' lives.

EBM is a "patient-centred" rather than "physician-centred" brand of medicine. It deals with clinical problems and questions that arise in the course of caring for individual patients. The practice of EBM is always triggered by a patient encounter which generates questions about the effects of therapy, the utility of diagnostic tests, the prognosis of disease, or the etiology of a disorder.

Table 4 describes the five steps that complete the EBM process:

Table 4: Steps in EBM

STEP	PURPOSE
State the question	To construct a well built, i.e., answerable, clinical question derived from the case at hand
Do the evaluation	To select the appropriate resource(s) and conduct the necessary search in order to track down the best evidence of outcomes that is presently available
Judge the utility of the available resources	To critically appraise the evidence gathered for its validity (i.e., how close it is to the truth) and applicability (i.e., its usefulness) in the case at hand.
Get back to the patient	To apply the evidence in the case at hand, by using it to "hone" the physician's clinical expertise and by taking the patient preferences into account.
Perform a self-evaluation	To evaluate the physician's performance with each patient

What Table 4 demonstrates is that, formally or informally, most of the activities that characterize EBM are used by clinicians ever since the early days of medicine. In fact, "western" medicine, as recently as 50 years ago, was EBM. Today's "alternative" and/or "traditional" types of medicine (e.g., herbal medicine, Ayurveda etc) are also EBM-like in the sense that their practitioners use their cumulative experience to formulate a clinical strategy for each case at hand rather than their knowledge of pathophysiology. In any case, such knowledge did not exist at least until the middle of the 17th century: William Harvey, e.g., described the circulation in 1628; Anthony van Leeuwenhoek invented the microscope in 1673, and Luigi Galvani described "animal electricity" in 1780. Finally, there are few practicing clinicians who do not use the literature, at least occasionally, to guide their decisions. What EBM adds to the traditional clinical approach is the formalization of the literature consultation process and the addition to it of the necessary filtering of the literature so that the decisions taken are always based on both the "strongest" and the "most relevant" evidence.

That being as it may, critics perceive an overt reliance of EBM on literature which has prompted them to call EBM "cook book medicine". They view EBM guided decisions as based solely on the evidence rather than on sound clinical judgment. The answer is that EBM does not supersede or annul individual clinical expertise but it represents a substantial part of clinical decision making [29, also http://www.hsl.unc.edu/lm/ebm/index.htm cited Dec 29, 2004]. Evidence supports and supplements individual clinical expertise and helps the physician to satisfy patient preferences.

Another concern is that EBM relies on population studies to treat individuals (also at http://www.hsl.unc.edu/lm/ebm/index.htm cited Dec 29, 2004); that it takes the results of studies of large groups of people and tries to apply them to individuals who may have unique circumstances or characteristics, not found in the study groups. This is valid criticism insofar as it is not always possible to decide whether or not the information and results are applicable to the individual patient. In addition, discussing the results with the patient, as it is required by the EBM process, opens up the possibility for the patient to misunderstand the evidence and, as a result, to hinder the process of clinical decision making. In addition, some times there are no randomized controlled trials or "a gold standard" that applies to the clinical question at hand. In this case the clinician has the burden to decide how strong his evidence should be and to look for the best compromise as far as the strength of evidence is concerned.

The strength the different types of evidence can be thought of as a stepped pyramid (Fig 1). The stronger the evidence, the higher the level on the pyramid it occupies. The base of the "evidence pyramid" rests on the basic medical sciences (Anatomy, Biochemistry, Microbiology, Pathology, Pharmacology, Physiology, etc), the different clinical disciplines (Internal Medicine, Surgery, etc) and the different medical specialties. Clinical research most often starts from an observation or some compound suspected to have medicinal value or, finally, from a "raw" idea. All these have to be investigated at the level of pathophysiology, a process that starts with laboratory models, proceeds with animal testing, and finally ends with tests on humans. Human testing usually begins with volunteers and goes through several phases of clinical trials before the drug or diagnostic tool can be authorized for use within the general population. Randomized controlled trials are then done to further test the effectiveness and efficacy of a drug or therapy.

If the physician does not find the best level of evidence to answer his question, then he should consider moving down the pyramid and use other types of studies to supplant his clinical judgment. After all, in some cases there is no real evidence to support clinical judgment. In these cases the clinician should rely upon his knowledge of pathophysiology to guide him through. A simple definition for the type of evidence that forms each of the steps of the "evidence pyramid" is given in Table 5 along with indications as to the "strength" of each type of evidence. A guide as to how to "climb down" the pyramid steps in order to find the evidence best fitting a question is given in Table 6. Finally, one should be aware of Practice Guidelines. These are systematically developed statements that review, evaluate the evidence and make explicit recommendations. When available, they are of assistance to both practitioner and patient, helping to make decisions for specific clinical circumstances.

Fig 1: The "evidence pyramid" which is used to illustrate the evolution of the literature and indicate the strength of evidence available. As one moves up the pyramid the amount of available literature decreases while its relevance to the clinical setting increases. Adopted and adapted from http://www.hsl.unc.edu/lm/ebm/index.htm cited Dec 29, 2004

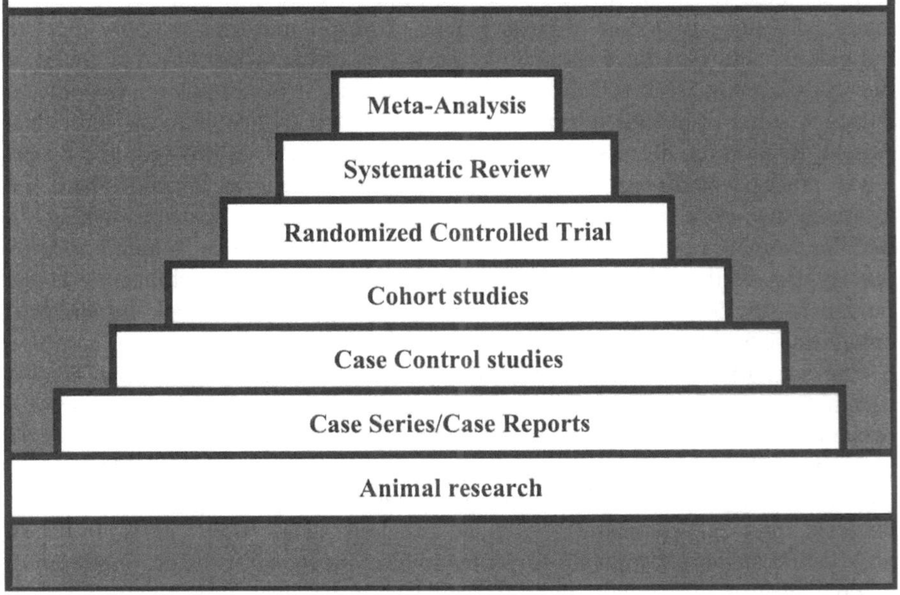

Table 5: The constituting steps of the "evidence pyramid"	
TYPE OF EVIDENCE	**INFORMAL DEFINITION & INDICATIONS AS TO THE EVIDENCE'S "STRENGTH"**
Meta-analysis	It uses statistical techniques to combine the results of several studies into one large study.
Systematic Reviews	They focus on a clinical topic and answer specific questions. They are based on extensive literature searches in order to identify studies with sound methodology. These studies are then reviewed, assessed, and summarized.
Randomized Controlled Trials (RCT)	They are carefully planned studies of the effect of a therapy or a test on patients. They attempt to reduce the potential for bias and allow for comparison between intervention and control groups.
Cohort Studies	They use large population samples and follow patients with a specific condition or patients who receive a particular treatment over time and compare them with another group that is similar but has not been affected by the condition being studied.
Case Control Studies	They compare patients who have a specific condition with people who do not. They are less reliable than randomized controlled trials and cohort studies because statistical relationships do not imply causal links.
Case Series/ Case Reports	They are collections of reports on the treatment of individual patients (a report refers to a single patient). Since they cannot use controls with which to compare outcomes, they have no statistical validity.
Animal research	Delineation of the mechanisms of action of drugs and treatments and studies on the pathophysiology of disease.

Table 6: Climbing down the "evidence pyramid"	
Therapy	RCT>cohort > case control > case series
Diagnosis	prospective, blind comparison to a gold standard
Etiology/Harm	RCT > cohort > case control > case series
Prognosis	cohort study > case control > case series
Prevention	RCT>cohort study > case control > case series
Clinical Exam	prospective, blind comparison to gold standard
Cost	economic analysis

Why EBM combines with TM to give EBT; implications for healthcare delivery, the teleconsultants and the patients.

The ultimate application of EBM is at the level of the individual clinician's decisions about his patient. EBM, therefore, is an explicit approach to clinical problem solving which requires the use of current best evidence in making medical decisions about each individual patient. It is also a way of professional development that relies on continual professional learning. Finally EBM is based on the assessment, by the physician of the validity of the information he gathers and his judgement as to its relevance to the individual patient.

It is clear that although EBM has been criticized for the fact that most of its actions or steps are in use by clinicians ever since the early days of medicine, in fact it would have been impossible for EBM to exist at any time prior to the 1980s. As late as the 1960s scientific (medical) information production was still manageable. Starting in the 1970s, however, it became large enough as to overwhelm the most studious and willing physician. Had the Internet and the associated databases and search engines not come of age, practicing EBM would not be what it is today. In 1979, for example, Professor Archie Cochrane was complaining that "It is surely a great criticism of our profession that we have not organized a critical summary, by specialty or subspecialty, adapted periodically, of all relevant RCTs" [12]. In other words, in 1979, even for a visionary like professor Cochrane, it was impossible to perceive that critical summaries "of all relevant RCTs" would be carried out by individual physicians, for each individual patient they treated; instead, the task seemed so huge that only a collective, slowly adapting effort to identifying "valid information" seemed to be the answer.

In order to achieve evidence-informed decisions, by searching secondary databases as well as the primary literature for relevant articles, by assessing the validity and usefulness of those articles and by judging the relevance of them to the individual patient, the health practitioner should be familiar with the precepts and IT tools available for practicing EBM. It is such a familiarity that makes it possible to bring the enormous relevant literature under control, and, as databases improve, to answer clinical questions at the point of care in real time. Interestingly enough, modern TM uses the same "wires" or "information highway lanes" to bring the patient next to the teleconsultant and the meeting of these two "ways of practicing medicine" gives rise to EBT.

Overcoming the (technologically trivial) problem of (virtually) getting the patient next to his attending teleconsultant, however, is not the only common point that EBM and TM share. Today, TM is heralded as the way to provide health services in underserved regions all over the world. The reason is that good health of a population is synonymous with equality of access to healthcare and good health is fundamental for economic development. It is therefore of cardinal importance that an investment in health accompanies any economic development scheme: Clean water for sub-Saharan villages, extensive children vaccination programs in South America or other forms of public health interventions elsewhere, has always preceded economic development investment in the underdeveloped world. Since the main driving force behind TM is to provide health services in underserved regions all over the world, epidemiological information about distant geographic areas and information on the pathophysiology of less known diseases become important and have to be searched for. For example, malaria and tuberculosis are currently infecting large populations in Colombia and Brazil. Getting help to them but also containing the spread of these diseases to unaffected populations is of cardinal importance and an area where TM can help.

Again, the Internet and its associated information handling technologies are the best place to start (and in most cases, end) the search. But this is not the end of the story: Again, EBM is the only way that a teleconsultant can cope with such situations that tax the knowledge that an ordinary physician uses in his daily practice. Diseases that are characteristic of the so-called "western lifestyles," also appear in the less developed countries of the world. The treatment of cancer, cardiovascular diseases or pregnancy related problems is also of concern there, albeit in a different light and with respect to local population characteristics. The lifestyle related aggravating factors, for example, in the case of cardiovascular diseases, will definitely be different for a near-starvation reared patient in an African village than for a middle aged wealthy merchant from a neighboring city.

Closer at home, another area in which EBT can be of great value is home care for the elderly or the prison populations [7, 8]. The treatment of elderly patients suffering from disabling diseases such as Alzheimer's disease, heart failure, respiratory insufficiency or other chronic diseases, can be, in many instances, carried out at home at great savings in terms of resources and with increased efficiency and efficacy. Finally, EBT has an important role to play in providing health care aboard ships, planes, oil rigs, and even spacecraft. Given that medicine, in this case, is practiced with a very limited arsenal of drugs and with the assistance of lower skill paramedics, searching for best evidence to assist the teleconsultant in decision making becomes of cardinal importance.

Finally, one should not ignore the value of EBT in medical education [6]. An efficient and effective health-care infrastructure requires access to appropriate expertise coupled with continuing education of health-care professionals. The public, i.e. the final consumer of health services, has to also be educated especially in light of the fact that EBM requires informed patients if it is going to be successful. Education and rising public awareness about breast cancer, following Betty Ford's bout with the disease, e.g., has been credited with improving the chances of early detection of disease and reducing the subsequent treatment requirements in the US. Focusing on prevention through education about diet, smoking, hygiene etc. is thought to lead to a physically healthy society and is actively pursued as public policy. Finally, as far as the third world is concerned, education and training are among the most important factors in achieving sustainable development and they represent one of the development activities which stand to benefit most from appropriate use of telecommunications. TM services offer the opportunity for both training and education [5].

Above all, with the participation of local representatives, TM can create a forum for continuing medical education. Also, the necessary infrastructure can be used to access on-line services or participate in seminars through videoconferencing as well as the basis for the dissemination of preventative health-care information. Tele-education consists of at least three areas:

1. Distance education,
2. Access to remote information and
3. Community health education.

All three can be thought of as components of EBM and all of them can be accomplished through the Internet. Distance education usually involves a small rural teaching hospital linked to a major city teaching hospital. In this way, students at the rural site, e.g., can "attend" a lecture conducted by a professor at the big teaching hospital. Paramedics and junior hospital staff can witness or be informed about particular medical techniques and practices.

5.2 The technological scope and the medical extent of TM services

While medical science changes in terms of new drugs, non-invasive approaches to examination and more precisely controlled ways of treatment, the methods for delivering medical services are also changing. It is, increasingly, no longer necessary for the patient and the health care provider to be in the same room before a high quality medical consultation can take place. This is the high point in a series of advances, which started 70 years ago, when merchant mariners were treated by remote consultation delivered over "short waves". Advances in communications that came over the intervening years e.g., VHF, INMARSAT based satellite communications etc., as well as advances in the equipment attached at both ends of the TM communication channel, improved on the quality of care delivered through TM [3,4]. On land, the "plain-old-telephone-system" (POTS) enabled doctors to practice limited aspects of medicine over vast distances without travel, a benefit that permitted more persons to live and work in remote areas. Recent advances in digital and communications technologies rapidly expand the repertoire of health care applications that can be remotely administered. Satellites and optic fiber infrastructures, coupled with advances in the capture, storage, transmission, and display of electronic representations of medical information, allow doctors to do many things remotely. Last but not least, the Internet is emerging as a powerful transparent integration platform for distributed medical information handling and processing [30]. TM, therefore, is finally maturing as a practical method for health care delivery.

TM encompasses a diverse set of practices, technologies and applications [6, 8]. The most common TM activities are:

1. Consultations or second opinions.
2. Diagnostic test interpretation.
3. Chronic disease management.
4. Post-hospitalization or postoperative follow-ups

5. Emergency room triage.
6. Virtual "visits" by a specialist.

As recently as five years ago it was customary to characterize TM by the type of information sent (such as radiographs or clinical findings) and by the means used to transmit it. Although the underlying technology tends to homogenize the ways different types of information is transmitted, TM services are still routinely categorized as being of three main types depending of whether they are based on the transmission of data, audio or images. Within each of these broad types, several subtypes are recognized.

Information transmitted during TM transactions

Data

Data transmission includes data, in the form of relatively static information, such as a patient's medical record and dynamic information such as vital signs data (e.g. heart rate and blood pressure).

As far as static information is concerned, there is widespread use of e-mail for administrative purposes including the transmission of patient records, referral letters and test results between general practitioners (GPs) and hospitals. Many hospitals, clinics and other health institutions around the world use computer systems routinely and have stored their medical records and databases electronically. This allows doctors to retrieve information about their patients very quickly and also to keep patient records up to date: Teleconsultants can access patient records and update the data from a distance. Finally, e-mail tele-consultation has been used for treatment planning and, when necessary, for organizing the transfer (including international transfer) of patients from a medically underserved locale to a medical centre.

Of particular interest to EBT is the coming of age of many specialized medical databases, especially in the industrialized countries. Information contained in these databases, combined with the patient data and available (literally) on the same computer screen, can form the basis of practising EBT. In general access to these databases is via the Internet. In some instances, access is free, in others, the user pays for access. MEDLINE, for example, is the on-line medical literature retrieval service sponsored by the US National Library of Medicine, a part of the National Institute of Health. It is free to use and it contains details of over twelve million articles.

Telemetry, on the other hand, provides a means for monitoring human and animal physiological functions from a remote site and it includes examples of vital sign transmission [19]. One of the earliest telemetry applications was the monitoring of the physiological functions of astronauts while they were in space. More recently, telemetry systems have been proposed and, in some cases, adapted for use on board aircraft. The coming of age, however, of telemetry is identified with the advent of the Internet and the appearance of the first home based, vital sign, remote monitoring devices.

Audio

Despite the advent of various communication modalities, including the all pervasive Internet, still the simplest TM service is the consultation between health-care workers by telephone. The conventional telephone service (PSTN) is probably the most cost-effective means of facilitating consultations between remote and rural areas and urban hospitals within a country or with centres of excellence in other countries. The telephone is also widely used for consulting between doctor and patient.

Images

• *Teleradiology*

Medical images are an essential part of modern medicine. They may be still pictures, for example radiographs, or moving pictures, i.e. video. Teleradiology is, presently, the most widely used TM service and it refers to the transmission of radiological images from one location to another for the purpose of interpretation or consultation. As such, the term teleradiology covers the transfer of X-rays and computed tomography (CT) images, magnetic resonance imaging (MRI), ultrasound images, images from nuclear medicine scans, and from thermography, fluoroscopy and angiography. Each of these modalities produces anatomical or functional images of the patient. The different types of images produced and transferred within or between radiology departments include, but are not limited to:

1. Conventional X-ray images
2. Computed tomography (CT) scans.
3. Magnetic resonance images (MRI)
4. Ultrasound investigations: there are ultrasonography applications in cardiology, internal medicine, obstetrics, gynaecology and emergency medicine.
5. Nuclear medicine investigations including plain conventional camera imaging, single photon emission computed tomography (SPECT) and positron emission tomography (PET).
6. Thermography images
7. Fluoroscopy images
8. Angiography and digital subtraction angiography

- ***Telepathology***

Another major field of interest in TM is the practice of Telepathology. Pathology is the medical study of disease-related changes in cells and tissues. In telepathology, the pathologist examines tissue images on a monitor rather through the microscope. Pathology covers a very broad range of diseases and medical disciplines and this makes it impossible for any single pathologist to be expert in them all. Hence consultations are an important part of the practice in pathology and opinions from those who specialize in particular diseases are often of paramount importance. Furthermore, special studies on a pathology specimen are frequently called for, following the initial evaluation of a microscopic preparation, sometimes away from the referring site. This entails sending the pathology specimens to the consultative site for processing, a process that takes time, costs money and involves risk of specimen destruction or loss.

Telepathology can be used for obtaining a second opinion or for obtaining a primary diagnosis since it minimizes most of these limitations. In the past ten years, two main ways to do telepathology have been tried: remote examination of still microscopic images or remote examination of moving video images, sometimes with robotic control of the remote microscope. The verdict however is still not in since the transmission of moving video images, coupled with robotic control of the remote microscope is still expensive and requires very high-speed telecommunications links. On the other hand, still image transmission, though cheaper, has various disadvantages in practice.

- ***Teledermatology***

Dermatology deals with the skin and its diseases and it is probably the medical specialty that depends, most of all, on direct, optically aided or unaided, observation of the skin. Teledermatology involves dermatology and it focuses on the diagnosis and clinical management of patients at a distance. Like telepathology, it can be conducted using either still images (store-and-forward TM) or moving images (real-time or interactive TM). Acceptable diagnostic accuracy and clinical management has been achieved using low cost video equipment, while simple e-mail transmission of still pictures has successfully being used to diagnose and treat remote patients.

Store-and-forward TM versus real-time or interactive TM

As already hinted, the different TM applications can be grouped into two major categories, depending on the immediacy they require for the completion of the clinical task at hand: Store-and-forward TM and real-time or interactive TM. Store-and-forward TM programs operate in many clinical domains [2] and, despite the worldwide advent of the Internet, still today offer the best hope for extending TM to the poorest countries in Africa at a reasonable cost and with substantial benefits. However, studies assessing the efficacy of most store-and-forward TM programs are lacking. When available, the evidence is of insufficient quality to judge the efficacy of store-and-forward TM. The major exception is Teledermatology, which has been extensively evaluated as a store-and-forward TM specialty. In its case, the diagnostic accuracy and the resulting patient management decisions have been found comparable to those of in-person clinical encounters. It improves access to care and it has adequate patient acceptance.

Store-and-forward TM differs from face-to-face encounters in that a history and physical examination is not performed by the clinician. Instead, the clinician gets a report of the history and physical examination along with audio or video data (in an asynchronous manner). As mentioned, this method of patient-doctor encounter is well tolerated in the case of Teledermatology. However, it is by necessity the only way of patient-doctor interaction in the case of Maritime Emergency TM or in low bandwidth applications, mainly through the use of low orbit polar route satellites. Thus, despite the fact that store-and-forward TM is more time-consuming than in-person consultations, and that no formal assessment of the health outcomes of store-and-forward TM exist, the fact that no major change (apart from improvements in communications technology) has taken place in the way Maritime Emergency TM is performed since the 1920's while an estimated 15000 Maritime Emergency TM interventions occur every year, speaks well about store-and-forward TM. This, of course, does not answer the question of whether store-and-forward TM results in comparable patient or clinician satisfaction or in comparable costs of care.

As bandwidth improves, an increasing number of clinical TM services become candidates for and might be provided by clinician-interactive TM. Chief among them are history taking and physical examination, psychiatric examination, and ophthalmologic assessment. However, in contrast to store-and-forward Teledermatology, studies of clinician-interactive TM show that it is diagnostically inferior to in-person dermatology. On the other hand, studies in the domains of cardiology, emergency medicine, otolaryngology, certain ophthalmology conditions, and pulmonary medicine show equivalent diagnostic accuracy. On the question of access to care, clinician-interactive TM seems to provide improved access in the case of neurosurgery, medical-surgical evaluation, and cardiac care. Furthermore, despite the fact that the jury is still out on whether clinician-interactive TM services improve health outcomes, clinicians, patients, parents of patients and families of patients seem to be satisfied with their clinician-interactive TM services experiences. Finally, there is some evidence emerging that costs of care can be reduced via clinician-interactive TM

Success is a very elusive concept when one refers to TM. To make things clear, the vast majority of the over 1000 TM implementations that have been reported [19,22], criticized or variously tabulated in the literature, regards experiments in TM and pilot applications rather than situations where TM has been actually integrated in everyday practice. It is, therefore, difficult to talk about actual TM services. Instead, it is much more appropriate to talk about specific situations where TM has successfully met a definite need and where there is reasonable expectation that a service can be organized to meet long term needs in a sustainable fashion. Viewed from this standpoint, the following situations present the most promising fields for TM applications:

1. Emergency TM: Specially designed applications include the case of ships, oil-rigs and airlines; they also include remote scientific expeditions and monitoring stations. More general applications include isolated small islands and some military and army situations.
2. Primary care type applications: They include applications in home health (long term patients at home, geriatric facilities, old-age homes, asylums of all kinds) as well as populations which, for various reasons, are medically underserved (prisons, refugee camps, socially or racially isolated neighbourhoods). They also include specialist applications where long term, regular monitoring is required (e.g., ophthalmology monitoring in diabetic retinopathy)
3. Public health applications: They include applications such as population screening and health education.

Many other applications can be thought of and in fact have been implemented. Some of them concern consumer health services, drugs and pharmacy services, access to libraries etc.

5.3 How are EBT services delivered?

Accessing the sources of evidence

Practicing EBM is synonymous to searching the published literature (Second step of the EBM process; Table 4) to find answers to clinical questions that were formulated during the first step ("State the question"; Table 4). In most cases, a well-built clinical question leads directly to a good search strategy. Always, the goal is to locate a randomized controlled trial; it would provide good evidence to help answer the clinical question. Since, at present, there are, roughly, approximately 15 million published reports, journal articles, correspondence and studies available to clinicians, choosing the best resource to search is an important decision. Large databases such as MEDLINE are good conduits to the primary literature. Secondary resources such as ACP Journal Club, POEMS and Clinical Evidence, provide assessments of the original studies. The Cochrane Library provides access to systematic reviews which help summarize the results from a number of studies. The main getaways to the EBM literature and practice guidelines are summarized in Table 7.

Table 7		
No.	**SOURCE**	**CONTENT**
1	**Agency for Health Care Research and Policy (AHRQ)** http://www.ahrq.gov cited Dec 29, 2004	Contains information about EBM including downloading of full text articles in PDF. It also provides general knowledge concerning usual health problems and public health matters.
2	**Bandolier** http://www.jr2.ox.ac.uk/bandolier/index.html cited Dec 29, 2004	Monthly independent journal about Evidence based Healthcare. It contains reviews and analyses appearing in Pubmed and in the Cochrane Library.
3	**BestBETS** http://www.bestbets.org cited Dec 29, 2004	Developed by the Emergency Department of the Manchester Royal Infirmary in UK, it gives rapid answers to real life clinical questions. Focused on Emergency Medicine, it also contains a significant number of articles about cardiology, nursing, primary care and pediatrics. It links with other EBM websites.
4	**Centre for Evidence Based Medicine** http://www.cebm.net cited Dec 29, 2004	Developed by Oxford University, it contains information about EBM along with an EBM glossary, and FAQ about the practice of EBM
5	**CINAHL** http://www.urmc.rochester.edu/hslt/miner cited Dec29, 2004	The Edward G. Miner Library is a digital library containing many databases, Medline, e-journals, e-books and it is accessible from home. It contains resources for researchers, patients, students and professionals. In addition it contains an option for rare books and manuscripts in the area of medical, dental and nursing history.
6	**Cochrane Library and Collaboration** http://www.cochrane.org cited Dec 29, 2004	It has links to many sites concerning EBM. It contains over 350,000 controlled trials and 1500 systematic reviews. It is available both on CD-ROM and in the Internet (there are many databases included in the library). Search for words or for title is possible, while the on-line version of the library can be read in English, German, French, Chinese, Italian and Brazilian. Full text reviews can be downloaded.
7	**EBM Tool Kit** http://www.med.ualberta.ca/ebm/ebm.htm cited Dec 29, 2004	Developed at the University of Alberta, Canada, it contains an EBM glossary, links to other EBM sites, and strategies for more fruitful search such as a "basic search

		strategy", a "quick filter", and an "advanced search strategy"
8	**Evidence- Based Medicine** http://www.evidence-basedmedicine.com cited Dec 29, 2004	It is a bi-monthly journal, which includes articles concerning family practice, internal medicine, pediatrics, obstetrics, gynecology, psychiatry and surgery. It has many EBM Links and the ability to view the top 10 papers concerning EBM.
9	**Evidence-Based Medicine Education Center of Excellence** http://www.hsl.unc.edu/ahec/ebmcoe/pages/index.htm cited Dec 29, 2004	Developed by the University of North Carolina, it contains abstracts , links to the Cochrane Library and Pubmed databases, links to 2 e-journals and specific knowledge for learning and teaching EBM
10	http://healthweb.org cited Dec 29, 2004	Developed by the University of Illinois at Chicago, it links to EBM Websites, databases (like the Cochrane Library, the Pubmed, and the Trip Database), electronic journals and associations
11	**Health Information Research Unit – McMaster University** http://hiru.hirunet.mcmaster.ca cited Dec 29, 2004	Developed by the McMaster University, it contains links to the Canadian Network and to Cancer Care Ontario
12	http://www.hsl.unc.edu/services/tutorials/ebm/index.htm cited Dec 29, 2004	Contains an introduction to EBM along with an EBM glossary, a tutorial on the practice of EBM (including instruction on how to, e.g., conduct a literature search) and a presentation of a few cases for testing one's skills in using EBM.
13	**MEDLINE** http://www.uic.edu/depts/lib/lhsp/resources/med.shtml cited Dec 29, 2004	This is the Premiere Biomedical Database. It was developed in the University of Illinois at Chicago and it provides information about other EBM Databases, EBM publications and internet resources. It contains over 4000 international biomedical journals and provides access to PubMed and Ovid Medline
14	**National Guidelines Clearinghouse** http://www.guideline.gov cited Dec 29, 2004	Developed by the US Department of Health and Human Services, it contains abstracts and links to full text guidelines. It permits the comparison of two or more guidelines and resources for themes such as bioterrorism, bibliographies, and glossary for terms used in abstracts and frequently asked questions.

15	**Netting the Evidence** http://www.shef.ac.uk/~scharr/ir/netting cited Dec 29, 2004	Developed in Sheffield, UK, it contains journals, databases (including the Cochrane Database but not Pubmed), links to EBM Organizations and full text documents
16	**POEMS (Patient Oriented Evidence That Matters)** http://www.infopoems.com/ cited Dec 29, 2004	POEMS contains over 200 summaries of evidence based articles.
17	**TRIPDatabase** http://www.tripdatabase.com cited Dec 29, 2004	It is a monthly updated database which initially contained 1,100 links to EBM articles. It contains TripWire which is a way for users, to focus and specify their search.
18	**University of Washington Pediatrics EBM CAT-Bank** http://pedsccm.wustl.edu/EBJournal_Club.html cited Dec 29, 2004	It provides a free access to full-text articles about EBM and links to EBM databases, groups in the web, journals and systematic reviews, along with a user's guide to medical literature.
19	**University of Michigan Evidence-Based Pediatrics Critically Appraised Topics** http://www.med.umich.edu/pediatrics/ebm cited Dec 29, 2004	Developed by the Department of Pediatrics in the University of Michigan, it offers access to EBM links, a methodology for teaching EBM and a number of critically appraised topics in many medical specialties (cardiology, nephrology, neonatology, neurology, etc).
20	**US Preventive Services** http://odphp.osophs.dhhs.gov cited Dec 29, 2004	This page provides direct Internet access to the *Guide to Clinical Preventive Services* which is also available via the National Library of Medicine's HSTAT (Health Services/Technology Assessment Text) database at http://www.ncbi.nlm.nih.gov/books/bv.fcgi?rid=hstat (cited Dec 29, 2004) and the Office of Disease Prevention and Health Promotion at http://odphp.osophs.dhhs.gov/pubs/guidecps.(cited Dec 29, 2004) The latest information on the *Guide* is online at http://www.ahrq.gov/clinic/prevnew.htm (cited Dec 29, 2004)
21	http://www.york.ac.uk/inst/crd/search.htm cited Dec 29, 2004	It is a center for review and dissemination that offers reviews on specific topics, links to three databases (DARE, NHS, HTA), publications, and a dissemination service able to accept enquiries via e-mail in the case of a question by the reader.

Starting from one of the getaways listed in Table 7, or any other comparable source, one can collect and review both the titles and abstracts, that the search comes up with, and attempt to identify potentially relevant articles. What is fairly certain is that at the end of a diligent search there will be a number of articles and other primary sources of information current information, which can answer the clinical questions that were formulated during the first step of the EBM process. The next step is to read the article and evaluate the information keeping in mind that everything that will follow hinges upon three basic questions that need to be answered for every type of study:

1. Are the results of the study valid?
2. What are the results?
3. Will the results help in caring for the patient?

Normally, within a regular research paper or report, the answers to these questions are found in the methodology section. It is here where the investigators normally address issues of statistical or systematic bias. Randomization, blinding and proper accounting for all patients and materials help insure that the study results are not overly influenced by the investigators, the patients or other external factors. However, apart from these general admonitions as to the design of a study that aspires to provide evidence, there are different requirements that an EBM user of a study's conclusions should insist upon, depending on the type of the study. Summaries of these requirements for the results of a therapy study to be valid, for a diagnostic study to be valid, for a prognosis study to be valid, and for the results of an Etiology/Harm study to be valid are presented in Tables 8 through 11, respectively.

Table 8: Conditions that should be met for the results of a therapy study to be valid

No.	Requirement	Brief description
1	Randomized assignment of patients	Assignment of patients to either treatment or control groups must be done by a random allocation to ensure the creation of groups of patients, who will be similar in their risk of the events one wants to prevent. Randomization balances the groups for prognostic factors (such as disease severity) and eliminates over-representation of any one characteristic within the study group. Randomization should be concealed from the clinicians and researchers to help eliminate conscious or unconscious bias.
2	The patients who entered a trial must be properly accounted for at the trial's	The study should begin and end with the same number of patients and patients that dropped out of the study must be accounted for, otherwise the conclusions are invalid. In the case that patients drop out because of the adverse effects

	conclusion	of the therapy being tested and are not accounted for, the conclusions reached may be over confident as far as the efficacy of the therapy is concerned.
3	Complete follow-up	Studies should have better than 80% follow-up for their patients, while lost patients should be assigned to the "worst-case" outcomes and still support the original conclusion of the study, if we want to be sure of a study's conclusions.
4	Patients should be analyzed in the groups to which they were originally assigned during randomization	Patients who forget or refuse their treatment should not be eliminated from the study analysis because excluding them leaves behind those that are more likely to have a positive outcome. This introduces biases in the study and annuls the effects of randomization
5	Blinding	To eliminate bias and preconceived notions as to how the treatments should be working, the people involved in a study should not know which treatments are given to which patients. In double blinding neither the patient nor the clinician knows which treatment is being administered. When it is difficult or even unethical to blind patients to a treatment, then the results should be interpreted by a "blinded" clinician.
6	Similarity of groups at the start of the trial	Treatment and control groups must be similar for all prognostic characteristics except one: whether or not they received the experimental treatment.
7	Groups should be treated equally	Study groups must be treated in exactly the same manner except for administration of the experimental treatment. If there are interventions, other than the study treatment, which are applied differently to each group, these must be clearly described.

Table 9: Conditions that should be met for a diagnostic study to be valid

No.	Requirement	Brief description
1	Independent, blind comparison with a "gold" standard	A "gold" standard (e.g., an autopsy or biopsy) either provides objective criteria (e.g., a laboratory test not requiring interpretation) or sets a current clinical standard (e.g., 3D sonohysterography) for diagnosis. Patients in the study should have undergone both the diagnostic test in question and "gold" standard test.

		Clinicians evaluating the tests should be blinded, i.e., the results of one test should not be known to the clinicians who are conducting or evaluating the other test.
2	The sample must include a wide spectrum of patients who will undergo the specific testing in clinical practice	The spectrum of patients must include those with mild and severe cases, early and late cases, and patients who were treated as well as patients who were untreated for the target disease. The test should also be applied to patients with disorders that are commonly confused with the target disease.
3	Replication	The study methodology should be presented in enough detail so that it can be repeated within the appropriate setting. This includes detailed specification of dosage levels, patient preparations, timing, etc.

Table 10: Conditions that should be met for a prognosis study to be valid

No.	Requirement	Brief description
1	Randomized assignment of patients, who are at a similar point in the course of the disease.	Patients must be included in the study at a uniformly early point in the disease, ideally, when the disease first manifests itself clinically.
2	Complete follow-up	Patients should be followed until they fully recover or one of the disease outcomes occurs. A long enough follow-up is necessary in order to develop a valid picture. Usually this means that at least 80% of participants are followed up until the occurrence of a major study end point.
3	Using objective and unbiased outcome criteria	If outcomes include a wide range of conditions between death and full recovery, these must be clearly defined, specific criteria should be proposed for each possible outcome of the disease and be used during patient follow-up. Investigators deciding on the clinical outcomes must be "blinded" to the patient characteristics and prognostic factors in order to eliminate possible bias in their observations.
4	Adjustment for important prognostic factors	Patients' clinical characteristics must be similar. This means that sometimes adjustments have to made based on age, gender, or sex to get a true picture of the clinical outcome.

Table 11: Conditions that should be met for the results of an Etiology/Harm study to be valid		
No.	**Requirement**	**Brief description**
1	Clearly identified comparison groups.	The choice of comparison groups must ensure that they are similar with respect to important determinants of outcome, other than the one of interest. Comparability must be clearly demonstrated. Characteristics of the exposed and non exposed patients need to be carefully documented.
2	Exposures and outcomes must be measured in the same way in the groups being compared	The measurements should avoid any kind of bias, whether from recall bias (by patient motivation to help) or by interviewer bias (probing by interviewers for the "right" answer). Using objective data, such as medical records, can help eliminate bias.
3	Complete follow-up	Non-availability of patients for complete follow-up comprises the validity of the study since these patients may have very different outcomes than those that stayed with the study.
4	Correct temporal relationships must exist in terms of cause and effect	The intervention, whether therapeutic or harmful, must have happened before the adverse outcome occurred.
5	Existence of dose-response gradients	The utility of the results depends on whether it can be demonstrated that the adverse effect increases when the intensity or duration of the exposure to the harmful agent is increased. When the object of a study is to prove the beneficial effects of exposure to a therapeutic or prevention agent, then an increase in the intensity or duration of the exposure, should make it less likely for an adverse event to occur.

The evaluation of medical literature is a complex undertaking. Answers to questions of validity are not always clearly stated in the literature and many times the clinicians have to decide on their own about the validity of the evidence that is turned up by their search.

However, assuming that the physician reaches a valid conclusion on the validity of the evidence he unearths, it is still necessary to examine the results of his search are applicable to his individual patient. This process is summarized in the following three questions that have to be answered:

1. Does the study represent people similar to the specific patient?

2. Does the study cover the aspect of the problem that is most important to the specific patient?
3. Does the study suggest a clear and useful plan of action?

Once the teleconsultant can answer all three of these questions affirmatively, then he can proceed to implement the plan of action he selected for his patient.

Integrating best evidence into existing TM systems and TM protocols

The successful integration of best evidence into existing TM systems and TM protocols requires that a certain e-health model to the provision of health services is adopted first. The model must have clear clinical and geographic targets: The simultaneous applicability of current telehealth technologies and EBM, for example, to most types of TM has not been demonstrated as yet. The most promising areas for demonstrating the successful integration of EBM and TM are:

1. Internal medicine, especially when it comes to clinical applications such as infectious diseases that threaten to make a come back (e.g., malaria and tuberculosis), Gynaecology (e.g., ultrasound applications in pregnancy monitoring),
2. Urology and
3. Cardiovascular diagnosis etc.

It should be noted however, that this list is heavily biased by the authors' preferences and actual TM implementations and should not dissuade the interested reader from thinking or attempting to expand on it.

Potential benefits of the integration of best evidence into existing TM systems and TM protocols arise not only in the area of health provision but also in social development where, apart of diagnosis and therapy, EBM answers to questions of etiology/harm or prognosis of endemic diseases can contribute to the initiation and/or strengthening of local public health activities.

The general objectives of any integration of EBM and TM into EBT are:

1. To implement an e-health model that, apart from access, it improves the quality of health care resources.
2. To promote education, technology transfer and, where applicable, economic growth though the introduction and use of Internet and IT for health service improvement.
3. To foster social development through the improvement of disease control and health services.

The impact of any effort to implement EBT is threefold: Clinical, technological and social. In each case it depends on the particular TM application domain, the specific geographical area or, finally, the social condition that it serves.

The clinical impact of EBT centres on:

1. The efficient and cost effective use of high-tech and high quality medical resources, that are available in large cities, in order to improve the health services for residents in remote and/or underserved regions.
2. The reduction of morbidity and mortality in underserved regions achieved through the provision of the means for early detection and treatment of diseases (including contagious diseases such as Malaria and tuberculosis) and the use of communication and e-health technologies.
3. The improvement of primary healthcare achieved through the use of high-tech but relatively low cost peripherals by local general practitioners or paramedics under the supervision of remotely located experts.
4. Contributing to the advancement of medical research, diagnosis and treatment methods, through the efficient collection and sharing of data on treatment outcomes and patient demographics.

The technological impact of EBT centres on the development of intelligent user interfaces, both for the health professionals and the patients. Such interfaces will help meet the main challenge of EBT which is to make electronically accessible the guidelines, the diagnosis and treatment results and the necessary databases for practicing EBM in the targeted regions.

Finally, the social impact of EBT is expected to become evident in reducing the gap between underserved regions and large cities in medical service levels. In this respect it should be noted that the simplicity of TM networks, that the present and future growth of the Internet implies, and the adaptation of EBT to local needs confirms that much can be done to give access to health care, where little had been available before. Traditionally, TM has been described as benefiting populations in remote, rural areas. However, since economic growth is associated with a decreasing dependence on agriculture, it is inevitable that rural populations will decline and urbanization will be the first step towards industrialization in most underdeveloped countries. This makes past TM demonstrations irrelevant to the envisaged growth of TM in the future: Past TM demonstrations do not relate to the delivery of health care for the populations of the urban areas, which is exactly where TM may have a profound effect on the overall delivery of health care, especially to under-served urban populations of the developing countries.

For example, it has been demonstrated that in Albania, access to specialty care services is far more important to the underserved urban populations than reducing the cost of medical services. This has resulted in a situation where there is a strong financial incentive for foreign medical establishments to use TM to gain entrance to the Albanian health services market and to promote patient migration to neighbouring countries where high quality medical care is available. Based on that, one can conclude that, so long as what is considered commonplace, even in moderately developed countries, is not available to the urban populations of developing countries, we can expect that EBT will have a serious role to play both in terms of avoiding unnecessary medical acts and in raising the level of healthcare available to the underprivileged urban populations of the developing countries.

EBT contributions to the different specialties

Table 12 summarizes the results of a Medline search which attempted to evaluate the interest TM has generated over the past 15 years in the different medical specialties. This was done in an effort to assess both the penetration of TM into the different medical fields of potential application and to confirm the choices of the present study as to what is really important in developing an EBT. Not surprising, out of 2630 scientific papers that were identified as contributed by the different specialties, radiology, surgery, pathology, dermatology and cardiology occupied the top 5 spots totaling amongst the 2067 scientific papers or more than 78.5% of the total. Interestingly, the term EBT brought forth a surprisingly small number of citations, 77 in all, indicating that EBT is indeed a new field of scientific endeavor. Interestingly enough, among them figure articles on the safety and effectiveness of minor injuries telemedicine [10], on following-up patients and assessing outcomes in teledermatology [21] and on telehealth responses to bio-terrorism and emerging infections [32] to randomly name a few of the most recent ones. This is an indication that EBT is spreading to all fields that classical TM covered. At the same time concerns about TM and EBT are voiced and discussed [20].

Table 12: Interest TM has generated in the different medical specialties	
Specialty	**No. of Medline Citations**
Cardiology	166
Dermatology	235
Endocrinology	13
ENT	11
Geriatrics	21
Gynecology-Obstetrics	48
Internal Medicine	92
Neurology	57
Oncology	86
Orthopedics	35
Pain	44
Pathology	460
Pediatrics	126
Radiology	619
Surgery	617
Total	**2630**

5.4 Conclusions and Future directions

Since the 1990s TM has made a lot of progress, both technologically and scientifically. There have been more than 1000 TM experiments or reports on the operation of TM pilot sites that have been conducted during the last 15 years. There were more than 6546 publications on TM listed in PubMed as of Sept.15, 2004 containing the word "telemedicine". There were also a total of 15334 citations of articles on TM and Telehealth included in the bibliographic database of Telemedicine Information Exchange (TIE - http://tie.telemed.org/) on the same date. In addition, the TIE database is reporting that new citations were coming in at the rate of 85 citations per month during August and September 2004.

These figures demonstrate that TM works, and it can be used beneficially from clinical and economic standpoints. On the other hand, most of these programs are experimental in nature, their longevity not guaranteed (or even anticipated once their funding is exhausted) and, even when they are designed to be part of the everyday delivery of healthcare services, it is not clear, how many may fail to survive beyond initial funding or enthusiasm. Furthermore, the evidence for the efficacy of TM is also not clear due to the fact that the methodology of TM evaluations made so far precludes definitive statements. Given that the nature of most TM applications, to date, have been experimental in nature, most of them are based on small sample sizes that do not allow reasonably certain statistical analysis while the settings, by definition in most cases, differ substantially from the equivalent clinical ones. Last but not least, many of the studies focus on patient populations that might be less likely than others to benefit from improved health services, such as people who have complex chronic diseases and are the subjects of home care arrangements.

However, the momentum for TM that was demonstrated has kept TM experiments and implementations going despite any objections that could or have been raised. Today, we have to admit that TM is at a key transition point or juncture. Attention is now shifting toward consolidating what were often isolated initiatives into larger networks and to the "mainstreaming" of TM as a core mode of service delivery, turning it from something "special" into "business as usual". There are many TM proponents that argue that the whole issue of TM evaluation is unimportant or at least premature. With the advent of high Internet speeds, mobile telephony and wireless data exchange, the technologies and methodologies that support TM, as a whole, will become ubiquitous and will not require any specific evaluation methodologies. Indeed, as TM looses its newcomer's luster, matures, and becomes increasingly commonplace it will eventually be as commonplace as the telephone and as standard as any other aspect of healthcare. This trend is further enhanced from the fact that TM implies longer term financial impacts at the level of the hospital organizations, at the level of the healthcare services or at the level of national and international health policy. These impacts will come from the same source (the move towards an Information Society) as practically everything else that at this instant, i.e. the first quarter of the 21st century, is changing the way we perform our daily chores and is driving the process of globalization.

Against this background we can conclude that EBT is small but growing. The more than 1000 TM experiments that have been reported in the literature over the last 15 or so years, demonstrate that TM can work. At the same time, their growing number is a clear sign that TM can be used beneficially from clinical and economic standpoints. Although the evidence for the efficacy of TM technology is not in yet [1], EBT is considered as the natural offspring of developments in the area of healthcare delivery.

Along the same lines, it is expected that the future focus of TM will shift to diseases with a high burden of illness and barriers to access to care. This will substantially add to the momentum of incorporating EBM into TM, i.e. to the emergence of EBT. At the same time, evidence based methodologies can be brought into the self assessment of the whole field of TM: Systematic observation of the effect of a telemedicine service will eventually begin with the use of patient registries. RCTs that assess patient outcomes and costs related to entire episodes of care will come into the vogue as demonstration projects will be phased out. Basic research in TM will also start replacing applied (technological) research as TM will mature and the needs to refine target populations for services, refine interventions and develop standardized tools to measure effectiveness and harm, become pressing.

References

1. Agency for Healthcare Research and Quality. Telemedicine for the Medicare Population. Evidence Report/Technology Assessment: Number 24. AHRQ, Rockville, MD. Publication Number 01-E011 (2001). This paper is available at http://www.ahrq.gov/clinic/epcsums/telemedsum.htm (cited Dec 29, 2004).

2. Anogianakis, G., and Maglavera, S.: Medical teleconsultation and emergency aid services to European fishing vessels. Journal of Telemedicine and Telecare (1996) 2 (Suppl 1) S1:118-19.

3. Anogianakis, G., Maglavera, S., Pomportsis, A., Bountzioukas, S., Beltrame, F. and Orsi, G.: Medical emergency aid through telematics: design, implementation guidelines and analysis of user requirements for the MERMAID project. Stud Health Technol Inform (1997) 43 Pt A: 74-8.

4. Anogianakis, G., Maglavera, S. and Pomportsis, A.: Relief for maritime medical emergencies through telematics. IEEE Trans Inf Technol Biomed (1998) 2:254-60.

5. Anogianakis, G.: Utilising multimedia for training merchant mariners as paramedics. Studies in Health Technology and Informatics (2000) 72: 66-72.

6. Anogianakis, G., Ilonidis, G., Anogeianaki, A., Milliaras, S., Klisarova, A., Temelkov, T. and Vlachakis-Milliaras, E.: A clinical and educational telemedicine link between Bulgaria and Greece. Journal of Telemedicine and Telecare (2003a) 9(Suppl 2): S2-4.

7. Anogianakis, G., Ilonidis, G., Milliaras, S., Anogeianaki, A. and Vlachakis-Milliaras, E.: Developing prison telemedicine systems: the Greek experience.Journal of Telemedicine and Telecare (2003b) 9(Suppl 2) : S:4-7.

8. Anogeianaki, A., Anogianakis, G., Ilonidis, G. and Milliaras, S.: The Korydallos, Greece, prisons telemedicine system experience: why technology alone is not a sufficient condition. Studies in Health Technology and Informatics (2004)98:16-8.

9. Appleby, J., Walshe, K. and Ham, C.: Acting on the evidence. NAHAT, Birmingham, UK. NAHAT Research Paper (1995) No. 17.

10. Benger, JR., Noble, SM., Coast, J. and Kendall, JM.: The safety and effectiveness of minor injuries telemedicine Emerg Med J (2004) 21(4):438-45.

11. Brauer, GW.: Telehealth: the delayed revolution in health care. Medical Progress Through Technology (1992) 18: 153.

12. Cochrane, AL.: 1931-1971: A critical review, with particular reference to the medical profession. In: Medicines for the year 2000, Office of Health Economics, London(1979)

13. Cook, DJ. and Levy, MM.: Evidence –based medicine. A tool for enhancing critical care practice. Crit Care Clin (1998) 14:353-8.

14. European Commission: Directorate General XIII. Research and technology development on telematics systems in health care: AIM Annual Technical Report on RTD: Health Care (1993) p. 18.

15. Geddes, JR. and Harrison, PJ.: Closing the gap between research and practice. Br J Psychiatry (1997) 171: 220-225.

16. Glasziou, P., Del Mar, C. and Salisbury, J.: Evidence - based Medicine Workbook. London, BMJ Books (2003).

17. Goldberg, MA., Sharif, HS., Rosenthal, DI., Black-Schaffer, S., Flotte, TJ., Colvin, RB. and Thrall, JH.: Making global telemedicine practical and affordable: demonstrations from the Middle East. American Journal of Roentgenol (1994) 163 (6): 1495-1500.

18. Hicks, N.: Evidence based healthcare. Bandolier (1997) 4 (39): 8.

19. International Telecommunications Union Impact of telecommunications in health-care and other social services. ITU-D Study Groups, First Study Period (1995-1998), Report on Question 6/2, Telecommunication Development Bureau, Geneva, CH (1997).

20. Kienzle, HF.: Fragmentation of the doctor-patient relationship as a result of standardisation and economisation Z Arztl Fortbild Qualitatssich (2004) 98(3):193-9.

21. Krupinski, EA., Engstrom, M., Barker, G., Levine, N. and Weinstein, RS.: The challenges of following patients and assessing outcomes in teledermatology J Telemed Telecare (2004)10(1):21-4.

22. Lacroix, A.: International concerted action on collaboration in telemedicine: G8 sub-project 4 Stud Health Technol Inform (1999) 64:12-9.

23. Marwick, C.: Proponents Gather to Discuss Practicing Evidence-Based Medicine. JAMA (1997) 278: 531-532.

24. McKibbon, KA., Wilczynski, N., Hayward, RS., Walker-Dilks, CJ. and Haynes RB.: The medical literature as a resource for evidence based care. Working Paper from the Health Information Research Unit, McMaster University, Ontario, Canada (1995).

25. Muir Gray, JA: Evidence-based healthcare: how to make health policy and management decisions. London: Churchill Livingstone (1997).

26. National Institute of Public Health, First Annual Nordic Work-shop on how to critically appraise and use evidence in decisions about healthcare. Norway (1996).

27. Preston, J., Brown, FW. and Hartley, B.: Using telemedicine to improve health care in distant areas. Hosp Community Psychiatry (1992) 43(1): 25-32.

28. Rosenberg, W. and Donald, A.: Evidence based medicine: an approach to clinical problem solving. BMJ (1995) 310 (6987):1122-1126.

29. Sackett, DL., Rosenberg, WM., Gray, JA., Haynes, RB, and Richardson, WS.: Evidence based medicine: what it is and what it isn't. BMJ (1996) 312 (7023): 71-72.

30. Stalidis, G., Prentza, A., Vlachos, IN., Anogianakis, G., Maglavera, S. and Koutsouris, D.: Intranet health clinic: Web-based medical support services employing XML. Stud Health Technol Inform (2000) 77: 1112-6.

31. World Health Organization. Advisor on Informatics of the World Health Organization; Report by the WHO Director General to the 99th Session of the Executive Board, 6 January 1997 (1997). (Ref: EB99/30).

32. Yellowlees, P. and MacKenzie, J.: Telehealth responses to bio-terrorism and emerging infections J Telemed Telecare (2003) 9 Suppl 2:S80-2.

6. Current Status of Computerized Decision Support Systems in Mammography

G.D. Tourassi, Ph.D.

Department of Radiology, Box 3302 DUMC, Duke University Medical Center, Durham, NC 27710

Abstract

Breast cancer is one of the most devastating and deadly diseases for women today. Despite advances in cancer treatment, early mammographic detection remains the first line of defense in the battle against breast cancer. Patients with early-detected malignancies have a significantly lower mortality rate. Nevertheless, it is reported that up to 30% of breast lesions go undetected in screening mammograms and up to 2/3 of those lesions are visible in retrospect. The clinical significance of early diagnosis and the difficulty of the diagnostic task have generated a tremendous interest on developing computerized decision support systems in mammography. Their main goal is to offer radiologists a reliable and fast "second opinion". Several systems have been developed over the past decade and some have successfully entered the clinical arena. Although several studies have indicated a positive impact on early breast cancer detection, the results are mixed and the decision support systems are under ongoing development and evaluation. In addition, there are still several unresolved issues such as their true impact on breast cancer mortality, the overall impact on the recall rate of mammograms and thus the radiologists' workload, the reproducibility of the computerized second opinions, the ability of a knowledgeable radiologist to effectively process these opinions, and ultimately clinical acceptance. Furthermore, the medical and legal implications of storing and/or dismissing computerized second opinions are currently unknown. Given the number of unresolved issues, the clinical role of the decision support systems in mammography continues to evolve. The purpose of this article is to review the present state of computer-assisted detection (CAD) and diagnosis (CADx) in mammography. Specifically, the article will describe the principles of CAD/CADx, how it is currently applied in mammography, examine reported limitations, and identify future research directions. Research work is presented towards the application of knowledge-based systems in mammography to address some of the current CAD limitations. Finally, the natural extension of CAD to telemammography is discussed.

Keywords: breast cancer; mammography; computer-assisted diagnosis

G.D. Tourassi: *Current Status of Computerized Decision Support Systems in Mammography*, StudFuzz **184**, 173–173 (2005)
www.springerlink.com

6.1 INTRODUCTION

Breast cancer is one of the most devastating and deadly diseases for women today. In 2002, it is estimated that approximately 258,000 new cases of breast cancer were diagnosed in the United States [1]. It is also estimated that 40,200 women died from breast cancer in 2001 [2]. The above statistics suggest that, on average, one woman died of breast cancer every 13 minutes in 2001. Similar projections regarding breast cancer incidence and mortality have been made for 2003 [3].

Early detection is a critical defense strategy in the battle against breast cancer. Patients with early-detected malignancies have a significantly lower mortality rate [4-6]. At present, mammography is considered the most reliable technique for early breast cancer detection. Nevertheless, mammographic interpretation is a challenging clinical task and radiologists' variability is well-documented [7,8]. It is reported that up to 30% of breast lesions go undetected in screening mammograms [9-11] and up to 2/3 of those lesions are visible in retrospect [12]. Although many missed cancers in screening mammograms are due to sub-optimal visual perception [10], a significant portion of them (over 60%) are visually scrutinized as much if not more than the reported cancers [11,12]. These findings suggest that both perceptual and interpretation errors are limiting factors in mammography.

The clinical significance of early diagnosis and the difficulty of the diagnostic task have generated a tremendous interest on developing computerized decision support systems in mammography. Their main goal is to offer radiologists a reliable and fast "second opinion" regarding the presence and type of possible breast abnormalities in a mammographic study. The research field is known as Computer Assisted Detection and Diagnosis (CAD/CADx). The CAD abbreviation typically comprises a wide range of computer algorithms designed to detect and characterize potential abnormalities in a mammogram. The suspicious mammographic regions detected by a CAD system serve as cues to the radiologists.

Although several studies showed that CAD technology has a positive impact on early breast cancer detection [7,9,13,14], there are also studies with conflicting findings [15,16]. In addition, a wide range of critical issues has been brought to focus. For example, in screening mammography a cueing CAD tool is expected to operate at a high sensitivity level (detection rate). Consequently, such tool is compromised by a higher false-positive rate. The impact of false-positive CAD cues on the recall rate of mammograms is under investigation [7,13,14,17,18]. Generally, it is assumed that the radiologists will be able to discard easily most of the false-positive cues. However, some studies have challenged this belief. These studies also showed that low-performing CAD tools degrade radiologists' performance in non-cued areas [19]. Therefore, it is recommended that a cueing CAD tool should be used by an experienced interpreter to effectively process all cues [20]. Nevertheless, dismissing CAD cues is a complex process heavily dependent on physicians' attitudes towards CAD and their level of experience. Furthermore, the medical and legal implications of dismissing CAD cues are currently unknown [20]. Finally, the CAD issue that has attracted the least attention is reproducibility. A limited study indicated that CAD reproducibility was clinically insufficient [21]. Although more recent studies have shown improvement in reproducibility [22,23], insufficient reproducibility means that the storage of CAD cues as parts of the patient's medical record would increase the legal implications. Given the number of unresolved issues, the clinical role of CAD in mammography is the topic of continuous debate.

Since mammography is becoming increasingly digital, there is little doubt that CAD is here to stay but its clinical role will continue to evolve to optimize the cost-benefit aspects associated with the application of computerized decision systems in breast cancer diagnosis. In the following sections, a review of mammography and related decision support systems is presented.

6.2 MAMMOGRAPHY

6.2.1 Technique

A mammogram is a non-invasive, low-dose, radiographic exam of the breast and thus far, the most effective screening study for breast cancer. The American Cancer Society recommends women to have a 'Baseline Mammogram' before the age of 40 years. Then, regular screening is recommended every two years till the age of 50 years. Since age is a well-known risk factor for breast cancer, annual screening is recommended for women older than 50 years old. Contrary, regular screening before the age of 40 is a topic of debate. Since younger breasts are more dense, mammography is not very sensitive. Consequently, the National Cancer Institute (NCI) encourages women who have had breast cancer and those who are at increased risk due to a genetic history of breast cancer to seek expert medical advice about the frequency of screening.

Screening mammograms are typically performed using screen-film systems. During mammography, each breast is first compressed to improve the quality and diagnostic value of the acquired image. Breast compression is necessary to even out the breast thickness. The process ensures that all of the breast tissue is visualized and small lesions are not obscured by overlapping breast tissue. Typically, two standard projections are acquired per breast: a) the craniocaudal view (CC) and b) the mediolateral oblique view (MLO). The two views are designed to provide supplemental information by covering as much of the breast parenchyma as possible. Furthermore, the more subtle manifestations of breast cancer are often visible in only one view. It has been documented that the misinterpretation error is significantly reduced with two view compared to single view mammograms [24]. The effectiveness of a mammographic study can be further improved by acquiring additional views of the breast, by magnifying suspicious mammographic regions, and by using multimodality strategies (ultrasound, MRI). Often, such additional studies are required when there are suspicious findings and/or in women with dense breasts where the compression factor is not satisfying. After acquisition, the breast images are typically viewed on film at a view box or as soft copy on a digital mammography workstation. Figure 1 shows a typical two-view per breast mammographic study from a publicly available resource, the Digital Database of Screening Mammography (DDSM) [25].

The most recent development in mammography is the full-field digital mammography (FFDM) [26]. Replacing the screen-film systems with the digital mammography detectors allows for higher contrast resolution, thus facilitating the detection of subtle, low contrast abnormalities. There are several comparative studies in process to determine if FFDM can substantially improve breast cancer detection compared to screen-film mammography [27,28]. The results are preliminary and remain conflicting. Regardless, the CAD algorithms and clinical role of CAD are identical in either screen-film or digital mammography.

(a) Right CC

(b) Left CC

(c) Right MLO

(d) Left MLO

Figure 1: Two-view per breast mammographic study from the Digital Database of Screening mammography (DDSM).

6.2.2 Mammographic signs of breast signs

The three most common types of breast abnormalities are: 1) microcalcifications, 2) masses and, 3) architectural distortion. Each type of abnormality manifestates mammographically with unique morphological and textural characteristics. These characteristics dictate the type of algorithm that forms the foundation of the various decision support systems that exist in mammography. The following is a brief description of each type of mammographic abnormality.

6.2.2.1 Calcifications

Calcifications are small calcium deposits that can be produced from cell secretion or from necrotic cellular debris. They appear as small bright spots on a mammogram. About 25% of all breast cancers manifestate as clusters of microcalcifications [29]. They may appear with or without an associated lesion. Figure 2 shows example DDSM mammograms with annotated clusters of microcalcifications. Typically, their number, morphology, and distribution provide clues as to whether they can be associated with a benign or malignant process. As a general rule, round or oval shaped calcifications that are uniform in shape are more likely to be benign. Contrary, calcifications that are irregular in shape, size, with linear or branching distribution raise highly the suspicion of malignancy. It has been described that calcifications associated with a malignant process resemble small fragments of broken glass.

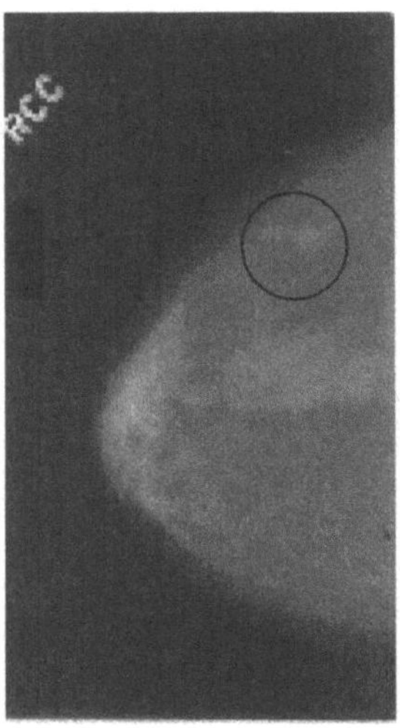

(a) Right CC

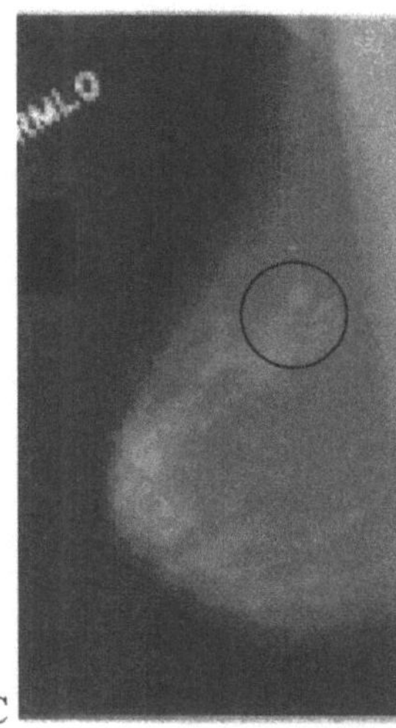

(b) Right MLO

Figure 2: DDSM mammogram with annotated malignant microcalcification cluster.

6.2.2.2 Masses

A breast mass is a localized sign of breast cancer (Figure 3). If it appears in only one view, then it is considered a focal density. Masses come in a wide range of shapes, sizes, and contrast. They can be extremely subtle, often obscured by normal tissue. Thus, they are far more challenging to detect than calcifications. Studies have shown that breast masses comprise the overwhelming majority of missed cancers [9,10]. Similar to calcifications, clinicians try to assess the likelihood of malignancy depending on the morphological characteristics of the mass (size, shape, margin, density).

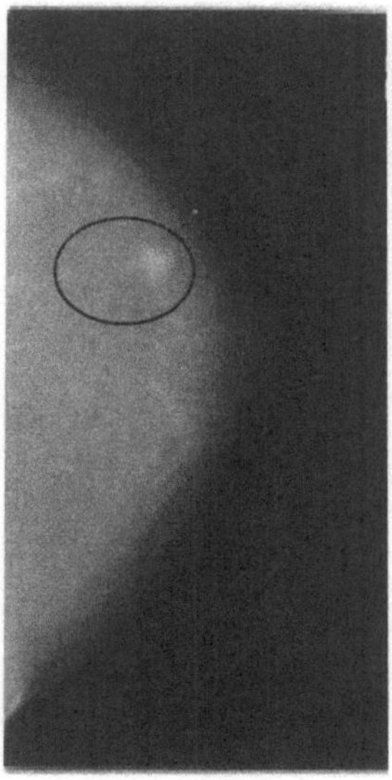
(a) Left CC
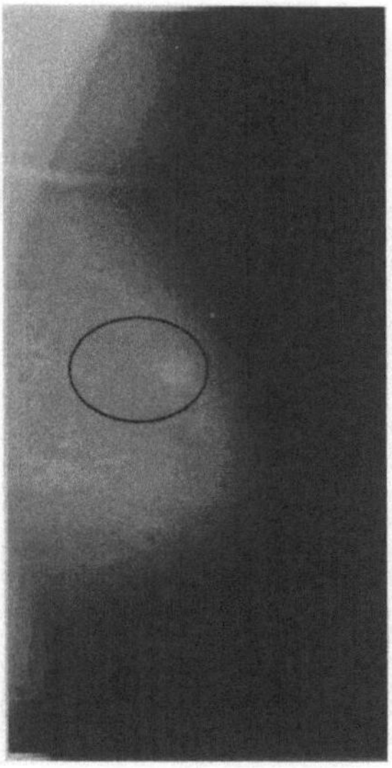
(b) Left MLO

Figure 3: DDSM mammogram with annotated malignant mass.

6.2.2.3 Architectural Distortion

Architectural distortion (AD) is the third most common mammographic manifestation of nonpalpable breast cancer (other than a focal mass or a microcalcifiction cluster) [30-32]. According to the Breast Imaging and Reporting System (BI-RADS), AD is described as follows: "The normal architecture is distorted with no definite mass visible. This includes spiculations radiating from a point, and focal retraction or distortion of the edge of the parenchyma. Architectural distortion can also be an associated finding." [33]. Since cancer infiltration disrupts the normal parenchyma architecture, AD is considered an early sign of cancer. However, surgical scars, fibrocystic changes, and simply superimposition of breast tissues may generate similar parenchymal distortions [34,35]. Consequently, AD is the most challenging breast cancer manifestation to detect [34]. Figure 4 highlights four examples of AD. Note that in some cases AD appears as a focal retraction and in others as radiating lines.

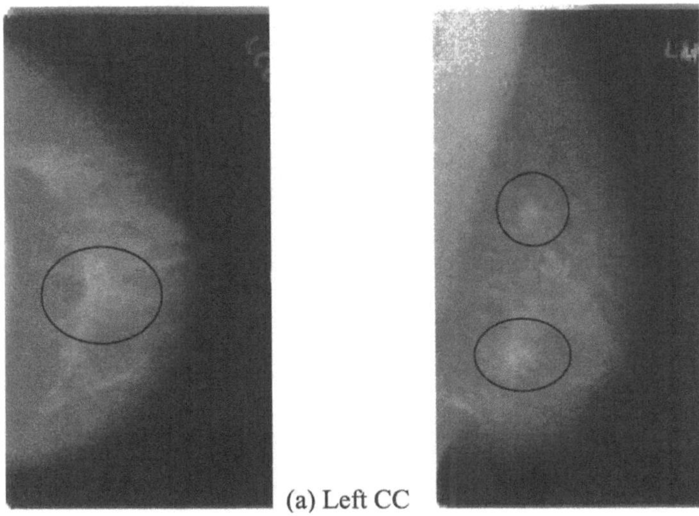

(a) Left CC (b) Left MLO

Figure 4: DDSM mammogram with 3 annotated areas depicting malignant architectural distortion.

6.3 DECISION SUPPORT SYSTEMS

6.3.1 What is CAD?

The field of Computer-aided Detection and Diagnosis in mammography deals with the development of computer tools for automated diagnostic interpretation of mammograms. CAD techniques typically follow a two-stage approach. Initially, image processing is performed to identify suspicious mammographic regions. Subsequently, morphological and/or textural features are automatically extracted from these regions. The features are merged with linear classifiers or artificial intelligence techniques to further refine the detection and diagnosis (benign vs. malignant) of potential abnormalities.

Regardless of the CAD algorithm, the decisions of a CAD system are expected to serve as second opinions to the clinicians. Consequently, the ultimate goal of CAD is to reduce the perceptual and cognitive error associated with clinicians' interpretation of screening mammograms. A CAD system is successful when it directly addresses a clinical challenge.

6.3.2 Overview of CAD algorithms

CAD research has been very active in mammography over the past 15 years.

Although a wide range of CAD techniques have been proposed and explored, most CAD systems follow a similar multistage process. The process is highlighted in Figure 5.

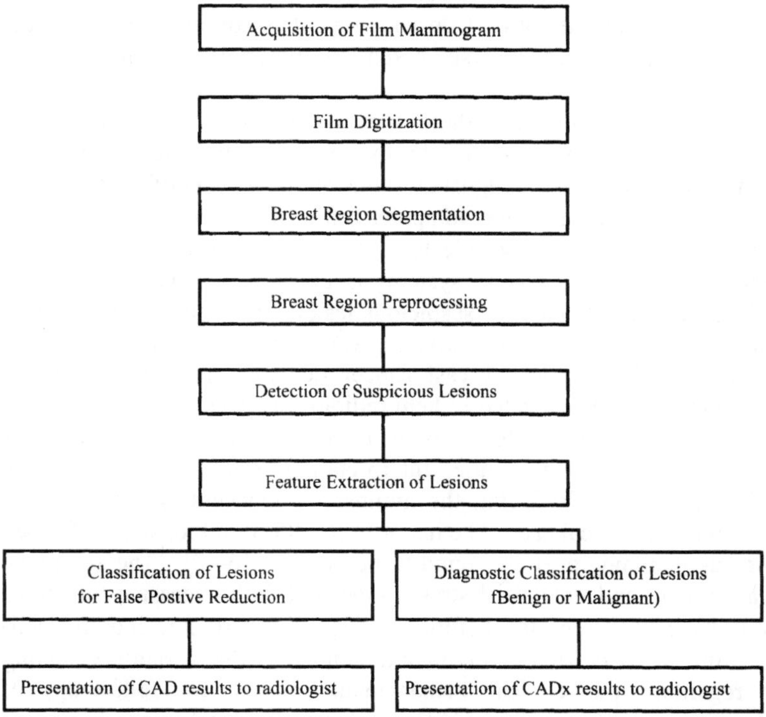

Figure 5: Diagram of hierarchical steps followed in CAD/CADx systems in mammography

In stage 1, the film mammogram is digitized at a high resolution. The resolution requirement depends on the smallest abnormality to be detected but most studies perform digitization at 50 m or 100 m per pixel. As a general rule, a much smaller pixel size is required for the detection of microcalcifications than masses. Then, to improve computational efficiency the breast region is automatically extracted. An accurate segmentation of the breast is often challenging however due to the poor visibility of the breast boundary. The nonuniform background region includes information plates and unexposed film regions that further complicate the task. In addition, the large size of a mammographic study (50-100 MB of data are associated with a patient) require a fast and efficient segmentation algorithm. There is a variety of breast segmentation techniques proposed [36-41]. These methods include primarily thresholding, gradient analysis, edge-detection, region-growing techniques, wavelet analysis, active contour models, and neural networks. In addition, some preprocessing is often performed in the breast region to correct the low contrast around the breast skin line due to the smaller breast thickness [42-44].

With the breast region identified and its contrast corrected, the search process begins in stage 2. Regardless of the specifics of the image processing algorithms, the search process aims to identify suspicious lesions within the masked breast. However, due to the difficulty of the detection task, this step typically results in a large number of suspicious lesions. Consequently, it is common to follow the detection process with further analysis based on morphological and textural features for false positive reduction.

Feature-based analysis comprises stage 3 of a CAD system and it aims to reduce false positive detections in CAD. Furthermore, it is used for diagnosis in CADx systems to determine the malignancy status of lesions identified during the detection process. The results of the computerized analysis are presented to the radiologist who is ultimately responsible for patient management. Note that the clinical purpose of CAD and CADx systems is different. A CAD system is expected to help radiologists identify suspicious lesions that need further follow-up with additional imaging. Consequently, a CAD system is designed to address the perceptual error that burdens breast cancer detection in mammograms. Contrary, a CADx system is expected to help radiologists determine if an already detected lesion requires biopsy to determine its malignancy status. Thus, a CADx system is designed to reduce the interpretation error associated with mammographic diagnosis. Reducing the number of unnecessary biopsies is a different yet important clinical task. The majority (65-85%) of biopsies performed due to suspicious mammograms are found to be benign [46-49]. The economic cost, physical burden, and emotional stress associated with excessive biopsy of benign lesions have been reported before [50-57]. Furthermore, another well-documented problem associated with mammography is the variability among radiologists regarding the clinical management (biopsy vs. follow-up) of suspicious breast lesions [9,58,59]. CADx systems could substantially reduce observer variability in diagnosis and patient management in breast cancer screening programs.

The remaining section focuses on stages 2 and 3 by highlighting computer vision techniques that have been proven successful in a variety of CAD/CADx systems for mammography.

6.3.2.1 CAD techniques for calcifications

There is a wide variety of image processing algorithms applied for the detection and diagnostic characterization of microcalcification clusters in mammograms. All algorithms aim to describe the morphology, texture, and spatial distribution of individual calcifications.

Microcalcifications appear as tiny, bright spots embedded in the complex breast parenchyma background. Because of their relative higher contrast, the detection of calcifications is considered a relatively easier task than the detection of masses. Detection techniques presented include contrast enhancement, segmentation algorithms, texture analysis, k-nearest neighbor clustering, wavelets, fractal modeling, and neural networks [60-74]. Since the published studies are based on different databases, direct performance comparison among the various techniques is not feasible. Overall, reported detection performance ranges from 85% to 98% with a false positive rate of about 0.5 clusters per image.

Contrary to detection, the diagnostic characterization of detected microcalcification clusters is a far more challenging task. The diagnostic analysis relies heavily on morphological and spatial descriptors that are typically merged into a classifier such as neural networks, fuzzy logic, and decision trees [74-78]. Similar to the detection problem, reported diagnostic performance ranges widely. An extensive survey of CAD/CADx techniques for microcalcifications appears in Reference 79.

6.3.2.2 CAD techniques for masses

Although larger in size, the mammographic detection of breast is a more challenging task than the detection of microcalcifications. Since breast parenchyma presents a rather complex background, overlapping tissues often appear as suspicious masses confusing both mammographers and computer vision algorithms. Consequently, there is an extensive literature on the development of CAD techniques for mass detection in mammograms. The techniques involve a variety of algorithms with a similar underlying philosophy; to extract features that characterize the mass size, shape, contour, orientation, and density. Subsequently, based on these features a decision is made regarding the presence and malignancy status of a suspicious lesion [80-90]. Thus far, a less explored detection and classification strategy involves knowledge-based approach based on template matching techniques. Such approach eliminates optimization issues regarding the search and selection of significant features. Several investigators have shown promising results [91-94], although creating a comprehensive database of mass templates is nontrivial. Overall, the reported detection performance of the various CAD algorithms is lower than that for calcifications ranging from 75% to 90% with a higher false positive rate. However, determining the malignancy status of a detected mass is an easier task with reported performance of ROC area index above 0.90 [88-90].

6.3.2.3 CAD techniques for architectural distortion

Since calcifications and masses are the most prevalent mammographic signs of breast cancer, CAD/CADx research has focused strongly on those. However, to date, few CAD schemes have been specifically evaluated for detecting architectural distortion (AD). In 2001, Birdwell et al. [10] reported that after retrospective CAD analysis of 115 breast cancers missed during screening mammography, their CAD tool correctly identified 83% (5/6) of missed malignancies that presented as architectural distortions. In 2002, Evans et al. [95] reported that 85% (17/20) of invasive lobular carcinoma that presented as AD were successfully marked by a single CAD system. In a recent study [96] focusing specifically on CAD performance for detecting AD, the two most widely available CAD systems demonstrated only limited success. The evaluation study was based on 45 mammographic cases with AD deemed present and actionable by a panel of expert mammographers. Both systems showed less than 50% case sensitivity (49% and 33% respectively) with 0.7-1.27 false positive marks per image. Image sensitivity was even lower (38% and 21% respectively).

From the image processing point of view, the detection of AD is most challenging. Radiating lines is the pronounced morphological characteristic of AD. Thus far, there are only a handful of studies dedicated to the detection of linear structures in mammograms: the multiscale directional line operator [97], the radial-edge gradient detection [98,99], the directional second order Gaussian derivatives [100,101], the curvi-linear structure detection technique [102,103], and skeleton analysis [104]. These techniques aim to detect linear structures and characterize their strength and orientation. Since mammograms contain a variety of normal linear structures (e.g., vessels, ducts, fibrous tissue, skinfolds), the techniques are typically used for false positive reduction in a mass detection scheme. If a detected focal density is not associated with strong radiating lines, then it can be safely eliminated as a benign finding. In addition, techniques have been proposed for characterizing radiating spicules as part of mass classification schemes [105,106]. However, the above techniques have not been specifically designed to address AD but rather to identify spicules, a strong sign of malignancy. Furthermore, AD often manifestates as focal retraction. Recent studies have tried to address this type of abnormality as well [107]. Template matching techniques have also been proposed for the task [108]

Due to the reportedly suboptimal detection performance, CAD techniques for AD is considered as one of the future research directions in the field. The significance of the clinical problem and the potential benefit of CAD was recently emphasized in a study that showed that earlier detection of architectural distortion is associated with a possible gain in prognosis [109].

6.3.2.4 Other applications of CAD in mammography

Other than detection and diagnosis, there have been several attempts to develop decision support systems that assess breast parenchymal density in a screening mammogram. The prevalence of dense breast tissue in a mammogram is often cited as a risk factor for breast cancer. Dense structures in a mammogram that are radiographically visible include ducts, lobular elements, and fibrous connective tissue, though fibroglandular tissue is typically regarded as the major component of density variation between mammograms. Visual assessment of breast density is subjective burdened with large inter and intra-observer variability. Several studies have indicated the merit of quantifying tissue composition in digital mammograms [110-117].

6.3.3 Issues in the development and evaluation of decision support systems in mammography

Regardless of the computer vision algorithms, the development and evaluation of a CAD/CADx system always starts at a laboratory setting with retrospective analysis of a specific set of mammograms. Due to the great variability of patient populations and the appearance of screening mammograms, there can be tremendous differences in the reported performance of such system. Critical issues that affect the results of a laboratory study are: i) database (size, case difficulty, disease prevalence), and ii) performance evaluation techniques. The following section presents a brief overview of current practices regarding these issues.

6.3.3.1 Effect of database

Direct comparison of various CAD/CADx systems is often impossible because these systems are developed and evaluated on different datasets. Screening mammograms present a wide range of interpretation difficulty. For example, mammograms that contain primarily fatty breast parenchyma are always easier to interpret than mammograms with primarily dense breast tissue. Similarly, lesion size affects detectability. Thus, if a dataset contains relatively large breast lesions, the CAD study will produce overoptimistic results. Although many investigators devote time in painstakingly developing their own dataset, it is recognized that not everyone has access to clinical data. Furthermore, it is critical to create benchmark databases that are publicly available and allow for direct comparisons among the various studies [118]. Thus far, there are two such databases for screening mammography.

1*) The Digital Database of Screening Mammography (DDSM):* DDSM was collected at the University of South Florida under the DOD Breast Cancer Research Program grant number DAMD17-94-J-4015 [25]. It is available at http://marathon.csee.usf.edu/Mammography/Database.html. It is by far the largest database and the most commonly used by the image analysis research community as a benchmark database for CAD for mammography. The database contains 2,620 complete screening mammographic studies. The mammograms were obtained at several clinical sites. Each study includes two images (standard craniocaudal and mediolateral oblique views) of each breast. For each case there is also associated patient information: age at time of study, ACR breast density rating, subtlety rating for abnormalities, description of abnormalities (mass, calcification) and image information (scanner and spatial resolution). Images containing suspicious areas have associated pixel-level "ground truth" information about the locations and types of suspicious regions. The database includes normal, cancer, and benign cases. A normal screening mammogram is one in which no further "work-up" was required and the patient had a normal exam at least four years later. A cancer case is a screening exam with at least one biopsy-proven malignancy. A benign case is a screening exam in which something suspicious was found, but was determined to not be malignant (by pathology or additional imaging). The database includes also a few "benign without callback" cases. These are screening exams in which no additional films or biopsy was done to confirm the benign finding. These cases contained something interesting enough for the radiologist to mark. DDSM includes three volumes, each containing mammograms digitized with a different digitizer (LUMISYS, HOWTEK, and DBA). They were digitized at approximately 50 microns and 12-bit depth pixels.

2) *The Mammography Image Analysis Socitey database (MIAS)*: Only a limited version of this database is publicly available (http://peipa.essex.ac.uk/ipa/pix/mias). The Mini MIAS contains approximately 300 screening mammograms with a variety of breast lesions present. Ground truth is provided for all cases. The database contains only MLO views, digitized with a scanning microdensitometer (Joyce-Loebl, SCANDIG3) to 50 micron x 50 micron resolution and 8-bit pixel depth. The images were then reduced to 200 micron. More information regarding the MIAS database is provided in [119].

The DDSM is far more popular since it provides a large number of cases from various geographical locations. In addition, the database provides physicians' assessment of case difficulty. Finally, the variety of digitizers facilitates studies to assess the impact of the digitization scheme on the overall performance of the CAD system. However, regardless of the database choice, the investigators need to carefully determine the impact of the database size and the sampling scheme they adopt in the development and evaluation of their techniques. The data sampling issue has been carefully addressed in the literature and it is beyond the scope of this review. Overall, the investigators need to ensure that their training and test sets are well-balanced containing cases of various difficulty and a comprehensive collection of mammograms with breast cancer signs and normal breast parenchyma.

6.3.3.2 Performance evaluation techniques

Depending on the decision problem, two different techniques are typically used to report CAD/CADx performance. Detection performance is reported using Free-response Receiver Operating Characteristic (FROC) curves. Diagnostic performance is reported using Receiver Operating Characteristics (ROC) analysis. Both techniques are designed to summarize performance independently of decision thresholds or disease prevalence.

1)*Receiver Operating Characteristics (ROC):*

Based on the classical signal detection theory, ROC analysis is the most popular methodology for the evaluation of the diagnostic performance of decision support systems in mammography. The underlying assumption is that the decision problem is binary with two mutually exclusive states (i.e., benign vs. malignant, true lesion vs. false positive). Conventionally, an ROC curve plots the true positive fraction (or sensitivity) vs. the false positive fraction (or [1 - specificity]) for a wide and continuous range of decision thresholds and provides a more meaningful and valid measure of diagnostic performance. Furthermore, ROC curves can be used to determine optimum decision levels that maximize accuracy, average benefit or other measures of clinical efficacy. The area Az under the ROC curve is the most commonly used evaluation index. The more the curve is shifted to the upper left corner of the graph (specificity = sensitivity = 1) the better the diagnostic performance. The area index varies between 0.5 (representing chance behavior) and 1.0 (representing perfect performance). Generally, a higher value of the area index indicates better performance. In mammographic applications, it is often critical to operate the decision support system at a high sensitivity level (e.g. >90%). Consequently, the partial ROC area index is often more meaningful. The partial ROC area index focuses on the part of the ROC curve that corresponds to clnically relevant operating points. Figure 6 shows typical ROC curves.

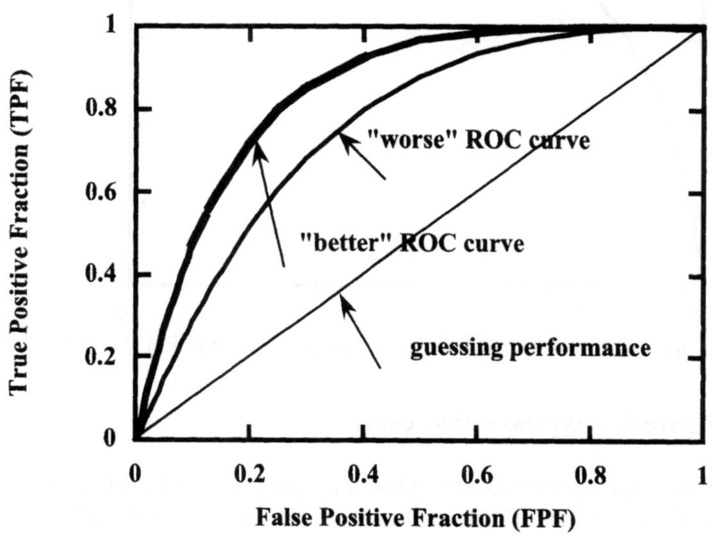

Figure 6: Typical ROC curves.

2)*Free-response Receiver Operating Characteristic (FROC):*

FROC analysis extends the ROC philosophy to detection tasks where more than one lesions maybe present in one image. Given an image, the decision maker (i.e., the mammographer or the CAD system) is allowed to mark multiple image locations as suspicious. Consequently, there may be more than one true detections and/or false positive detections per image. An FROC curve plots the sensitivity vs. the average number of false positive detections per image. Contrary to ROC analysis, the maximum number of FP responses is not fixed. Therefore, the x axis does not represent a fraction between 0 and 1 as in ROC curves. Figure 7 shows a typical FROC curve. It needs to be emphasized that in mammographic applications the researchers tend to report results either per case or per image. Since a screening mammographic study contains two images per breast, some published studies consider a lesion correctly detected if it is detected in at least one of the two images. Other investigators prefer to analyze each image independently, a decision often driven by the need for higher statistical power for the reported result. Although there is no preferred strategy, it needs to be carefully considered when comparing results between two different studies.

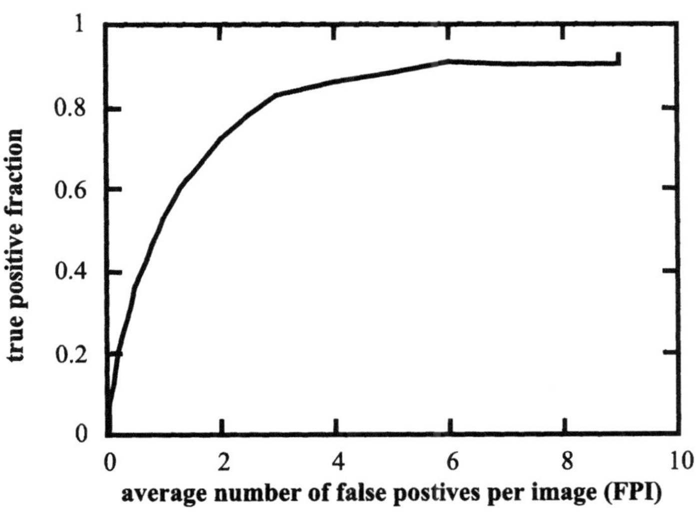

Figure 7: A typical FROC curve.

An extensive literature on the theoretical background, the statistical properties, and current status of the ROC and FROC methods can be found in [120-124]. In addition, two excellent software online resources for ROC and FROC analysis are available at http://xray.bsd.uchicago.edu/krl/KRL_ROC/software_index.htm and http://jafroc.radiology.pitt.edu/index.htm respectively.

6.3.4 Preclinical presentation and evaluation of a promising decision support system

After the initial development and laboratory evaluation of a promising decision support system, the next step is a preclinical evaluation to determine what is the most efficient way to integrate the system in the clinical arena. Thus far, the general strategy is to view such system as a reliable second opinion. Therefore, the preclinical evaluation aims to determine if this computer aid can truly improve the overall performance of physicians in their clinical work. Depending on the decision problem (detection or diagnosis), there are several important questions that need to be assessed:

1) Does the decision support system affect the overall detection rate of breast cancer?
2) Does the decision support system affect the actionability of a questioned mammographic region? This is truly a multiscale question aiming to address if the system can help physicians increase the actionability rating of correctly detected and localized cancerous lesions but decrease the actionability rating of benign regions and mammographic regions falsely identified as containing lesions.
3) Does the decision support system affect the diagnostic characterization of correctly detected breast lesions? If yes, then the system may reduce the number of unnecessary biopsies.
4) How does the decision support system affect the reading time of screening mammograms?

The above questions are critical and designing evaluation studies to address them helps investigators determine the most efficient role of the decision support system. The most popular strategy is to design observer studies where physicians retrospectively review blindly mammograms with previously established ground truth (i.e., biopsy or long-term follow-up). The physicians review the cases in two separate modes. In mode 1, the physician is asked to read the case indicating any mammographic location that attracts his/her visual attention and is considered as a potential abnormality. For each suspicious image location, the physician maybe asked to a provide likelihood ratings regarding the presence of a lesion, its malignancy status, and the actionability status of the lesion (i.e., what is the likelihood that you will send the lesion for additional imaging or biopsy). In mode 2, the physician will review the case utilizing the decision support system as a second opinion. The system typically indicates mammographic locations that potentially contain abnormalities. For those locations, the system may also assign a likelihood rating regarding the malignancy status of the suspicious lesion. The physician will be asked to review the case taking into account the opinions of the decision support system and report their findings. If the physicians' clinical performance is better under reading mode 2 than mode 1, then the study suggests that the CAD system has beneficial effect.

Human observer studies are very time-consuming and often burdened by biases that need to be carefully accounted in the subsequent data analysis. For example, to avoid context bias and fatigue bias, the observer study is always performed in sessions over a period of several months. The available test cases are randomly divided into smaller, equal-sized sets. Each reading session includes only one set. To reduce learning effects, the order of reading sessions is always varied among observers. Furthermore, within each reading session, the presentation order of the cases is randomized differently for each one of the observers to further avoid context bias. Since each case is reviewed using two modes, a mandatory delay of several weeks between consecutive readings of the same case needs to be imposed to avoid memorization bias.

6.4 COMMERCIAL CAD SYSTEMS

Thus far, there are four commercial decision support systems in mammography that gained approval from the Food and Drug Administration (FDA) and have made it successfully into clinical practice. All four have been developed to perform essentially the same task; to highlight mammographic areas that are suspicious for breast cancer and might otherwise be missed. They all operate on the same decision making principles highlighted in Figure 5 with variations of course in the type of image processing and classification algorithms employed. The first and by far most popular commercial CAD product is the R2 ImageChecker (R2 Technology Inc., Los Altos, CA, USA). The CAD system initially digitizes the mammographic films to 50 microns resolution and 12bit pixel depth. Detected masses and calcifications are marked with different symbols and serve as prompts to the mammographers. Other popular systems are SecondLook (CADx Medical Systems Inc., Quebec, Canada), the MammoReader (Intelligent Systems Software, Inc., Clearwater, FL), and MAMMEX TR™ (SCANIS Inc., Foster City, CA, USA). Overall the systems operate at the same level: 98% sensitivity for calcifications, 88% sensitivity for masses, and on average 1.5 false positive marks per case.

6.5 THE EVOLVING ROLE OF CAD IN MAMMOGRAPHY

6.5.1 How can we facilitate clinical acceptance?

The ultimate goal of decision support systems in mammography is to identify breast cancer at an earlier stage so that patient treatment is more effective and therefore patient prognosis is better. Although these systems have made it successfully into the clinical arena, comparative studies have shown mixed results often suggesting that the contribution of CAD may not be as significant as earlier studies have indicated in laboratory settings. However, it is well recognized that larger, prospective studies are still required since the results of a study can be severely biased by disease prevalence, case difficulty, observer study design, and long-term follow-up. Prospective studies can accurately assess if earlier diagnosis did indeed have quantifiable positive impact in patients that there would have been otherwise missed by the radiologist.

Unfortunately, one critical parameter in these studies that is difficult to assess and control is the radiologists' attitude towards the decision support systems.

Thus far, the decision support systems are designed to examine independently each mammogram and provide a second opinion to the radiologist who is responsible for the patient's care. Since several studies have verified the importance of double reading [125], the decision support is asked to play the role of an effective second reader. The double reading strategy relies on the premise that lesions missed by one radiologist will be detected by the second reader. However, if there is a disagreement, the two readers may discuss the case to decide the optimal strategy for the particular patient. In their present role, commercial CAD systems in mammography cannot fulfill this requirement. Consequently, clinical acceptance of these systems in the real world has been very challenging. A common criticism is that even if accurate, such systems operate as black boxes unable to justify any decision they make. Radiologists are often reluctant to accept CAD decisions. Such reluctance jeopardizes any potential benefit of using the CAD system as a second reader to improve breast cancer detection. Contrary, if a radiologist is too eager to accept every CAD opinion without further thinking, this strategy has also two very negative outcomes. First, the radiologist will send many more patients to unnecessary additional imaging and/or biopsy alarmed by the CAD prompts jeopardizing the cost and time benefit of using CAD as a second opinion. Second, a less recognized detrimental effect is that by relying too much on the CAD prompts, the radiologist may alter his/her search pattern by carefully reviewing only mammographic areas that have been marked as suspicious by the CAD tool. Consequently, small, low contrast lesions may be missed by both the radiologist and the CAD. Future CAD research needs to focus on developing successful integration strategies to optimize the clinical role of CAD and maximize patient benefit. Consequently, the role of CAD will continue to evolve in mammography.

6.5.2 Interactive CAD/CADx systems

One of the latest attempts in CAD/CADx research is the development of interactive systems that allow radiologists formulate their own questions and get accurate answers with adequate explanation to facilitate clinical acceptance. Knowledge-based (KB) CAD systems appear to fulfill the need for interactive and interpretive decision systems in mammography. Generally, KB systems aim to provide evidence-based decision support using a knowledge databank. A KB system typically relates a new case to similar cases stored in its knowledge databank. Based on the similar cases, a diagnosis is assigned to the new case by analogy or by copying the answer if the match is close enough. The main benefits of using KB-CAD systems in mammography are the following: (1) KB-CAD systems take full advantage of growing digital image libraries without further re-training of the CAD system and, (2) they are interactive allowing physicians to formulate their own questions and get interpretable answers (e.g., the CAD response is often analogous to the odds-ratio). A recently published editorial in *Radiology* recognized content-based image retrieval as a new research direction in radiology [125]. However, the computational demands of maintaining, indexing, and querying a large image databank have limited the application of these tools in mammography. Furthermore, defining similarity between two images is nontrivial. Common practice is to select important image features and feature-based distance metrics to determine similarity.

6.6 APPLICATION OF A KB-CAD SYSTEM

A specific KB-CAD research effort is highlighted here for the detection and diagnosis of masses in mammography. Tourassi et al. recently proposed a CAD system that follows a knowledge-based decision approach [93,94]. The system assigns a likelihood measure regarding the presence of a mass in a mammographic region selected for evaluation. The likelihood measure is estimated based on the region's global similarity with other cases stored in a digital image library. Typically, content-image retrieval techniques rely on feature-based similarity measures. However, the selection and optimization of suitable features is nontrivial. Contrary, the proposed system moves from a feature-based similarity assessment to a featureless approach. The researchers exploit information theory to formulate metrics that measure the global similarity of two mammographic cases. The metrics are based on image entropy. If two images are related, then one image should contain important diagnostic information about the other. The metrics are calculated using the actual images.

The following is a brief description of the system. The CAD system has three critical components: (1) the knowledge databank, (2) the template-matching algorithm and, (3) the knowledge-based decision algorithm (Figure 8). The knowledge databank contains mammographic regions of interest (ROIs) of known pathology. Each ROI stored in the databank serves as a template. A query suspicious mammographic region is compared to the stored templates using the template-matching algorithm. A decision algorithm effectively combines the similarity indices and pathology status of the stored templates into a prediction regarding the presence of a mass in the query region.

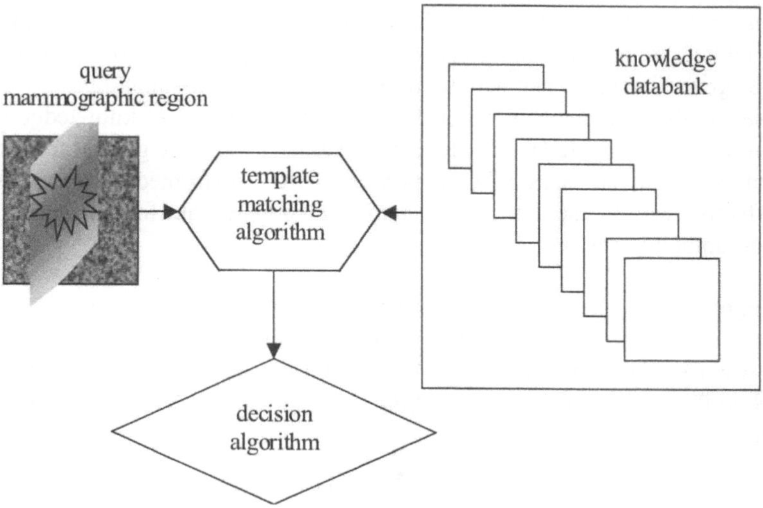

Figure 8: Knowledge-based CAD system

To measure the similarity between a query and a template, the mutual information between the two images is calculated. Mutual information (MI) is a measure of general interdependence between random variables [126]. Since MI makes no assumptions about the nature of the relationship between variables, it is quite general and often regarded as a generalization of the linear correlation coefficient.

The concept of MI can be easily extended to images. If X and Y represent two medical images, their MI I(X;Y) is expressed as:

$$I(X;Y) = \sum_x \sum_y P_{XY}(x,y) \log_2 \frac{P_{XY}(x,y)}{P_X(x) P_Y(y)} \qquad [1]$$

where $P_{XY}(x,y)$ is the joint probability density function (pdf) of the two images based on their corresponding pixel values. Equation 1 assumes that the image pixel values are samples of two random variables x and y respectively. $P_X(x)$ and $P_Y(y)$ are the marginal pdfs. The basic idea is that when two images are similar, pixels with a certain intensity value in one image should correspond to a more clustered distribution of the intensity values in the other image. The more the two images are alike, the more information X provides for Y and vice versa. Therefore, the MI can be thought as an intensity-based measure of how much two images are alike. In the template-matching context, the MI increases when the query image X and the template image Y depict similar structures. Then, the pixel value in image X is a good predictor of the pixel value at the corresponding location in image Y. Theoretically, MI is a more effective and robust similarity metric than traditional correlation [126]. Correlation techniques assume a linear relationship between the intensity values in the two images. This assumption is often violated in medical images, especially in the presence of tumors. MI measures general dependence without making any a priori assumptions.

Subsequently, the decision algorithm is implemented. A knowledge-based decision index is computed using the level of similarity and the ground truth of the best-matched archived cases. Two experiments were performed to determine the most effective way to use the CAD system as a computer aid for the detection of mammographic masses.

Experiment 1: First, the knowledge databank contained only mammographic ROIs that depicted a mass. Given a query mammographic ROI Q_i, a decision index $D_1(Q_i)$ was calculated based on the MI between the query ROI and each known *mass* M_j in the knowledge databank. $D_1(Q_i)$ was the average MI of the k best mass matches:

$$D_1(Q_i) = \frac{1}{k}\sum_{j=1}^{k} MI(Q_i, M_j) \qquad [2]$$

Theoretically, a query ROI depicting a mass should match better with the databank of mass ROIs than a query ROI depicting normal breast tissue, thus resulting in a higher $D_1(Q_i)$.

Experiment 2: Second, the knowledge databank included both normal and mass ROIs. Given a query mammographic ROI Q_I, a decision index $D_2(Q_i)$ was calculated as the difference of two terms. The first term measures the average MI between the query ROI and its k best mass matches M_j. Similarly, the second term measures the average MI between the query ROI and its k best normal N_j matches. Theoretically, a query ROI depicting a mass should have a higher $D_2(Q_i)$.

$$D_2(Q_i) = \frac{1}{k}\sum_{j=1}^{k} MI(Q_i, M_j) - \frac{1}{k}\sum_{j=1}^{k} MI(Q_i, N_j) \qquad [3]$$

The diagnostic performance of the CAD system was evaluated using a leave-one-out sampling scheme. Given a database of 1,465 mammographic regions of interest (ROIs), each ROI was excluded once. In experiment 1, the remaining mass cases were used to establish the knowledge databank. In experiment 2, the remaining 1,464 cases were used to establish the databank. The experiments were repeated until every ROI served as a query ROI. The calculated decision indices D_1 and D_2 were analyzed based on Receiver Operating Characteristic (ROC) analysis methodology (i.e., ROCKIT software package by Metz *et al.*). For both indices, ROC performance was estimated for varying values of the top best matches (parameter k). In addition, the decision indices were calculated using all archived cases (k=ALL).

Table 1 shows the overall ROC area index (A_Z) of the CAD system for each one of the decision indices D_1, D_2 and for varying number (k) of the top matches considered.

Table 1
ROC performance of the CAD scheme for two decision indices (D_1, D_2) and for varying number of the top matches considered (k=1,10,100, 200, ALL).

	1	10	`100	200	ALL
D_1	0.71±0.01	0.71±0.01	0.72±0.01	0.73±0.01	0.75±0.01
D_2	0.71±0.01	0.79±0.01	0.85±0.01	0.86±0.01	0.87±0.01

Several observations can be made based on Table 1. First, the CAD system has a significantly better ROC performance when the decision index is calculated using the knowledge databank that includes both mass and normal cases (D_2). Second, CAD performance improves as more archived cases are considered in the calculation of the decision index D_2. The CAD system achieves its best ROC performance (A_Z=0.87±0.01) when all archived cases are included in the calculation of D_2. Specifically, the system achieves 90% sensitivity while safely eliminating 65% of the normal regions. Contrary, when the detection decision is based only on the best mass matches (D_1), the ROC area index is statistically significantly lower (A_Z=0.75±0.01) but substantially less dependent on the parameter k.

The performance of the best CAD tool was analyzed separately for benign and malignant masses. The tool showed robust performance among the two groups of masses: A_Z(malignant masses vs. normal) = 0.88±0.01 and A_Z(benign masses vs. normal) = 0.86±0.01.

Since mass detection is more challenging in dense breasts, separate analysis was performed on the CAD performance for each subgroup of ROIs based on the DDSM density rating of the mammogram from which they were extracted. Table 2 summarizes those results. As expected, the detection performance of the CAD tool degraded dramatically in denser breasts. Degradation of CAD performance due to increased breast density has been reported before [127].

Table 2
ROC performance of the CAD scheme for various breast parenchyma densities. The detection task becomes progressively more challenging as density increases.

Density	Az
1: fatty breast	0.98±0.01
2: fibroglandular breast	0.91±0.01
3: heterogeneous breast	0.87±0.02
4: dense breast	0.64±0.05

Finally, to assess the effect of case difficulty, the best CAD performance was further analyzed for each subgroup of masses based on their DDSM subtlety rating. The subtlety rating is a subjective impression of the DDSM radiologist on the subtlety of the lesion. A higher subtlety rating indicates a more obvious lesion. Table 3 shows that the overall ROC area index of the CAD tool is fairly robust regardless of the reported subtlety of the mass ROIs. The only exception is the subgroup of masses with Subtlety rating 2. For this subgroup, the KB-CAD had a statistically significantly lower ROC performance than the other subgroups.

Table 3

ROC performance of the CAD scheme based on the perceived subtlety of the masses recorded by the DDSM radiologists.

Subtlety Rating	ROC Area
1	0.87±0.04
2	0.77±0.03
3	0.86±0.01
4	0.85±0.02
5	0.89±0.01

Based on the results, the proposed knowledge-based CAD technique can be easily translated into a real-time, interactive CAD system to help radiologists in the detection of masses in screening mammograms. Furthermore, the same idea can be extended from detection to diagnosis. The following highlights a simulation study on how the radiologist's input can be included in the image retrieval process by using relevance feedback.

Relevance feedback is a form of interaction between the user and the retrieval system [128]. It aims to improve the quality of retrieval by letting the user disregard some retrieved cases as "not similar enough". Relevance feedback is used to optimize the set of query features and their relative importance when measuring the similarity index. In the simulation study, a relevance feedback algorithm was implemented using the reported BIRADs findings for the query (Q) and retrieved R masses. The BIRADs features are a common lexicon used by radiologists when they report their mammographic findings [129]. The BIRADs findings become part of the patient's record.

The relevance feedback algorithm estimates the relevance factor (RF) between two masses as a weighted sum of the absolute differences of their shape and margin BIRADs descriptions. The difference in mammographic density is also considered in the calculation of the relevance factor:

$$RF(QR)=1-\left[w_1*|diff\_density|+w_2*|diff\_shape|+w_3*|diff\_margin|\right] \qquad [4]$$

The relevance factor is designed to be equal to 1 if two masses have identical BIRADs features and 0 if they have completely opposite BIRADs features.

The RF is used in the formulation of a new decision index:

$$DI(Q_i)=\frac{1}{k}\sum_{j=1}^{k}RF(Q_i,M_j)*MI(Q_i,M_j)-\frac{1}{k}\sum_{j=1}^{k}RF(Q_i,B_j)*MI(Q_i,B_j) \qquad [5]$$

The new decision index assigns higher importance to retrieved masses with similar BIRADs features as those of the query mass.

DI can be used as the decision variable for ROC analysis. A study was performed using a database of 365 mammographic masses. Each mass was excluded once to serve as a query case. The remaining masses were used to establish the databank of cases with known ground truth. The experiments were repeated until every mass served as a query mass. ROC performance was estimated for varying values of the parameters k, w1, w2, w3. The estimated ROC area index AZ was used as the reported index of performance.

In addition, in order to evaluate independently the significance of the three BIRADs features, a feed-forward backprogagation neural network (BP-ANN) was constructed. The ANN had a three-layer architecture and it was trained to determine the malignancy status of a mass using the Levenberg-Marquardt algorithm [130,131]. Specifically, the ANN input layer had three nodes. Each input node corresponded to each one of the BIRADs features. The hidden layer had six nodes and the output layer had a single, decision node. As with the CBIR classifier, the ANN was evaluated based on the leave-one out crossvalidation method.

The following table summarizes the performance of the CBIR system as measured by the ROC area index AZ for varying number of the weight parameters. For comparison, the ROC performance of the BP-ANN was 0.79±0.02.

Table 4

ROC performance of the CBIR-CADx with and withour relevance feedback for variable number of top retrievals (k), The weights wi represent the relative importance of the BIRADs mammographity density, mass shape, and mass margin parameters for relevance feedback.

	k=1	k=10	k=100	k=ALL
NO RF	0.52±0.03	0.53±0.03	0.57±0.03	0.62±0.03
w_1=1.0 w_2=0.0 w_3=0.0	0.50±0.03	0.63±0.03	0.60±0.03	0.60±0.03
w_1=0.0 w_2=1.0 w_2=0.0	0.70±0.02	0.78±0.02	0.79±0.02	0.75±0.02
w_1=0.0 w_2=0.0 w_2=1.0	0.66±0.03	0.81±0.03	0.83±0.03	0.83±0.03
w_1=0.0 w_2=0.5 w_2=0.5	0.68±0.03	0.80±0.03	0.84±0.03	0.85±0.03
w_1=0.5 w_2=0.5 w_2=0.0	0.70±0.02	0.75±0.02	0.78±0.02	0.79±0.02
w_1=0.3 w_2=0.3 w_2=0.3	0.70±0.02	0.83±0.02	0.85±0.02	**0.86±0.02**

As the table shows the CBIR-CADx performance varies substantially depending on the decision index and the number of retrieved cases (K). Overall, performance improves as more retrieved cases are considered in the calculation of the decision index. Furthermore, performance improves when all BIRADs features contribute equally in the assessment of retrieval relevance. Finally, the CBIR-CADx with RF system achieves a statistically significantly better performance compared to ANN alone or the CBIR system without RF. These results indicate that combining a feature-based relevance feedback technique with a non-feature based image retrieval approach improves dramatically the overall diagnostic performance.

6.7 EXTENSION TO TELEMAMMOGRAPHY

One of the most exciting future research directions for computerized decision support systems is their incorporation to telemammography. Due to the high volume and diagnostic challenge of mammographic studies, telemammography facilitates widespread accessibility to breast screening programs. Mobile mammography screening units are able to reach women in remote areas that are more reluctant to seek specialized routine health care. Their overall goal is to provide screening services to patients who are geographically separated from medical specialists. With continous advances in the field of telecommunications, telemammography allows high quality interpretation of screening mammograms at remote locations where radiology coverage and expertise are deficient.

The direct benefits of online screening and telediagnostic service for breast cancer cannot be overemphasized; i) improved health care access, ii) time-critical care, iii) reduced cost reduction through resource sharing of expensive equipment and personnel. However, since online transmission and interpretation of all screening mammograms can be costly, decision support systems are essential to reduce the number of transmitted mammograms. Such utilization shifts the clinical focus of CAD systems. Since fewer than 10 in 1,000 screening mammograms turn out to contain cancerous signs, it would be clinically critical to automatically identify a large portion of normal mammograms. Then, these undoubtedly normal mammograms can be moved to off-line reading to contain the cost of telemammography. Such application would require a decision support system that operates at 100% sensitivity (detection rate). Although operating at such high sensitivity will create a large number of false positive interpretations, it is still a critical step that can substantially reduce the transmission and online reading costs by eliminating a large portion of the truly normal mammograms. Some investigators have recently recognized the practical significance of developing CAD tools for the automated recognition of normal mammograms. Subsequently, the screening mammograms that were identified as abnormal during the first stage can be further analyzed with more elaborate CAD/CADx tools before they are transmitted to a central location for diagnostic interpretation by experienced mammographers. Such strategy can improve the quality of health care through faster and better diagnosis for women at remote locations as remote experts can be consulted for complicated cases of abnormal findings. Patients can receive screening results at the time of their screening visit.

In conclusion, the recent advances of digital mammography, the enormous amount of mammograms produced by screening programs, the success of CAD, and the recognized benefit of double reading leave little doubt that CAD enhanced telemammography will soon become clinical reality.

6.8 CONCLUSIONS

Computerized decision support systems have become a clinical reality with several commercial systems already in the market and in use around the world. However, the field is considered still in its infant stage. At the present time, the decision support systems are used as second opinion for screening purposes. Although several retrospective studies have shown positive impact, newer prospective studies have questioned the magnitude of the benefit CAD offers in mammography. However, it is universally recognized that the initial role of CAD as a silent second reader may be rather limited. Clearly, CAD performance is as important as understanding how radiologists interact with the CAD system, especially since it is suspected that the system may alter the radiologist's visual search and decision-making practices [132]. The ever-increasing digital nature of radiology dictates that computerized decision support systems are here to stay.

But the field is at crossroads. Current research efforts have started shifting the focus from improving diagnostic performance to improving the user-computer interaction. Research efforts in both directions will ultimately define the optimal role and true benefit of decision support systems in mammography.

REFERENCES

1. American Cancer Society, 2002. "Cancer Facts and Figures 2002", American Cancer Society, Atlanta, GA.
2. R.T. Greenlee, M.B. Hill-Harmon, T. Murray, M. Thun, "Cancer statistics, 2001," Ca: Cancer J Clin 51, 15-36 (2001).
3. A. Jemal, T. Murray, A. Samuels, et al. "Cancer statistics, 2003," Ca: Cancer J Clin 53, 5-26 (2003).
4. L. Tabar, C. Fagerberg, A. Gad, et al. "Reduction in mortality from breast cancer after mass screening with mammography," Lancet 1, 829-832 (1985).
5. I. Jatoi, A.B. Miller, "Why is breast-cancer mortality declining?," Lancet Oncology 4, 251-254 (2003).
6. D.B. Kopans, "The most recent breast cancer screening controversy about whether mammographic screening benefits women at any age: nonsense and nonscience," AJR Am J Roentgenol 180, 21-26 (2003).
7. W.A. Berg, C. Campassi, P. Langenberg, M.J. Sexton, "Breast imaging reporting and data system: Inter- and intraobserver variability in feature analysis and final assessment," AJR Am J Roentgenol 174, 1769-1777 (2000).
8. C.A. Beam, E.F. Conant, E.A. Sickles, "Factors affecting radiologist inconsistency in screening mammography," Acad Radiol 9, 531-540 (2002).
9. R.E. Bird, T.W. Wallace, B.C. Yankaskas, "Analysis of cancers missed at screening mammography," Radiology 184, 613-617 (1992).
10. R.L. Birdwell, D.M. Ikeda, K.F. O'Shaughnessy, E.A. Sickles, "Mammographic characteristics of 115 missed cancers later detected with screening mammography and the potential utility of computer-aided detection," Radiol 219, 192-202 (2001).
11. B.C. Yankaskas, M.J. Schell, R.E. Bird, D.A. Desrochers, "Reassessment of breast cancers missed during routine screening mammography: A community-based study," AJR 177, 535-541 (2001).
12. L.J.W. Burhenne, S.A. Wood, C.J. D'Orsi, S.A. Feig, D.B. Kopans, et al., "Potential contribution of computer-aided detection to the sensitivity of screening mammography," Radiol 215, 554-562 (2000).
13. T.W. Freer, M.J. Ulissey, "Screening mammography with computer-aided detection: Prospective study of 12,860 patients in a community breast center," Radiol 220, 781-786 (2001).
14. M.A. Helvie, L. Hadjiiski, E. Makariou, et al., "Sensitivity of noncommercial computer-aided detection system for mammographic breast cancer detection: pilot clinical trial," Radiol 231:208-214 (2004).
15. D. Gur, H. Sumkin, H.E. Rockette, M. Ganott, C. Hakim, L.A. Hardesty, T.S. W.R. Poller, R. Shah, L. Wallace, Rockette, "Changes in breast cancer

detection and mammography recall rates after the introduction of a computer-aided detection system," J National Cancer Institute 96(3): 185-190 (2004).
16. P.M. Taylor, J. Champness, R.M. Given-Wilson, H.W.W. Potts, K. Johnston, "An evaluation of the impact of computer-based prompts on screen readers' interpretation of mammograms," Brit J Radiol 77: 21-27 (2004).
17. B. Zheng, M.A. Ganott, C.A. Britton, C.M. Hakim, L.A. Hardesty, T.S. Chang, H.E. Rockette, D. Gur, "Soft-copy mammographic readings with different computer-assisted detection cuing environments: Preliminary findings," Radiol 221, 633-640 (2001).
18. C. Marx, A. Malich, M. Facius, U. Grebenstein, D. Sauner, S.O.R. Pfleiderer, W.A. Keiser, "Are unnecessary follow-up procedures induced by computer-aided diagnosis (CAD) in mammography? Comparison of mammographic diagnosis with and without use of CAD" Eur J Radiol 51(1):66-72 (2004).
19. B. Zheng, R.G. Swenson,, S. Golla, C.M. Hakim, R. Shah, L. Wallace, D. Gur, "Detection and classification performance levels of mammographic masses under different computer-aided detection cueing environments, " Acad Radiol 11(4): 398-406 (2004).
20. C.J. D'Orsi, "Computer-aided detection: There is no free lunch," Radiol 221, 585-586 (2001).
21. A. Malich, T. Azhari, T. Bohm, M. Fleck, W.A. Kaiser, "Reproducibility - an important factor determining the quality of computer aided detection (CAD) systems," Eur J Radiol 36, 170-174 (2000).
22. B. Zheng, L.A. Hardesty, W.R. Poller, J.H. Sumkin, S. Golla, "Mammography with computer-aided detection: Reproducibility assessment - Initial experience, " Radiol 228(1): 58-62 (2003).
23. C.G. Taylor, J. Champness, M. Reddy, P. Taylor, H.W.W. Potts, R. Given-Wilson, "Reproducibility of prompts in computer-aided detection (CAD) of breast cancer," Clin Radiol 58(9): 733-738 (2003).
24. E.A. Sickles, "Findings at mammographic screening on only one standard projection: outcomes analysis," Radiol 208: 471-475 (1998).
25. M. Heath, K. Bowyer, D. Kopans, et al, "Current Status of the Digital Database for Screening Mammography," in Digital Mammography, Kluwer Academic Publishers (1998). Available: http:// marathon.csee.usf.edu/Mammography/Database.html
26. L. Irwig, N. Houssami, C. van Vliet, "New technologies in screening for breast cancer: a systematic review of their accuracy," Brit J Cancer 90 (11): 2118-2122 (2004).
27. C.M. Kuzmiak, G.A. Millnamow, B. Qaqish, E.D. Pisano, E.B. Cole, M.E. Brown, "Comparison of full-field digital mammography to screen-film mammography with respect to diagnostic accuracy of lesion characterization in breast tissue biopsy specimens, " Acad Radiol 9: 1378-1382 (2002).
28. P. Skaane, A. Skjennald, "Screen-film mammography versus full-field digital mammography with soft-copy reading: Randomized trial in a population-based screening program - The Oslo II study," Radiol 232: 197-204 (2004).
29. R.R. Mills, R. Davis, A.J. Stacey, "The detection and significance of calcifications in the breast: a radiological and pathological study," Brit J Radiol 49: 12-26 (1976).

30. E.A. Sickles, "Mammographic features of 300 consecutive nonpalpable breast cancers," AJR 146, 661-663 (1986).
31. A.M. Knutzen, J.J. Gisvold, "Likelihood of malignant disease for various categories of mammographically detected, nonpalpable breast lesions," Mayo Clin Proc 68, 454-460 (1993).
32. J. Johnston, C. Clee, "Analysis of 308 localization breast biopsies in a New Zealand hospital," Austral Radiol 35,148-151 (1991).
33. American College of Radiology, Breast Imaging Reporting and Data System (BI-RADS), 3rd ed. Reston, VA: American College of Radiology, (1998).
34. D. Kopans. *Breast imaging*, 2nd ed. Philadelphia: Lippincott-Raven, (1998).
35. P. Samardar, E. Shaw de Paredes, M.M. Grimes, J.D. Wilson, "Focal asymmetric densities seen at mammography: US and pathologic correlation," Radiographics 22, 19-33 (2002).
36. R.J. Ferrari, R.M. Rangayyan, J.E.L. Desautels, R.A. Borges, A.F. Frere, "Identification of the breast boundary in mammograms using active contour models," Med & Biol Eng Comp 42: 201-208 (2004).
37. T. Ojala, J. Nappi, O. Nevalainen, "Accurate segmentation of the breast region from digitized mammograms," Comp Med Imag Graphics 25: 47-59 (2001).
38. U. Bick, M.L. Giger, R.A. Schmidt, R.M. Nishikawa, D.E. Wolverton, K. Doi, "Automated segmentation of digitized mammograms," Acad Radiol 2, 1-9 (1995).
39. S.L. Lou, H.D. Lin, K.P. Lin, D. Hoogstrate, "Automatic breast region extraction from digital mammograms for PACS and telemammography applications," Comp Med Imag Graphics 24: 205-220 (2000).
40. A.J. Mendez, P.G. Tahoces, M.J. Lado, M. Souto, J.L. Correa, J.J. Vidal, "Automatic detection of breast border and nipple in digital mammograms," Comp Meth & Prog Biomed 49:253-262 (1996).
41. H.E. Rickard, G.D. Tourassi, A.S. Elmaghraby, "Self-organizing maps for masking mammography images," presented at the 2003 ITAB Conference, Birmingham, UK, 24-26 April.
42. U. Bick, M.L. Giger, R.A. Schmidt, R.M. Nishikawa, K. Doi, "Density correction of peripheral breast tissue on digital mammograms," Radiographics 16: 1403-1411 (1996).
43. J.W. Byng, J.P. Critten, M.J. Yaffe MJ, "Thickness-equalization processing for mammographic images, " Radiol 203: 564-568 (1997).
44. A.P. Stefanoyiannis, L. Costaridou, S. Skiadopoulos, G. Panayiotakis, "A digital equalisation technique improving visualisation of dense mammary gland and breast periphery in mammography, " Eur J Radiol 45:139-149 (2003).
45. D. D. Adler, and M. A. Helvie, "Mammographic biopsy recommendations," Current Opinion in Radiology 4, 123-129 (1992).
46. D. B. Kopans, "The positive predictive value of mammography," AJR Am J Roentgenol 158, 521-526 (1992).
47. S. Ciatto, L. Cataliotti, and V. Distante, "Nonpalpable lesions detected with mammography: review of 512 consecutive cases," Radiology 165, 99-102 (1987).

48. A.M. Knutzen and J.J. Gisvold, "Likelihood of malignant disease for various categories of mammographically detected, nonpalpable breast lesions," Mayo Clin Proc 68, 454-460 (1993).
49. L.W. Bassett, D.H. Bunnell, J.A. Cerny, and R.H. Gold, "Screening mammography: referral practices of Los Angeles physicians," AJR Am J Roentgenol 147, 689-692 (1986).
50. F. M. Hall, "Screening mammography - potential problems on the horizon," NEJM 314, 53-55 (1986).
51. F. M. Hall, J. M. Storella, D. Z. Silverstone, and G. Wyshak, "Nonpalpable breast lesions: recommendations for biopsy based on suspicion of carcinoma at mammography," Radiology 167, 353-358 (1988).
52. D. Cyrlak, "Induced costs of low-cost screening mammography," Radiology 168, 661-3 (1988).
53. E.A. Sickles, "Periodic mammographic follow-up of probably benign lesions: results in 3,184 consecutive cases," Radiology 179, 463-468 (1991).
54. X. Varas, F. Leborgne, and J.H. Leborgne, "Nonpalpable, probably benign lesions: role of follow-up mammography," Radiology 184, 409-414 (1992).
55. M.A. Helvie, D.M. Ikeda, and D.D. Adler, "Localization and needle aspiration of breast lesions: complications in 370 cases," AJR Am J Roentgenol 157, 711–714 (1991).
56. J.M. Dixon and T.G. John, "Morbidity after breast biopsy for benign disease in a screened population," Lancet 1, 128 (1992).
57. G.F. Schwartz, D.L. Carter, E.F. Conant, F.H. Gannon, G.C. Finkel, and S.A. Feig, "Mammographically detected breast cancer: nonpalpable is not a synonym for inconsequential," Cancer 73,1660–1665 (1994).
58. H.J. Burhenne, L.W. Burhenne, D. Goldberg, T.G. Hislop, et al., "Interval breast cancer in screening mammography program in British Columbia: analysis and calcification," AJR Am J Roentgenol 162, 1067-1071 (1994).
59. J. Elmore, M. Wells, M. Carol, H. Lee, et al., "Variability in radiologists' interpretation of mammograms," New England J Med 331, 1493-1499 (1994).
60. H-P Chan, K.N. Doi, C.J. Vyborny, K.L. Lam, R.A. Schmidt, "Computer-aided detection of microcalcifications in mammograms - methodology and preliminary clinical-study," Invest Radiol 23: 664-671 (1988).
61. J. Dengler, S. Behrens, J.F. Desaga, "Segmentation of microcalcifications in mammograms," Trans Med Im 12: 634–642 (1993).
62. N. Petrick, H.-P. Chan, B. Sahiner and D. Wei, "An adaptive density-weighted contrast enhancement filter for mamographic breast mass detection," IEEE Trans Med Im 15: 59–67 (1996).
63. T.O. Gulsrud and J.H. Husøy, "Optimal filter-based detection of microcalcifications," IEEE Trans Biomed Eng 48: 1272–1280 (2001).
64. R.N. Strickland and H.I. Hahn, "Wavelet transforms for detecting microcalcifications in mammograms," IEEE Trans Med Im 15: 218–229 (1996).
65. S.Y. Yu, L. Guan, " A CAD system for the automatic detection of clustered microcalcifications in digitized mammogram films," IEEE Trans Med Imag 19, 115-126, (2000).

66. B. Zheng, W. Qian and L.P. Clarke, "Digital mammography: mixed feature neural network with spectral entropy decision for detection of microcalcifications," IEEE Trans. Med. Imaging 15: (1996).
67. W. Zhang *et al.*, "Computerized detection of clustered micro-calcifications in digital mammograms using a shift-invariant artificial neural network," Med. Phys. 23: 517–524 (1994).
68. W. Zhang, K. Doi, M.L. Geiger *et al.*, "An improved shift-invariant artificial neural network for computerized detection of clustered microcalcifications in digital mammograms," Med. Phys. 23: 595–601 (1996).
69. L. Bocchi, G. Coppini, J. Nori, G. Valli, "Detection of single and clustered micro calcifications in mammograms using fractals models and neural networks," Med Eng & Phys 26: 303-312 (2004).
70. M.A. Gavrielides, J.Y. Lo, R. Vargas-Voracek, C.E. Floyd, "Segmentation of suspicious clustered microcalcifications in mammograms," Med Phys 27, 13-22 (2000).
71. M.A. Gavrielides, J.Y. Lo, C.E. Floyd, "Parameter optimization of a computer-aided diagnosis scheme for the segmentation of microcalcification clusters in mammograms," Med Phys 29: 475-483 (2002).
72. H.D. Cheng, Y.M. Lui, R.I. Freimanis, "A novel approach to microcalcification detection using fuzzy logic technique, " IEEE Trans Med Imag 17: 442-450 (1998).
73. H-P Chan, B. Sahiner, K.L. Lam, N. Petrick, M.A. Helvie, M.M. Goodsitt, D.D> Adler, "Computerized analysis of mammographic microcalcifications in morphological and texture feature spaces," Med Phys 25: 2007-2019 (1998).
74. F. Schmidt, E. Sorantin, C. Szepesvari, E. Graif, M. Becker, et al. " An automatic method for the identification and interpretation of clustered microcalcifications in mammograms," Phys Med Biol 44, 1231-1243 (1999).
75. D.L. Thiele, C. Kimme-Smith, T.D. Johnson, M. McCombs, L.W. Bassett, " Using tissue texture surrounding calcification clusters to predict benign vs malignant outcomes, Med Phys 23,549-545 (1996).
76. B. Zhang, Y.H. Chang, X.H. Wang, W.F. Good, "Comparison of artificial neural network and Bayesian belief network in a computer-assisted diagnosis scheme for mammography," Proceedings of SPIE—The International Society for Optical Engineering, 3661:1553–1561, San Diego, CA, USA, (1999).
77. L.O. Hall, "Learned fuzzy rules versus decision trees in classifying microcalcifications in mammograms," Proceedings of SPIE—The International Society for Optical Engineering, 2761: 54–61, Orlando, FL, USA, (1996).
78. M. Kallergi, "Computer-aided diagnosis of mammographic microcalcification clusters," Med Phys 31: 314-326 (2004).
79. H.D. Cheng, X.P. Cal, X.W. Chen, L.M. Hu, X.L. Lou, "Computer-aided detection and classification of microcalcifications in mammograms: a survey," Pattern recognition 36: 2967-2991 (2003).
80. W. Qian, L.H. Li, L.P. Clarke, " Image feature extraction for mass detection in digital mammography: Influence of wavelet analysis," Med Phys 26,402-408 (1999).

81. B. Zheng, Y.H. Chang, X.H. Wang, W.F. Good, D. Gur, "Feature selection for computerized mass detection in digitized mammograms by using a genetic algorithm," Acad Radiol 6, 327-332 (1999).
82. W. Qian, L.H. Li, L.P. Clarke, R.A. Clark, J. Thomas, "Digital mammography: comparison of adaptive and nonadaptive CAD methods for mass detection," Acad Radiol 6, 471-480 (1999).
83. H.P. Chan, B. Sahiner, M.A. Helvie, N. Petrick, M.A. Roubidoux, et al. " Improvement of radiologists' characterization of mammographic masses by using computer-aided diagnosis: an ROC study," Radiol 212, 817-827 (1999).
84. Z. Huo, M.L. Giger, C.J. Vybotny, D.E. Wolverton, R.A. Schmidt, K. Doi, "Automated computerized classification of malignant and benign masses on digitized mammograms," Acad Radiol 5, 155-168 (1998).
85. W. Qian, X.J. Sun, D.S. Song, R.A. Clark, " Digital mammography: Wavelet transform and Kalman-filtering neural network in mass segmentation and detection," Acad Radiol 8, 1074-1082 (2001).
86. S. Paquerault, N. Petrick, H.P. Chan, B. Sahiner, M.A. Helvie, " Improvement of computerized mass detection on mammograms: Fusion of two-view information," Med Phys 29, 238-247 (2002).
87. A.H. Baydush, D.M. Catarious, C.K. Abbey, C.E. Floyd, "Computer aided detection of masses in mammography using subregion Hotelling observers," Med Phys 30: 1781-1787 (2003).
88. H.D. Cheng, M. Cui, " Mass lesion detection with a fuzzy neural network," Pattern Recognition 37:1189-1200 (2004).
89. C.E. Floyd, Jr., J.Y. Lo, G.D. Tourassi, "Breast Biopsy: Case-Based Reasoning Computer-Aid Using Mammography Findings for the Breast Biopsy Decisions", AJR 175, 1347-1352 (2000).
90. A.O. Bilska-Wolak and C.E. Floyd, Jr., "Development and evaluation of a case-based reasoning classifier for prediction of breast biopsy outcome with BI-RADSTM lexicon", Med Phys 29, 2090-2100 (2002).
91. M. Lai, X. Li, W.F. Bischof, "On techniques for detecting circumscribed masses in mammograms," IEEE Trans. Med Imaging 8: 377–386 (1989).
92. Y-H Chang, L.A. Hardesty, C.M. Hakim, T.S. Chang, B. Zheng, W.F. Good, D. Gur, "Knowledge-based computer-aided mass detection on digitized mammograms: a preliminary assessment," Med Phys 28, 455-461 (2001).
93. G.D. Tourassi, R. Vargas-Voracek, D.M. Catarious, C.E. Floyd, "Computer-assisted detection of mammographic masses: A template matching scheme based on mutual information," Med Phys 30:2123-2130 (2003).
94. G.D. Tourassi, C.E. Floyd Jr., "Computer-assisted diagnosis of mammographic masses using an information-theroretic image retrieval scheme with BIRADs-based relevance feedback," presented at the 2004 SPIE Medical Imaging Conference, San Diego, CA, 14-19 February (2004).
95. W. Evans, L.W. Burhenne, L. Laurie, K. O'Shauhnessy, R. Castellino, "Invasive lobular carcinoma of the breast: mammographic characteristics and computer-aided detection," Radiol 225, 182-189 (2002).
96. J.A. Baker, E.L. Rosen, E.I. Gimenez, R. Walsh, M.S. Soo, "Computer-aided detection in screening mammography: Sensitivity of commercial CAD systems for architectural distortion." AJR 181: 1083-1088 (2003).

97. R. Zwiggelaar, T.C. Parr, J.E. Schumm, I.W. Hutt, C.J. Taylor, S.M. Astley, C.R.M. Boggis, "Model-based detection of spiculated lesions in mammograms," Medical Image Analysis 3, 39-62 (1999).
98. Z. Huo, M.L. Giger, C.J. Vyborny, et al. "Analysis of spiculation in the computerized classification of mammographic masses," Med Phys 22, 1569-1579 (1995).
99. W.P. Kegelmeyer, J.M. Pruneda, P.D. Bourland, A. Hillis, et al., " Computer-aided mammographic screening for spiculated lesions," Radiol 191, 331-337 (1994).
100. N. Karssemeijer, G.M. te Brake, "Detection of stellate distortions in mammograms," IEEE Trans Med Imag 15, 611-619 (1996).
101. G.M. te Brake, N. Karssemeijer, "Single and multiscale detection of masses in digital mammograms," IEEE Trans Med Imag 18, 628-639 (1999).
102. N. Cerneaz, M. Brady, "Finding curvi-linear structures in mammograms," Lecture Notes in Computer Science 905, 372-382 (1995).
103. C. Steger, "Extracting curvi-linear structures: a differential geometric approach," Lecture Notes in Computer Science 1064, 630-641 (1996).
104. H. Kobatake, "Detection of spicules on mammograms based on skeleton analysis," IEEE Trans Med Imag 15, 235-245 (1996).
105. R. Rangayyan, N. El-Faramawy, J. Desautels, O. Alim, "Measures of acutance and shape for classification of breast tumors," IEEE Trans Med Imaging 16, 799-810 (1997).
106. H. Bornefalk, "Use of phase and certainty information in automatic detection of stellate patterns in mammograms," presented at the 2004 SPIE Medical Imaging Conference, San Diego, CA, 14-19 February (2004).
107. T. Matsubara, T. Ichikawa, T. Hara, et al. "Automated detection methods for architectural distortion around skin line and within mammary gland on mammograms," International Congresss Series 1256:950-955 (2003).
108. G.D. Tourassi, C.E. Floyd Jr., "Performance Evaluation of an Information-Theoretic CAD Scheme For the Detection of Mammographic Architectural Distortion," presented at the 2004 SPIE Medical Imaging Conference, San Diego, CA, 14-19 February (2004).
109. M.J.M. Broeders, N.C. Onland-Moret, H.J.T.M. Rijken, J.H.C.L. Hendriks, A.L.M. Verbeek, R. Holland, "Use of previous screening mammograms to identify features indicating cases that would have a possible gain in prognosis following earlier detection," European Journal of Cancer 39: 1770–1775 (2003).
110. N Karssemeijer, "Automated classification of parenchymal patterns in mammograms," Phys Med Biol 43: 365–378 (1998).
111. J.W. Byng, M.J. Yaffe, R.A. Jong, R.S. Shumak, G.A. Lockwood, D.L. Tritchler, N.F. Boyd, "Analysis of mammographic density and breast cancer risk from digitized mammograms," Radiographics 18: 1587-1598 (1998).
112. R. Sivaramakrishna, N.A. Obuchowski, W.A. Chilcote, K.A. Powell, "Automatic segmentation of mammographic density," Acad Radiol 8: 250-256 (2001).

113. X. H. Wang, W. F. Good, B. E. Chapman, Y-H. Chang, W. R. Poller, T. S. Chang, L. A. Hardesty, "Automated assessment of the composition of breast tissue revealed on tissue-thickness-corrected mammography," American Journal of Roentgenology, 180: 257-262 (2003).
114. K. Bovis and S. Singh, "Classification of mammographic breast density using a combined classifier paradigm," Medical Image Understanding and Analysis (MIUA) Conference, Portsmouth, July 2002.
115. Y.-H. Chang, X.-H. Wang, L. A. Hardesty, T. S. Chang, W. R. Poller, W. F. Good, and D. Gur, "Computerized assessment of tissue composition on digitized mammograms," Acad Radiol, 9: 899-905 (2002).
116. C. Zhou, H.-P. Chan, N. Petrick, M. A. Helvie, M. M. Goodsitt, B. Sahiner, and L. M. Hadjiiski, "Computerized image analysis: estimation of breast density on mammograms," Medical Physics 28: 1056-1069 (2001).
117. H.E. Rickard, G.D. Tourassi, A.S. Elmaghraby, "Unsupervised tissue segmentation in screening mammograms for automated breast density assessment," presented at the 2004 SPIE Medical Imaging Conference, San Diego, CA (2004).
118. National Cancer Institute – Biomedical Imaging Program. BIP database resources. Available at *www3.cancer.gov/steer_iasc.htm.*
119. J. Suckling, J. Parker, D. Dance, S. Astley, I. Hutt, C. Boggis. I. Ricketts, E. Stamatakis, N. Cerneaz, S. Kok, P. Taylor, D. Betal and J. Savage. "The mammographic images analysis society digital mammogram database." Exerpta Medica. International Congress Series 1069: 375-378 (1994).
120. N.A. Obuchowski, "Receiver operating characteristic curves and their use in radiology," Radiol 229: 3-8 (2003).
121. D.P. Chakraborty, "Maximum likelihood analysis of free-response receiver operating characteristic (FROC) data," Med Phys 16:561-568 (1989).
122. D.P. Chakraborty, L. Winter, "Free-response methodology: alternate analysis and a new observer-performance experiment," Radiol 174: 873-881 (1990).
123. D.P. Chakraborty, "Statistical power in observer-performance studies: Comparison of the Receiver-Operating characteristic and free-response methods in tasks involving localization," Acad Radiol 9:147-156 (2002).
124. D.B. Kopans, "Double reading," Radiol Clinics of North America 38:719 (2000).
125. M.W. Vannier, R.M. Summers, "Sharing Images," Radiology 228, 23-25 (2003).
126. T.M. Cover, J.A. Thomas, *Elements of Information Theory* (John Wiley & Sons, New York 1991).
127. W.T. Ho, P.W.T. Lam, "Clinical Performance of Computer-Assisted Detection (CAD) System in Detecting Carcinoma In Breasts Of Different Densities," Clin Radiol 58, 133-136 (2003).
128. A. Del Bimbo, *Visual Information Retrieval*, Morgan Kaufmann Publishers, San Francisco (1999).
129. American College of Radiology, "Breast Imaging Reporting and Data System," Reston, VA: American College of Radiology, (1996).

130. D.E. Rumelhart, G.E. Hinton, R.J. Williams, "Learning internal representations by error propagation," in *Parallel Distributed Processing: Explorations in the Microstructures of Cognition (Vol. 2).* edited by D.E. Rumelhart and J.L. McClelland (The MIT Press, Cambridge, MA, 1986), 318-362.
131. M.T. Hagan, M. Menhaj, "Training fedd-forward networks with the Marquardt algorithm," IEEE Trans Neural Networks 5(6):989-993 (1994).
132. E.A. Krupinski, "Computer aided detection in clinical environment: benefits and challenges for radiologists," Radiology 231:7-9 (2004).

7. Medical Diagnosis and Prognosis Based on the DNA Microarray Technology

Y. Fukuoka[1], H. Inaoka[1-2] and I. S. Kohane[3-5]

1 School of Biomedical Science, Tokyo Medical and Dental University, 2-3-10 Kandasurugadai, Chiyoda-ku, Tokyo 101-0062, Japan
2 Institute of Biomaterials and Bioengineering, Tokyo Medical and Dental University, 2-3-10 Kandasurugadai, Chiyoda-ku, Tokyo 101-0062, Japan
3 Informatics Program, Children's Hospital, Harvard Medical School, Boston, MA, USA
4 Division of Health Sciences and Technology, Harvard University and MIT, Cambridge, MA, USA
5 Harvard Partners Center for Genetics and Genomics, Boston, MA, USA

7.1 Introduction

Immense genomic data have been accumulated through various research activities such as the Human Genome Project. A genome is the entire collection of information on the DNA molecules of each organism. The application of information technology to data mining analyses of genomic data is known as bioinformatics, which could be a most rewarding field for a computer scientist. This chapter describes DNA microarray technology, one of the hot topics in bioinformatics.

The DNA microarray technology makes it possible to simultaneously monitor expression patterns of thousands of genes [1-11]. A gene is expressed to produce the protein encoded by the gene. When a lot of the protein is produced, the gene is said to be highly expressed. In contrast, when no protein is produced, the gene is not expressed. Because there are many different types of proteins, each of which plays an important role in the cell, expression levels of genes are affected by a large number of biological and environmental factors. Accordingly, investigating a genome-wide expression pattern, i.e. how much of each gene product is made, provides important insight into pathological as well as biological conditions of the samples (cells, patients etc.).

Although the applications of DNA microarrays include basic biological research, disease diagnosis and prognosis, drug discovery and toxicological research, this chapter will focus on medical applications. The primary objective of such applications is identification of genes whose expression patterns are highly differentiating with respect to disease conditions (e.g. tumor types) and thus DNA microarrays are widely used to explore molecular markers of various diseases: cancer [12-30] and others [31-32]. Because an immense quantity of data is being accumulated with this novel technology, powerful and effective analysis methods

Y. Fukuoka, H. Inaoka and I.S. Kohane: *Medical Diagnosis and Prognosis Based on the DNA Microarray Technology*, StudFuzz **184**, 209–236 (2005)
www.springerlink.com

are required to mine invaluable information from the data. A number of computational techniques have been applied to extract the fundamental expression patterns inherent in patients' data [3-11].

The purpose of this chapter is to cover a broad range of topics relevant to medical diagnosis and prognosis based on the DNA microarray technology. The chapter consists of two parts: technical foundations of DNA microarrays and their applications to clinical medicine. The first part deals with the principles of DNA microarrays, issues on experimental designs in medical research with microarrays and methodology for data processing. This part also provides a brief and necessary description of basic molecular biology. The second part can be further divided into two subparts: the first half provides an overview of applications of DNA microarrays to clinical medicine and the second half describes some examples from the first half in more detail.

7.2 Technical foundation of DNA microarrays

7.2.1 Basic molecular biology

Understanding the DNA microarray technology requires a basic understanding of the fundamentals of molecular biology. This subsection provides a brief and necessary description of DNA (deoxyribonucleic acid), RNA (ribonucleic acid), gene, protein, gene expression and hybridization. Readers familiar with these concepts may skip this subsection.

DNA is a large polymer constructed by sequentially binding nucleotides, which are the basic building blocks consisting of a sugar (deoxyribose), a phosphate and one of four types of bases: adenine (A), cytosine (C), guanine (G) and thymine (T). The four bases are divided into two classes according to their chemical structures. One class, purine, involves A and G while the other, pyrimidines, includes C and T. When two strands of DNA are hold together via hydrogen bonds between laterally opposed bases, A specifically binds to T and C specifically binds to G. In principle there is no other combination and thus, it is said that A is complimentary to T and C is complimentary to G. The order of the bases along the DNA is referred to as the sequence of the DNA, which determines the information stored in the region of the DNA. The two-paired bases are called a base pair. The length of a DNA/RNA fragment is measured in base pair (bp).

A gene, which is the basic unit of heredity, is a discrete functional region within DNA. The DNA sequence of a gene is copied (or transcribed) onto RNA, which is a polymer similar to DNA[1]. This is the first step of gene expression, in which a DNA strand is used as a template for assembling the RNA. In the second step, a protein is synthesized based on the sequence of the assembled RNA, called

---

[1] The main differences between DNA and RNA are i) in RNA, the sugar is ribose and ii) uracil (U) is used instead of T.

messenger RNA (mRNA). Thus the flow of information is from DNA to RNA and then RNA to a protein. This is known as the central dogma of molecular biology.

Hybridization is a process by which two complementary, single stranded DNA/RNA form a stable double helix. When two complementary DNA/RNA strands are close to each other, these strands hybridize. The DNA microarray technique employs hybridization reactions between single-stranded fluorescent molecules contained in the sample and single-stranded sequences on the array surface.

7.2.2 Basic protocol of DNA microarray experiment

This subsection describes the essential ideas for measuring gene expression levels with microarrays. A DNA microarray is, in general, a substrate on which single-stranded molecules with various sequences are deposited (Fig. 1). We will refer to a single-stranded molecule on the substrate as a probe. A probe has the complementary sequence to its target DNA/RNA[2] which will hybridize to the probe. For one type of probe, enormous copies of the molecule having the same sequence are deposited in a spot on the array surface. A typical microarray contains hundreds or thousands of such spots arranged regularly and, accordingly, the microarray technology enables us to measure expressions levels of a huge number of genes simultaneously.

DNA microarrays measure gene expression levels based on the abundance of mRNA molecules in the specific type of cells being analyzed. A basic procedure for measuring expression levels with the DNA microarray is divided into three major steps as summarized in Table 1.

First, the sample cells are separated and the mRNAs in the cells are extracted. Each of the mRNAs is converted into the form of complementary DNA (cDNA) using the reverse transcription enzyme. At this stage, the amount of the cDNAs is insufficient to detect using a fluorescent labeling technique. The numbers of the target cDNAs must be increased via a polymerase chain reaction (PCR) before labeling. This process is called amplification. In some cases, the amplification process is carried out using an *in vitro* transcription (IVT) reaction and in these cases, the target molecules are complementary RNAs. Then the targets are labeled with fluorescent dyes.

In the next step, the labeled targets are reacted with the probes on the microarray. Once the targets hybridize to the probes, the unbound molecules are washed away. After the washing process, the targets bound to the probes can be visualized by fluorescent detection (Fig. 2).

---

[2] An expressed sequenced tag (EST) is another type of targets. ESTs, which are partial sequences of complementary DNAs, provide information on transcribed DNA sequences. They can be employed as targets for microarrays. However, for the sake of simplicity, when we talk the number of probes in what follows, the term "gene" will refer to both genes and ESTs.

The fluorescent image is scanned into a computer via an image scanner. In the image processing step, each spot is segmented and noise reduction as well as necessary processing for improving the image quality are carried out. (For more details of image processing, please consult Chapter 3 in [6] or Chapter 4 in [7].) The intensity of each spot can be related to the amount of the mRNA in the sample. The result of this step is a collection of numerical estimates representing the gene expression levels.

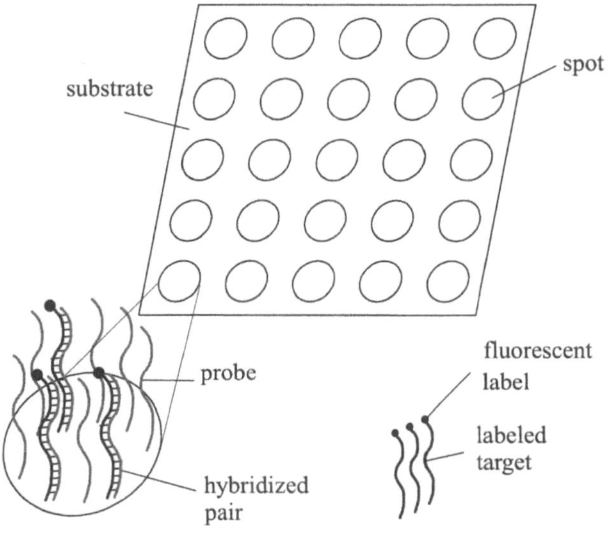

Fig. 1. A schematic illustration of a DNA microarray. Target molecules in a sample are labeled with a fluorescent dye and hybridize to probes having the complementary sequence to the target. The amount of the target molecules in the sample, i.e. the expression level of the gene, is estimated from the intensity of the light at the spot.

Tabel 1. A standard procedure for measuring gene expression levels with a DNA microarray

Sample preparation
cell separation
mRNA extraction
amplification
fluorescent labeling
Hybridization
hybridization between the labeled targets and the probes
washing to remove un-hybridized molecules
Data acquisition
scanning the fluorescent image
image processing
converting the intensities into expression levels

In a typical clinical study, expression levels are measured in several patients. For example, when the number of patients is ten, the entire procedure must be repeated ten times, yielding ten sets of expression profiles. These profiles are usually integrated into a single matrix form, in which a column represents an expression profile from a microarray and a row represents a change in the expression level of a gene among the ten patients (Table 2). It should be noted that each element in Table 2 represents the original value. A logarithmic transformation is often performed because original values can differ considerably in magnitude.

The data matrix given in Table 2 has n x 10 elements, where the number of the genes, n, is much greater than the number of the patients, 10. In contrast, a conventional clinical study likely involves hundreds of cases over which tens of variables are measured. This difference must be taken into account when analyzing microarray data [4].

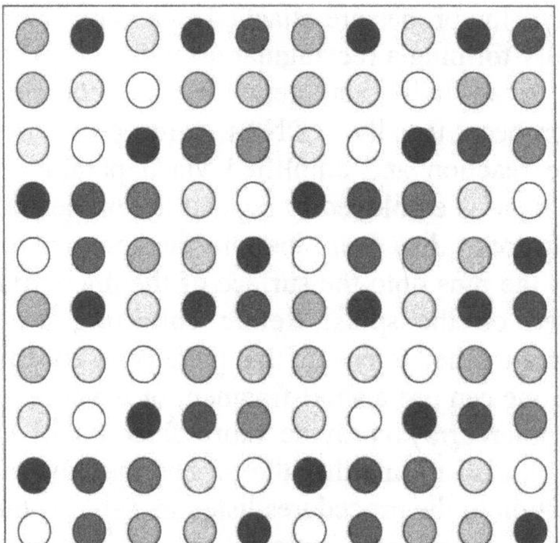

Fig. 2. A schematic example of an fluorescent image. The brightness of each spot represents the light intensity, which is related to the amount of the target molecules hybridized to the probe in the spot and thus the amount of the targets present in the sample. These intensities are converted into numbers after image processing.

Table 2. An example of expression data in a matrix form

	patient 1	patient 2	patient 3	patient 4	patient 5		patient 10
gene 1	159.8	18.1	63.3	80.5	53.2		64.2
gene 2	105.0	25.2	28.9	247.3	26.9		55.2
gene 3	62.7	18.5	67.0	53.7	27.8		22.0
gene 4	192.3	54.6	314.2	109.5	71.6		39.8
gene 5	716.1	366.3	651.4	663.2	836.5		716.1
gene 6	28.0	31.4	71.7	176.0	20.3	.	17.4
.							
.							
gene n	61.1	12.3	138.4	438.1	46.9		23.6

7.2.3 Two main types – cDNA microarray and oligonucleotide microarrays

Two main approaches are used for DNA microarray fabrication. The first type of fabrication involves two methods: deposition of PCR-amplified cDNA clones [1] and printing of synthesized oligonucleotides. In the other approach, *in situ* manufacturing, photolithography [2], ink jet printing [33] and electrochemical synthesis are employed. In what follows, we will focus on two widely-used types: cDNA microarrays [1] and oligonucleotide microarrays using photolithography [2]. The former is known as the Stanford type microarray. The latter is a ready-to-use, commercial microarrays called the Affymetrix type, oligonucleotide microarrays or GeneChip® and the necessary equipment for microarrays of this type is available from Affymetrix Inc.

Stanford type microarrays

In cDNA microarrays, the probes are attached to a number of spots arranged in a regular pattern usually forming a rectangular array (see Figs. 1 and 2). Each of the spots is dedicated to an individual gene. In the fabrication of this type of microarray, the probes, usually cDNAs, are previously prepared by a reverse-transcriptase reaction and amplified via a parallel PCR. A mechanical micro spotting technique is employed to deposit the probes onto the spots. In this technique, a spotting robot dips thin pins into the solutions containing the probe cDNAs and touches the pins onto the surface of the microarrays. In this way, the probes are deposited on the spots. Before collecting the next probes to be deposited, the pins are washed to ensure that there is no contamination.

In this approach, one can use a short fragment or a whole gene as a probe. This means that cDNA microarrays provide more freedom of choice in the probe selection. However, it also means that the probes must be prepared by the user. Accordingly, in addition to the procedures listed in Table 1, this approach requires some more steps: selection and preparation of probes and fabrication of microarrays.

This type of microarray is usually combined with comparative hybridization. This technique is often referred to as a dual channel experiment. In this method, the target molecules are extracted from two different specimens: for example, one is from tumor cells and the other is normal tissues. Hereafter, we call the former as the sample and the latter as the reference. In a dual channel experiment, two fluorescent dyes with different colors, usually a green-dye cyanine 3 (Cy3) and a red-dye cyanine 5 (Cy5), are employed to distinguish between the targets from the sample and the reference. After labeling with each dye, the targets from both specimens are mixed well and hybridized to a microarray (Fig. 3). This allows the simultaneous monitoring of expression levels in both specimens. In the image processing step, the light intensities are measured with the two colors taken into account.

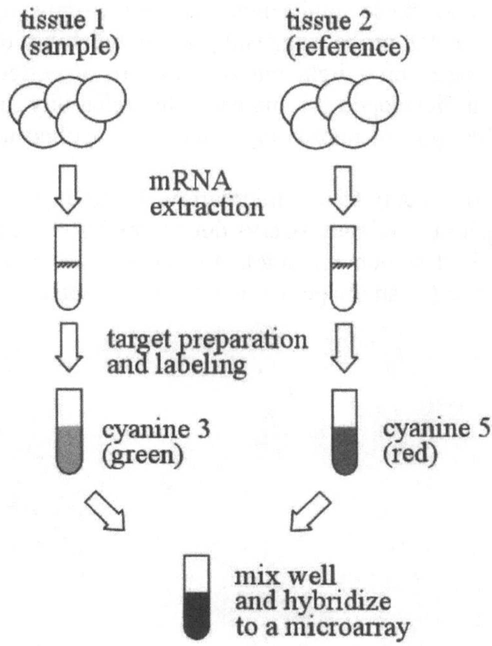

Fig. 3. Preparation of two specimens for a dual channel experiment

Affymetrix type microarrays

This type is a ready-to-use, commercial microarray known also as GeneChip® (Fig. 4). It employs the photolithographic technology used to build very large scale integrated (VLSI) circuits. During microarray fabrication based on *in situ* synthesis, the probes are photochemically synthesized on the substrate. If a probe should have a given base, the corresponding photolithographic mask has a hole allowing the base to be deposited at the probe position. Subsequent masks will produce the sequences in a base-by-base manner. Although this approach allows the fabrication of high density microarrays, the length of the sequence built on the microarray is limited because a probability of introducing an error at each step is not zero.

To compensate for the above disadvantage, a gene is represented by several short sequences. The selection of these sequences is performed based on sequence information alone. This approach can distinguish closely related genes because the particular sequences are chosen carefully to avoid unwanted cross-hybridization between the genes by excluding the identical sequences shared by those genes. There are probes with purposely mismatched sequences on this type of microarray. In a mismatch probe, the base at the center of the true sequence (perfect match) is replaced with its complementary base. For example, when the center of a perfect match is A (adenine), the corresponding mismatch has T (thymine) at the center. If a lot of molecules mistakenly hybridize to a mismatch probe, it is likely that those molecules also mistakenly hybridize to the corresponding perfect match probe, suggesting a low reliability of the probe pair. A statistical method based on a light intensity pattern of perfect and mismatch probe pairs has been developed to increase the reliability of the measured expression levels. This type of microarray can not be applied to a dual channel experiment.

Figure 4 shows (a) a ready-to-use microarray, GeneChip®, (b) an oven for maintaining the temperature of microarrays during the hybridization reaction, (c) an apparatus called fluid station for automatic biochemical processing (such as fluorescent labeling) and (d) an image scanner and a computer.

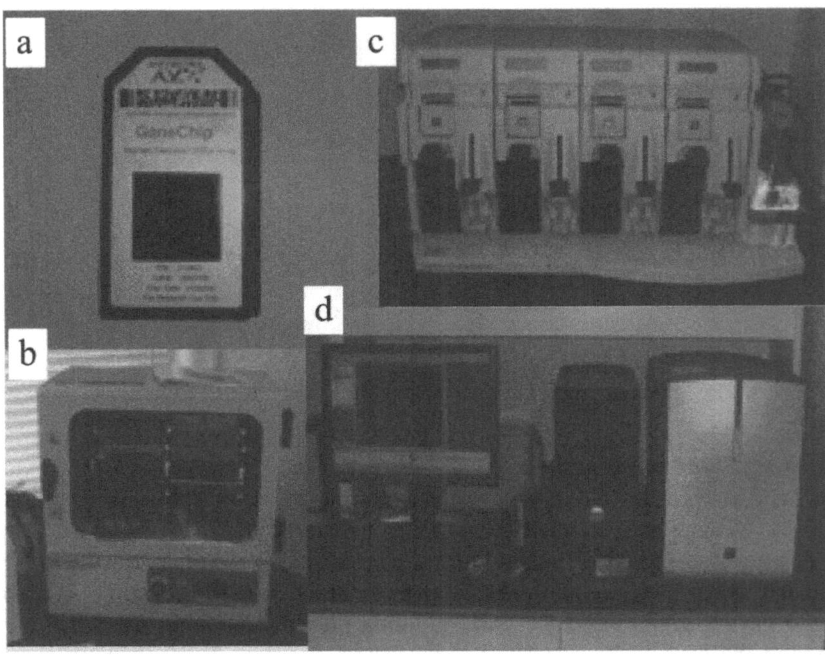

Fig. 4. Affymetrix GeneChip® and the analysis system. (a) A oligonucleotide microarray named GeneChip®, (b) a hybridization oven, (c) a fluid station and (d) an image scanner and a computer.

7.3 Experimental designs in medical research with DNA microarrays

This section provides an overview of DNA microarrays in the medical field. There are common experimental designs depending on the questions addressed in the research project. Four major experimental designs are illustrated in Fig. 5. The questions addressed are:

a) Is there any specific gene expression pattern associated with a certain disease?
b) Are there subcategories in a disease characterized by gene expressions patterns?
c) Are there recognizable differences in gene expression profiles between diseases?
d) What genes are differentially expressed before and after a specific treatment?

In what follows, these four experimental designs are referred to as a) molecular diagnosis, b) subtype discovery, c) disease classification and d) treatment response.

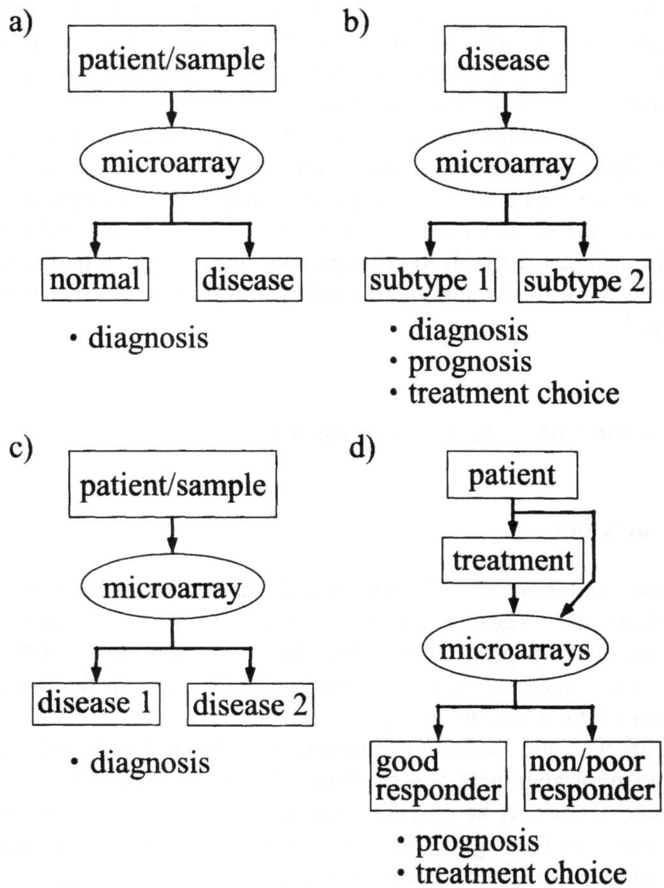

Fig. 5. Four major experimental designs: a) molecular diagnosis, b) subtype discovery, c) disease classification and d) treatment response. There is the primary question, addressed in a project, corresponding to each experimental design.

The primary objective of a project categorized as "molecular diagnosis" is to find an expression pattern observed only in a specific disease and distinguish a patient with the disease from those who are without it. As the name suggests, the main purpose of a study in the subtype-discovery category is to subdivide a clinically heterogeneous disease using the microarray technology. Given highly variable clinical courses, doctors may suspect that there are more than one type in the disease. In such a case, this experimental designed is employed. The resultant findings provide useful insights into the prognosis and the selection of the optimal treatment. This design can be also used for molecular classification of subtypes. The disease-classification design is used to explore molecular markers for the distinction between two or more diseases. The molecular-diagnosis design can be considered as a variant of this design. The prominent purpose of a research project using the treatment-response design is to find marker genes to quantitatively describe the effects of a treatment. This type of research provides valuable information to select the optimal treatment.

Regardless of the design, when the number of the conditions to be compared is two, the differentially expressed genes are important. The primary difference among the four designs is in the selection of samples. For instance, if the samples are obtained from normal and tumor tissues, the design is "molecular diagnosis." Accordingly, it is not difficult to combine two designs and actually, in [13] and [26], a combination of the subtype discovery and disease classification schemes was employed.

7.4 Processing of gene expression data

7.4.1 Preprocessing

In expression measurements with DNA microarrays, measurement variability and noise are inevitable. These could be introduced virtually at every step of a measurement: different procedures in the sample preparation, hybridization time and temperature, dust on a microarray, saturation in an fluorescent image, misalignment of spots, and so on [6].

These artifacts could lead us to spurious findings and poor hypotheses [4]. For instance, due to misalignment of some spots on a single microarray, the expression levels of some genes may be mistakenly underestimated for the microarray. If the expression levels of those genes for other patients are measured properly and the values are large, those genes seem to be well correlated. It is obvious that a strong correlation does not necessarily mean that those genes are regulated by the same mechanism. When analyzing microarray data, this fact should be taken into account.

Eliminating outliers is one possible remedy for the noisy nature of data[3]. Another approach is normalization. Variability in microarray data can be divided into two categories: systematic and random errors. The objective of normalization is to remove the systematic component. The normalization is also crucial when results of different data sets are combined. Although there is no standard method for normalizing microarray data, some methods are widely used: subtracting the mean expression levels of a microarray, dividing by the mean, using constantly-expressed genes as control and using regression models. For more details about the normalization procedures, please consult Chapter 12 in [6] or [34].

Among thousands of genes investigated with microarrays, the expression levels of some genes remain almost constant for all patients. In other words, the elements of a row in the data matrix (Table 2) are almost the same to each other. These genes are not informative and, accordingly, they should be excluded from the subsequent analysis. This exclusion procedure should be applied to the column vectors in the data matrix. This method is referred to as variation filter. There are some other filtering techniques for extracting only informative genes [4].

7.4.2 Data analysis

Although DNA microarrays have been widely applied to various biological as well as medical studies, there is no standard analytic method for the large amount of data. Computation techniques for data mining are applicable to expression data. Also, conventional statistical methods like primary component analysis (PCA) are applied to data analysis and visualization. However, the difference in the purposes of the studies may require different analysis methods.

The analysis methods can be divided into two categories: supervised and unsupervised methods. The former methods, which employ a training set to categorize expression data into predetermined groups, are applied to classification tasks. In the latter methods, the patterns inherent in the data are determined without any prior knowledge. Two unsupervised methods have been widely used to analyze expression data: the hierarchical clustering [35] and the self-organizing map (SOM) [36]. In addition to these, this subsection surveys various supervised and unsupervised methods for analyzing microarray data.

Unsupervised methods

Hierarchical clustering Hierarchical clustering [35] is an unsupervised method to analyze gene expression data. The object of this method is to create a dendrogram (Fig. 6) that assembles all elements (genes/patients) into a phylogenic-type tree. The basic idea is to iteratively group elements with similar patterns. A similarity metric is necessary to group elements. The Pearson

[3] Needless to say, carefully designed experiments are essential to reduce the measurement variability and noise. Also, if affordable, repeat (or replicate) measurements on the same sample is another possible solution for the random component of noise.

correlation coefficient r, given in Equation (1), is one of the common similarity metrics.

$$r = \frac{1}{N}\sum_{i=1}^{N}\left(\frac{x_i - \bar{x}}{\sigma_x}\right)\left(\frac{y_i - \bar{y}}{\sigma_y}\right) \tag{1}$$

Here, N denotes the number of the elements, $\bar{x}$ and $\bar{y}$ represent the average of x and y, respectively. σ_x and σ_y are the standard deviation of x and y.

First, the similarity scores for all possible pairs of the elements are calculated and the pair having the maximum value is identified. Then these two elements are joined to create a new node, representing their average. The similarity scores are recalculated and the same process is repeated until all elements form a single tree whose branch lengths represent the degree of similarity between the pairs. The resultant dendrogram is a good visualization tool, i.e. this method is particularly advantageous in visualization of similarities in expression patterns. Although the value of this method has been demonstrated in [15] and [35], it has shortcomings for gene expression analysis: lack of robustness and nonuniqueness. Despite these disadvantages, this method is popular for an analysis of expression data due to its simplicity.

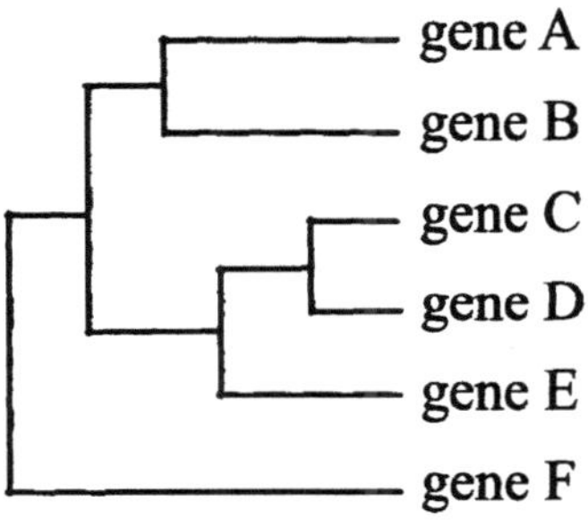

Fig. 6. An example of a dendrogram. This dendrogram indicates that genes C and D have similar expression patterns and that the expression pattern of gene F is very different from the patterns of the other genes. In this way, a dendrogram is a good visualization tool.

Self-organizing maps The self-organizing map (SOM), sometimes also referred as self-organizing feature map, was proposed by Kohonen [37-38]. The SOM is an unsupervised clustering method similar to k-means clustering. However, unlike the k-means method, the SOM facilitates easy visualization and interpretation. Kohonen has demonstrated that an SOM can be implemented as a feedforward artificial neural network (ANN) trained with an unsupervised learning algorithm. An ANN for a SOM is composed of input and competitive output layers (Fig. 7). The input layer has n units that represent n-dimensional input vector which is an expression profile of a gene/patient while the output layer consists of c units that represent c categories. The output units are arranged with a simple topology such as a two-dimensional grid. The two layers are fully connected, i.e., every input unit is connected to every output unit.

The connecting weights are modified to cluster input vectors into c classes. At the onset of a training process, the weights are initialized to small random values. On subsequent iterations, an input vector $\boldsymbol{P}_i$ is presented to the network in a random order and then the weights are adjusted on a winner-take-all basis. The winning unit is typically the unit whose weight vector $\boldsymbol{W}_j$ is the closest to $\boldsymbol{P}_i$. A weight vector $\boldsymbol{W}_j$ consists of the connecting weights from all input units to output unit $_j$.

$$\boldsymbol{W}_j = [W_{1j}, W_{2j}, \ldots, W_{nj}] \tag{2}$$

where W_{1j} denotes the weight from the first input unit to the j-th output unit. To achieve a topological mapping, not only $\boldsymbol{W}_j$, but also the weights of the adjacent output units in the neighborhood of the winner are adjusted. The weights are moved in the direction of $\boldsymbol{P}_i$ according to the following equation if unit k is in the neighborhood. Otherwise, the weight is not changed.

$$\boldsymbol{W}_k(t+1) = \boldsymbol{W}_k(t) + \alpha(t)\,(\boldsymbol{P}_i - \boldsymbol{W}_k(t)) \tag{3}$$

where $\alpha(t)$ is the learning rate at t-th iteration. The learning rate and the size of the neighborhood decrease with iteration number t.

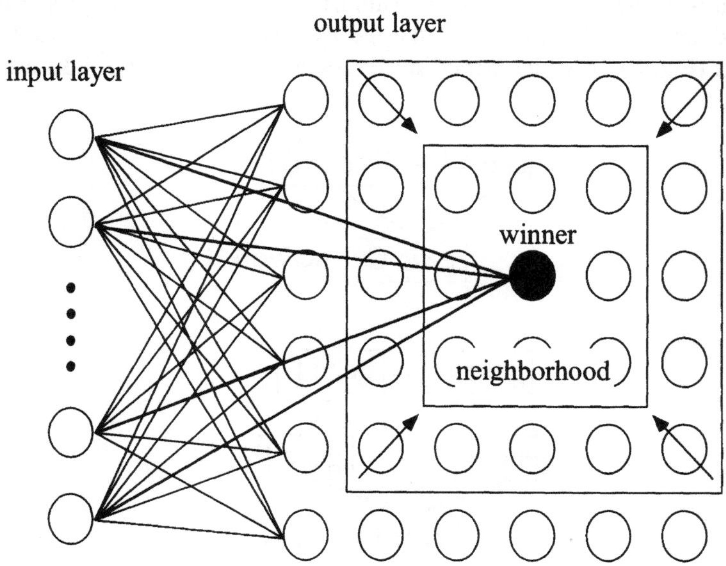

Fig. 7. An artificial neural network for self-organizing map

***k*-means method** The k-means algorithm is an unsupervised, iterative clustering method similar to the SOM [4], [39]. First, the number of the clusters, k, is determined. Then the k centers of the clusters (centroids) are initialized to randomly selected genes. Each gene is assigned to a cluster whose centroid is nearest to the gene. Then each centroid is updated with the average expression pattern of the genes in that cluster. These steps are repeated while the centroids move, i.e. the cluster memberships change. The k-nearest neighbours method can be considered as a supervised version of this algorithm. In the k-nearest neighbours method, k neighbours vote to classify a new sample into predetermined classes.

Network determination Various techniques are used to elucidate functional relationships of genes (termed gene regulatory networks): relevance networks [4], [11], [17], Boolean networks [40-41], bayesian networks [42] and petri networks [43]. Boolean networks are based on the Boolean algebra and describe logical relationships. Bayseian networks employ the bayseian probability theory and petri networks are bipartite digraphs. In what follows, we will focus on relevance networks.

Relevance networks offer an unsupervised method for constructing networks of similarity [4], [11], [17]. Multiple types of data can be used as demonstrated in [17], in which expression levels are combined with phenotypic measurements. In this method, expression levels of all genes are compared in a pair-wise manner. Although any similarity measure can be used when comparing the levels, usually, the Pearson correlation coefficient is calculated for every pair at this step. Then a threshold is determined and only the pairs having the coefficients greater than the threshold are linked. Groups of the genes linked together are displayed as networks (Fig. 8), in which genes are represented as nodes and links are shown with lines.

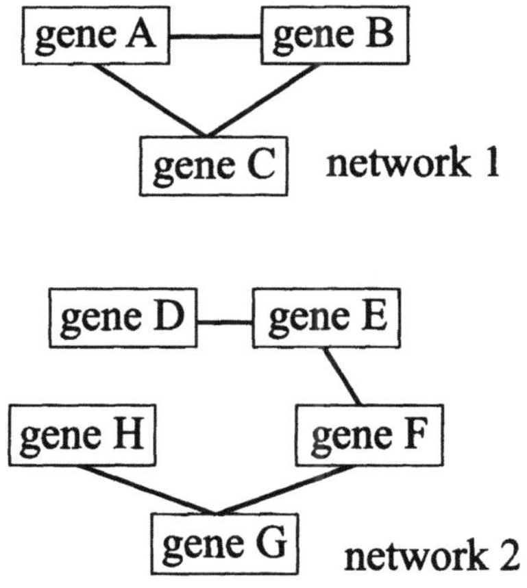

Fig. 8. Relevance networks. A node represents a gene, and a line denotes a functional relationship between the two genes.

Supervised methods

Artificial neural networks Artificial neural networks (ANNs) are powerful, supervised methods for various classification tasks [44] and widely applied to biomedical fields [45] and to gene expression data [18], [46-47]. Although some ANNs can be used as an unsupervised method, here we will focus on the most popular supervised approach.

The most popular learning algorithm for ANNs is the back-propagation (BP) method. The algorithm has been widely used to train multilayer, feedforward neural networks (Fig. 9). A feedforward network having three or more layers trained with this algorithm is often called multilayer perceptron. This algorithm can evolve a set of weights to produce an arbitrary mapping from input to output by presenting pairs of input patterns and their corresponding output vectors. It is an iterative gradient algorithm designed to minimize a measure of the difference between the actual output and the desired output.

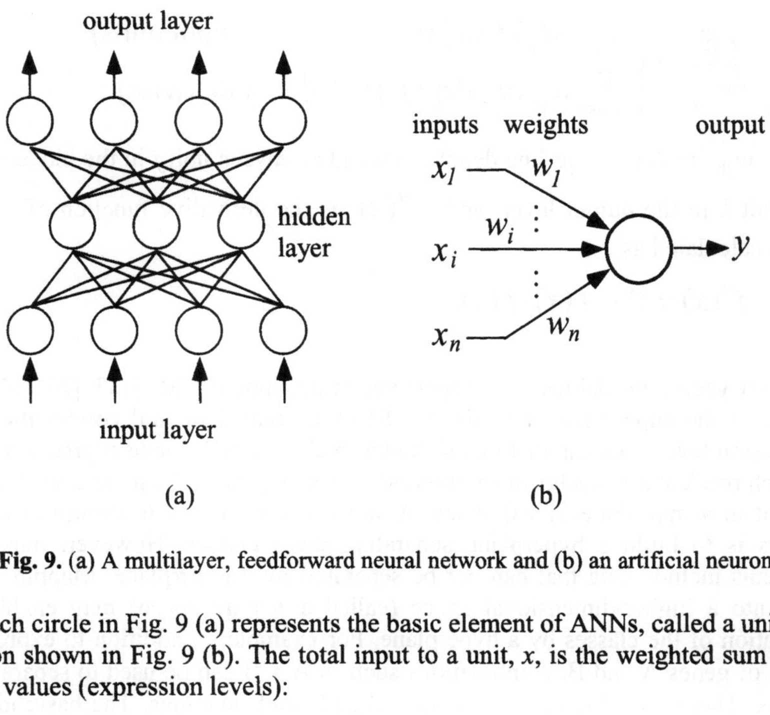

Fig. 9. (a) A multilayer, feedforward neural network and (b) an artificial neuron

Each circle in Fig. 9 (a) represents the basic element of ANNs, called a unit or a neuron shown in Fig. 9 (b). The total input to a unit, x, is the weighted sum of its input values (expression levels):

$$x = \sum_i w_i x_i \tag{4}$$

and its output, y, is determined by:

$$y = f(x) = \frac{1}{1 + \exp^{-x}} \tag{5}$$

Learning by the BP algorithm is carried out by iteratively updating the weights so as to minimize the quadratic error function E defined as:

$$E = \frac{1}{2} \sum (y_i^3 - d_i)^2 \tag{6}$$

where y_i^3 is the actual output of unit i in the output layer and d_i is its desired value. In a classification task, a class is represented with a combination of the desired values. A weight change, Δw, is calculated as:

$$\Delta w(t) = -\varepsilon \frac{\partial E}{\partial w} + \alpha \Delta w(t-1) \tag{7}$$

where

$$\frac{\partial E}{\partial w_{i,j}} = \begin{cases} (y_j^3 - d_j) f'(x_j^3) y_i^2 \cdots\cdots\cdots\cdots \text{(output units)} \\ (\sum_k w_{jk}\, \partial E / \partial x_k^3) f'(x_j^2) y_i^1 \cdots \text{(otherwise).} \end{cases} \tag{8}$$

Here, w_{jk} in the second line denotes a weight between unit j in the hidden layer and unit k in the output layer, and $f'(x)$ is the derivative function of $f(x)$ and is calculated as

$$f'(x) = (1 - f(x)) f(x). \tag{9}$$

Support vector machines A support vector machine (SVM) [11], [26], [48-49] is one of the supervised methods. An SVM is trained to find combinations of expression levels that can distinguish between classes in the gene expression data.

Each row/column vector in an expression matrix (Table 2) can be considered as a point in a multidimensional space. A straightforward way to discriminate two classes is to build a hyperplane separating these classes. However, most real problems include data that can not be separated by a hyperplane. Mapping such data into a higher-dimensional space (called a feature space) may enable the separation of the classes by a hyperplane. For example, in addition to expression levels of genes A and B, combinations such as A x B can be used to separate the classes. These combined functions are called kernel functions. The basic idea of SVMs underlies the mapping into the feature space and the kernel functions. SVMs avoid overfitting by separating the classes with the hyperplane having the maximum margin from the samples in the classes. More detailed description is found in [49].

Weight voting method The weight voting method [13] is a supervised method similar to the *k*-nearest neighbours algorithm.

When classifying two classes, an ideal marker gene is highly expressed in class 1, but is not expressed in class 2. In this method, a measure of correlation, $P(g, c)$, is calculated between a gene, g, and the ideal marker gene, c.

$$P(g,c) = \frac{\mu_1(g) - \mu_2(g)}{\sigma_1(g) + \sigma_2(g)} \tag{10}$$

where [$\mu_1(g)$, $\sigma_1(g)$] and [$\mu_2(g)$, $\sigma_2(g)$] represent the mean and standard deviation of g's expression levels in class 1 and 2, respectively. A large absolute value of $P(g, c,)$ indicates a strong correlation between g and c. The sign of $P(g, c)$ is positive or negative when g is highly expressed in class 1 or 2.

The genes are divided into two groups according to the sign of $P(g, c)$ and $n/2$ genes having the largest $|P(g, c)|$ are selected from each group. These n genes are informative for the classification. Two parameters (a_i, b_i) are defined for each informative gene.

$$a_i = P(i,c)$$
$$b_i = \frac{\mu_1(i) + \mu_2(i)}{2} \tag{11}$$

When a new sample is being classified, the vote of each informative gene is calculated as:

$$v_i = a_i(x_i - b_i) \tag{12}$$

where x_i denotes the expression level of the informative gene i in the sample. The total vote V_1 for class 1 is obtained by summing the absolute values of the positive votes over the informative genes, while the total vote V_2 for class 2 is obtained by summing the absolute values of the negative votes.

7.4.3 Validation

There is a central underlying assumption that genes that appear to be similarly expressed are functionally related. However, it should be emphasized that the clusters that we obtain through a computational analysis are only a reflection on the measurements made in a particular system. Also, we should understand that a gene can play different roles in different contexts. Without external knowledge, the results obtained from the expression data are of little use in generating new hypotheses. There exist some useful databases as the source of external knowledge. For example, one can acquire basic information on the genes of interest at GenBank[4] (or the web sites linked from it) and find publications about those genes through PUBMED[4].

---

[4] Both databases are accessible at http://www.ncbi.nlm.nih.gov/.

As described previously, the results may involve many spurious findings. Not all statistically significant changes in gene expression lead to a significant change in a biological/physiological system. Thus a validation process is required to eliminate those biologically or physiologically unimportant findings. There are two different approaches in the validation process: computational and biological validations. The former approach includes permutation testing, cross-validation and evaluating performance metrics (given in Table 3) [4]. In the biological validation, conventional biological techniques are used to test hypotheses derived from the data mining analysis. Both approaches are often combined to efficiently filter out spurious hypotheses. In those cases, the hypotheses that pass the computational validation process are tested biologically.

Table 3. Performance metrics

Sensitivity	$\dfrac{\text{Number of correctly classified event cases}}{\text{Total number of event cases}}$
Specificity	$\dfrac{\text{Number of correctly classified nonevent cases}}{\text{Total number of nonevent cases}}$
Accuracy	$\dfrac{\text{Number of correctly classified cases}}{\text{Total number of cases}}$

Cross-validation is a well-known technique for testing robustness of models obtained from a supervised method. This technique is useful when the number of available data is small because it repeatedly generates subsets of training and testing data and evaluates the performances of the resulting models from the subsets.

In the remainder of this subsection, we will explain permutation testing. When a hypothesis derived from a result of a microarray data analysis, one way to computationally validate the hypothesis is to take each of genes and randomly shuffle the expression levels. It should be noted that this permutation process never changes the basic statistics such as the mean and the variance. If the result of the analysis repeated using this permutated data set is nearly identical to the original one, the hypothesis may be false. If the result are very different from the original one, there is probably a certain biological process that yielded the original result.

As a concrete example, we take a hypothesis that neighbouring genes on DNA are likely to be co-expressed. If this is true, as the distance between two genes becomes short, they are more likely to be co-expressed. To test this hypothesis, we calculated the Pearson correlation coefficient for all possible gene pairs and a co-expression rate that is the fraction of the number of highly co-expressed pairs over the total number of pairs. (For more details about the analysis method, please consult [50].) This analysis was performed using both the original and permutated data sets. The results are shown in Fig. 10. The black and gray lines, respectively representing the original and permutated results, show very different behaviors. These results strongly suggest a certain biological mechanism that yielded the original result.

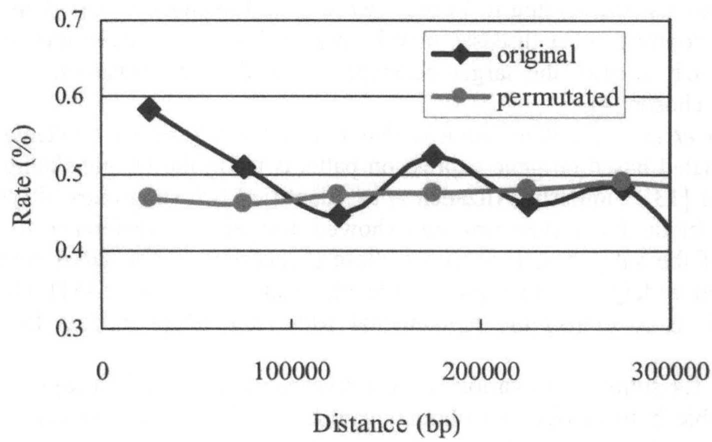

Fig. 10. An example of permutation testing. The black and gray lines show different behaviors, suggesting that a certain biological mechanism yielded the original result. For more details about the analysis method, please consult the main text and [50].

7.5 Application of DNA microarrays to medical diagnosis and prognosis

Each particular type of cell is characterized by a different pattern of gene expression levels although every cell in an individual contains the same genetic information on the DNAs. A human cell can be viewed as a functional unit containing thousands of genes, whose expression levels determine the functional state of the cell. Accordingly, one can hypothesize that most human diseases are accompanied by specific changes in gene expression levels and microarray-base analysis of disease tissues allows the identification of those changes.

This section surveys various applications of microarrays in the medical field. Common objectives of those applications are to discover molecular markers of diseases, to develop sensitive diagnostic and prognostic techniques, and to find drug candidates. In order to understand the biological phenomena behind a disease, expression levels need to be compared between healthy and ill individuals or at different time points for the same individual or population of individuals. It must be noted that we focus mainly on the analysis methods and experimental designs used in various studies although many biological and clinical findings have been described in the subsequent publications. Most of the datasets obtained in those studies are publicly available online.

7.5.1 Microarrays in cancer research

Although there exist a huge number of publications on the application of DNA microarrays to human subjects, most of studies are targeted at certain types of cancer. This is mainly because one can easily compare a tumor sample with the normal tissues surrounding it. In other words, the functionally important tissue is clear. In contrast, other diseases may involve a dysfunction over several organs, and in such a case, the target cell-type of expression measurement must be carefully chosen [4].

Golub *et al.* have demonstrated that two similar types of leukemia can be discriminated based on gene expression patterns using the weight voting method and SOM [13]. Similarly, Alizadeh *et al.* identified two subgroups of lymphoma with the hierarchical clustering and showed a significant difference in survival curves of the subgroups [15]. Since these pioneering works, DNA microarrays have been widely used to explore molecular markers of cancer [51]. One of the key goals is to extract the fundamental patterns inherent in data from tumor samples.

Table 1.4 summarizes various cancer researches using microarrays. As shown in the table both cDNA and oligonucleotide microarrays are widely used. The hierarchical clustering method has been used in many studies [14-16], [21], [23], [26-28], [30] mainly because of its simplicity and good visualization performance. Other computational techniques such as SOMs are applied to gene expression data from tumor samples.

Table 4. Maicroarray studies on various types of cancer

Ref	Type	Genes	Samples	Array type	Methods
13	leukemia	6,817	72	oligonucleotide	SOM, weight voting
14	colon	6,500	40/22	oligonucleotide	HC
15	lymphoma	17,593	128/96	cDNA	HC
16	melanoma	6,971	31	cDNA	HC
17	cell lines	6,416	60	oligonucleotide	relevance network
18	lymphoma	6,567	88	cDNA	ANN
19	multiple	16,063	218/90	oligonucleotide	SVM
20	multiple	16,063	190	oligonucleotide	kNN, weight voting
21	lung	12,600	186/17	oligonucleotide	HC
22	cell lines	6,817	60	oligonucleotide	weight voting
23	lymphoma	12,196	240	cDNA	HC
24	lymphoma	6,817	77	oligonucleotide	weight voting
25	leukemia	12,600	37	oligonucleotide	kNN
26	leukemia	6,817	360	oligonucleotide	SVM, HC, SOM
27	brain	6,817	99	oligonucleotide	kNN, PCA, HC
28	gastric	2,400	22	cDNA	HC
30	leukemia	12,599	120	oligonucleotide	HC

The column Ref shows the reference number. In the sample column, a notation a/b denotes the number of malignant and normal samples.
HC: hierarchical clustering, kNN: k-nearest neighbours, PCA: primary componet analysis

All four common experimental designs mentioned previously are used in these studies. The molecular-diagnosis design is used in [14] for colon tumor. Subtype discovery/classification was performed in lymphoma [15], [23-24], cutaneous malignant melanoma [16], lung cancer [21] and leukemia [26]. Disease classification was carried out for leukemia [13], [25-26], multiple cancers [19-20] and brain tumor [27]. Treatment responses or drug sensitivities were investigated in cancer cell lines [17], [22], and leukemia [30].

Although filtering techniques are employed to reduce the number of the genes for the analysis, it is still much greater than the number of the cases and this difference from typical clinical data must be taken into account when analyzing the data [4].

7.5.2 Microarrays for other diseases

Diabetes

Type 2 (non-insulin-dependent) diabetes mellitus is a metabolic disease involving abnormal regulation of glucose metabolism by insulin. Insulin resistance is a major risk factor for type 2 diabetes because it is a pre-diabetic phenotype. Under physiological conditions, insulin-stimulated glucose metabolism occurs mainly in skeletal muscle and fat cells. Accordingly, gene expression patterns of skeletal muscle tissues from 18 insulin-sensitive and 17 insulin-resistance equally obese Pima Indians were compared using oligonucleotide microarrays, including 40,600 genes [31]. With the Wilcoxon rank sum test (a non-parametric statistical test) on the expression data, 185 differentially expressed genes were found. Of these genes, 20 % were confirmed to be true positives through biological validation.

Muscular dystrophies

Gene expression profiling was performed to obtain insights into pathological processes involved in the progression of two muscular dystrophies [32]. Both dystrophies are with known primary biochemical defects, dystrophin deficiency (Dunchenne muscular dystrophy: DMD) and deficiency in α-sarcoglycan, a protein associated with dystrophin (α-SGD). For expression profiling with oligonucleotide microarrays (7,095 genes), muscle biopsies from five DMD patients, four α-SGD patients and five controls were used. The authors employed the replicate measurement scheme, i.e. each biopsy was divided into two fragments and the subsequent expression measurement was carried out using each fragment independently (in total 28 measurements). To minimize genetic variations between different individuals, they mixed the four or five samples from each of the three groups. This second scheme yielded six measurements because the mixed samples were obtained from each fragment. Differentially expressed genes between every pair of the three groups were identified and those genes were validated biologically.

7.5.3 Detailed reviews

Molecular classification of leukemia with SOMs and weight voting

Here we review applications of the weight voting method and SOMs to molecular classification of leukemia. In [13], Golub *et al.* employed the former method as a supervised technique for disease classification between acute lymphoblastic leukemia (ALL) and acute myeloid leukemia (AML) while they employed SOMs as an unsupervised method for subclass discovery. The data set consisted of expression levels of 6,817 genes obtained from 27 ALL patients and 11 AML patients.

Their supervised method is as follows. First, a filter is used to extract genes that were highly correlated with the distinction between ALL and AML. The filtering process extracted 1,100 genes. They selected 50 most informative genes for the weight voting method and carried out cross-validation tests. The 50-gene classifier was able to group all patients accurately. They examined a wide range of different number of informative genes (10 to 200 genes) with the method and all classifier achieved high accuracy.

Then subtype discovery was performed with SOMs. Before they applied the SOM to the expression data from the leukemia patients, they had tested their method using data sets of yeast cell cycle and hematopoietic differentiation [36]. In the yeast case, 828 genes that passed the variation filter were used as the input of the SOM, which had 6x5 output units arranged in a two-dimensional grid (see Fig. 7). Their results indicated that multiple clusters exhibited periodic behavior and that adjacent clusters had similar behavior. In the hematopoietic case, normalized expression levels of 567 genes were fed into the SOM having 4x3 output units. They reported that the clusters corresponded to patterns of clear biological relevance although they were generated without preconceptions. These results demonstrated their method's ability to assist in interpretation of gene expression.

First, to compare the performance of the SOM and the weight voting method, they employed a two-cluster SOM and trained it using the expression patterns of all 6,817 genes (i.e. no variation filter was used). The connecting weights were initialized with small random values at the onset of training, and the expression data were put into the SOM. On the subsequent training, an expression pattern of a gene was presented in a random order and the weights were updated according to Equation (3). The trained SOM assigned 25 patients (24 ALL, 1 AML) in one cluster and the other 13 samples (10 AML, 3 ALL) in the other class. This result indicated that the SOM was effective at automatically discovering the two types of leukemia.

Next, they employed a variation filter to exclude genes with small variation across the samples. The filtered data were fed into a four-cluster SOM for subtype discovery. The results suggested that there were two subtypes in ALL. A cluster was exclusively AML, another cluster contained a subtype of ALL and the other two contained the other subtype of ALL.

These results indicated that the SOM could distinguish ALL from AML and find subtypes of ALL. The success of the SOM methodology suggests that genome-wide profiling is likely to provide valuable insights into biological process that are not yet understood at the molecular level. This approach is applicable to other diseases and may become more common to analyze gene expression data in the near future.

Subtype discovery by hierarchical clustering in large B-cell lymphoma
Here we review an application of the hierarchical clustering algorithm to discover subtypes in lymphoma [15].

Diffuse large B-cell lymphoma (DLBCL) is a common subtype of lymphoma. Patients with DLBCL have highly variable clinical courses: 40 % of the patients respond well to current therapy and have prolonged survival, whereas the remainder have significantly worse prognosis. However, there had been no decisive classification scheme to categorize clinical and pathological entities before Alizadeh et al. devised a new method using DNA microarrays [15].

In [15], they focused on DLBCL to determine whether gene expression profiling could subdivide the clinically heterogeneous diagnostic category into molecularly distinct diseases with more homogeneous clinical behaviors. Ninety-six samples of normal and malignant lymphocytes were used. In addition to samples from DLBCL, they included samples from other types of tumors to evaluate the performance of the clustering algorithm. Fluorescent cDNA molecules, labeled with the Cy5 dye, were prepared from each sample. Reference cDNA molecules, labeled with the Cy3 dye, were prepared from nine different lymphoma cell lines. Each sample was combined with the Cy3-labeled reference and the mixture was hybridized to the microarray. The fluorescent ratio was quantified for each gene and reflected the relative abundance of the gene in each sample compared with the common reference mRNA pool. They measured expression profiles with cDNA microarrays with probes for 17,593 genes to explore molecular markers for subtypes. In total, 128 microarrays were used for the 96 samples.

A normalization by subtracting the mean levels and variation filtering [35] were carried out at the preprocessing stage. After filtering, 4,026 genes remained in the dataset and a hierarchical clustering was performed to group genes. The same algorithm was used to group the samples. The resultant dendrogram had some clusters corresponding to the different sample types, suggesting that the expression patterns reflected intrinsic differences between the tumor samples. An investigation of differences in the expression patterns for the DLBCL samples revealed the existence of two distinct clusters of the patients. A comparison of the clinical histories of the patients in both clusters indicated that the two clusters corresponded well to the two groups of the patients with the different mortality rates. Although no information on the identity was used in the clustering, the algorithm segregated the recognized classes of DLBCL.

7.6 Concluding remarks

This chapter described the technical foundations of DNA microarrays and their applications to medical diagnosis and prognosis. By providing massive, parallel platforms for acquisition of gene expression data, the DNA microarray technology enables systematic and unbiased approaches in biomedical research. Although this chapter tried to cover as many analysis methods and applications as possible, there are an enormous number of publications that we could not review here. Our survey in this chapter was limited to studies on humans. However, a considerable number of microarray studies have been carried out on animal models. The strategies described in this chapter are applicable to expression data from animal studies.

This chapter concludes with a view of future directions of the DNA microarray technology. First, as the cost of microarrays decreases, the quantity and quality of expression data will be undoubtedly increase. This will require more efficient and powerful computational methods for data mining. One of the ultimate goals in bioinformatics is automatic knowledge acquisition from expression data. We are currently far from this goal and some people are skeptical about its realization. However, steps must be taken towards the goal. An example of such a step is to develop an environment for assisting biological interpretation of expression data by associating information from various genomic databases. Although this chapter focused only on the DNA microarray technology, bioinformatics includes broad areas of topics and most genomic projects require well-trained bioinformaticians, who have strong backgrounds in computer science as well as biology. This chapter closes with an invitation to bioinformatics: Bioinformatics is one of the most challenging and rewarding fields for computer scientists and IT engineers.

References

1. Schena, M., Shalon, D., Davis, R.W., and Brown, P.O.: Quantitative monitoring of gene expression patterns with a complementary DNA microarray. Science, 270 (1995) 467-470.
2. Lockhart, D.J., Dong, H., Byrne, M.C., Follettie, M.T., Gallo, M.V., Chee, M.S., Mittmann, M., Wang, C., Kobayashi, M., Horton, H. and Brown, E.L.: Expression monitoring by hybridization to high-density oligonucleotide arrays, Nature Biotechnol., 14 (1996) 1675-1680.
3. Schena, M. ed.: DNA microarrays – a practical approach. Oxford University Press, New York (1999).
4. Kohane, I.S., Kho, A.T., and Butte, A.J.: Microarrays for an integrative genomics. MIT Press, Cambridge (2003).
5. Berrar, D.P., Dubitzky, W., and Granzow, M. eds.: A practical approach to microarray data analysis. Kluwer Academic Publishers, Boston/Dordrecht/London (2003).
6. Draghici, S.: Data analysis tools for DNA microarrays. Chapman & Hall/CRC, Boca Raton/London/New York/Washington DC (2003).

7. Stekel, D.: Microarray bioinformatics. Cambridge University Press, Cambridge (2003).
8. Lin, S.M., and Johnson, K.F. eds.: Methods of microarray data analysis. Kluwer Academic Publishers, Boston/Dordrecht/London (2002).
9. Lin, S.M., and Johnson, K.F. eds.: Methods of microarray data analysis II. Kluwer Academic Publishers, Boston/Dordrecht/London (2002).
10. Lin, S.M., and Johnson, K.F. eds.: Methods of microarray data analysis III. Kluwer Academic Publishers, Boston/New York/Dordrecht/London (2003).
11. Butte, A.: The use and analysis of microarray data, Nature Rev. Drug Discovery, 1 (2002) 951-960.
12. DeRisi, J., Penland, L., Brown, P.O., Bittner, M.L., Meltzer, P.S., Ray, M., Chen, Y., Su, Y.A. and Trent, J.M.: Use of a cDNA microarray to analyse gene expression patterns in human cancer, Nature Genet., 14 (1996) 457-460.
13. Golub, T.R., Slonim, D.K., Tamayo, P., Huard, C., Gaasenbeek, M., Mesirov, J.P., Coller, H., Loh, M.L., Downing, J.R., Caligiuri, M.A., Bloomfield, C.D. and Lander E.S.: Molecular classification of cancer: Class discovery and class prediction by gene expression monitoring. Science, 286 (1999) 531-537.
14. Alon, U., Barkai, N., Notterman, D.A., Gish, K., Ybarra, S., Mack, D., and Levine, A.J.: Broad patterns of gene expression revealed by clustering analysis of tumor and normal colon tissues probed by oligonucleotide arrays. Proc. Natl. Acad. Sci. USA, 96 (1999) 6745-6750.
15. Alizadeh, A.A., Eisen, M.B., Davis, R.E., Ma, C., Lossos, I.S., Rosenwald, A., Boldrick, J.C., Sabet, H., Tran, T., Yu., X., Powell, J.I., Yang, L., Marti, G.E., Moore, T., Hudson, J. Jr., Lu, L., Lewis, D.B., Tibshirani, R., Sherlock, G., Chan, W.C., Greiner, T.C., Weisenburger, D.D., Armitage, J.O., Warnke, R., Levy, R., Wilson, W., Grever, M.R., Byrd, J.C., Botstein, D., Brown, P.O. and Staudt, L.M.: Distinct types of diffuse large B-cell lymphoma identified by gene expression profiling. Nature, 403 (2000) 503-511.
16. Bittner, M., Meltzer, P., Chen, Y., Jiang, Y., Seftor, E., Hendrix, M., Radmacher, M., Simon, R., Yakhini, Z., Ben-Dor, A., Sampas, N., Dougherty, E., Wang, E., Marincola, F., Gooden, C., Lueders, J., Glatfelter, A., Pollock, P., Carpten, J., Gillianders, E., Leja, D., Dietrich, K., Beaudry, C., Berens, M., Alberts, D., Sondak, V., Hayward, N., and Trent, J.: Molecular Classification of cutaneous malignant melanoma by gene expression profiling. Nature, 406 (2000) 536-540.
17. Butte, A.J., Tamayo, P., Slonim, D., Golub, T.R., and Kohane, I.S.: Discovering functional relationships between RNA expression and chemotherapeutic susceptibility using relevance networks. Proc. Natl. Acad. Sci. USA, 97 (2000) 12182-12186.
18. Khan, J., Wei, J.S., Ringner, M., Saal, L.H., Landanyi, M., Westermann, F., Berthold, F., Schwab, M., Antonescu, C.R., Peterson, C., and Meltzer, P.S.: Classification and diagnostic prediction of cancers using gene expression profiling and artificial neural networks. Nature Med., 7 (2001) 673-679.
19. Ramaswamy, S., Tamayo, P., Rifkin, R., Mukherjee, S., Yeang, C.H., Angelo, M., Ladd, C., Reich, M., Latulippe, E., Mesirov, J.P., Poggio, T., Gerald, W., Loda, M., Lander, E.S., and Golub, T.R.: Multiclass cancer diagnosis using tumor gene expression signatures. Proc. Natl. Acad. Sci. USA, 98 (2001) 15149-15154.
20. Yeang, C.H., Ramaswamy, S., Tamayo, P., Mukherjee, S., Rifkin, R.M., Angelo, M., Reich, M., Lander, E.S., Mesirov, J., and Golub, T.R.: Molecular classification of multiple tumor types. Bioinformatics, 17 (2001) S316-S322.

21. Bhattacharjee, A., Richards, W.G., Staunton, J., Li, C., Monti, S., Vasa, P., Ladd, C., Beheshti, J., Bueno, R., Gillette, M., Loda, M., Weber, G., Mark, E.J., Lander, E., Wong, W., Johnson, B.E., Golub, T., Sugarbaker, D.J., and Meyerson, M.: Classification of human lung carcinomas by mRNA expression profiling reveals distinct adenocarcinoma subclasses. Proc. Natl. Acad. Sci. USA, 98 (2001) 13790-13795.
22. Staunton, J.E., Slonim, D.K., Coller, H.A., Tamayo, P., Angelo, M.J., Park, J., Scherf, U., Lee, J.K., Reinhold, W.O., Weinstein, J.N., Mesirov, J.P., Lander, E.S., and Golub, T.R.: Chemosensitivity prediction by transcriptional profiling. Proc. Natl. Acad. Sci. USA, 98 (2001) 10787-10792.
23. Rosenwald, A., Wright, G., Chan, W.C., Connors, J.M., Campo, E., Fisher, R.I., Gascoyne, R.D., Muller-Hermelink, H.K., Smeland, E.B., Jaffe E.S., Simon R., Klausner R.D., Powell J., Duffey P.L., Longo D.L., Greiner T.C., Weisenburger D.D., Sanger W.G., Dave B.J., Lynch J.C., Vose J., Armitage J.O., Montserrat E., Lopez-Guillermo A., Grogan T.M., Miller T.P., LeBlanc M., Ott G., Kvaloy S., Delabie J., Holte H., Krajci P., Stokke T., and Staudt, L.M.: The use of molecular profiling to predict survival after chemotherapy for diffuse large-B-cell lymphoma. New Eng. J. Med., 346 (2002) 1937-1947.
24. Shipp, M.A., Ross, K.N., Tamayo, P., Weng, A.P., Kutok, J.L., Aguiar, R.C.T., Gaasenbeek, M., Angelo, M., Reich, M., Pinkus, G.S., Ray, T.S., Koval, M.A., Last, K.W., Norton, A., Lister, A., Mesirov, J., Neuberg, D.S., Lander, E.S., Aster, J.C., and Golub, T.R.: Diffuse large B-cell lymphoma outcome prediction by gene-expression profiling and supervised machine learning. Nature Med, 8 (2002) 68-74.
25. Armstrong, S.A., Staunton, J.E., Silverman, L.B., Pieters, R., den Boer, M.L., Minden, M.D., Sallan, S.E., Lander, E.S., Golub, T.R., and Korsmeyer, S.J.: MLL translocations specify a distinct gene expression profile that distinguishers a unique leukemia. Nature Genet. 30 (2002) 41-47.
26. Yeoh, E.J., Ross, M.E., Shurtleff, S.A., Williams, W.K., Patel, D., Mahfouz, R., Behm, F.G., Raimondi, S.C., Relling, M.V., Patel, A., Cheng, C., Campana, D., Wilkins, D., Zhou, X., Li, J., Liu, H., Pui, C.H., Evans, W.E., Naeve, C., Wong, L., and Downing, J.R.: Classification, subtype discovery, and prediction of outcome in pediatric acute lymphoblastic leukemia by gene expression profiling. Cancer Cell. 1 (2002) 133-143.
27. Pomeroy, S.L., Tamayo, P., Gaasenbeek, M., Sturla, L.M., Angelo, M., McLaughlin, M.E., Kim, J.Y.H., Goumnerova, L.C., Black, P.M., Lau, C., Allen, J.C., Zagzag, D., Olson, J.M., Curran, T., Wetmore, C., Biegel, J.A., Poggio, T., Mukherjee, S., Rifkin, R., Califano, A., Stolovitzky, G., Louis, D.N., Mesirov, J.P., Lander, E.S., and Golub, T.R.: Prediction of central nervous system embryonal tumor outcome based on gene expression. Nature, 415 (2002) 436-442.
28. Lee, S., Baek, M., Yang, H., Bang, Y.J., Kim, W.H., Ha, J.H., Kim, D.K., and Jeoung, D.I.: Identification of genes differentially expressed between gastric cancers and normal gastric mucosa with cDNA microarrays. Cancer Lett., 184 (2002) 197-206.
29. Haviv, I., and Campbell, I.G.: DNA microarrays for assessing ovarian cancer gene expression. Mol.& Cell. Endocrinology, 191 (2002) 121-126.
30. Cheok, M.H., Yang, W., Pui, C.H., Downing, J.R., Cheng, C., Naeve, C.W., Relling, M.V., and Evans, W.E.: Treatment-specific changes in gene expression discriminate in vivo drug response in human leukemia cells. Nature Genet., 34 (2003) 85-90.

31. Yang, X., Pratley, R.E., Tokraks, S., Bogardus, C., and Permana, P.A.: Microarray profiling of skeletal muscle tissues from equally obese, non-diabetic insulin-sentive and insuline-resistant Pima Indians. Diabetologia, 45 (2002) 1584-1593.
32. Chen, Y.W., Zhao, P., Borup, R., and Hoffman, E.P.: Expression profiling in the muscular dystrophies: identification of novel aspects of molecular pathophysiology. J. Cell Biol., 151 (2000) 1321-1336.
33. Theriault, T.P., Winder, S.C. and Gamble, R.C.: Application of ink-jet printing technology to the manufacturing of molecular arrays. 101-120. In Schena, M. ed.: DNA microarrays – a practical approach. Oxford University Press, New York (1999).
34. Morrison, N., and Hoyle, D.C.: Normalization – Concepts and methods for normalizing microarray data. 76-90. In Berrar, D.P., Dubitzky, W., and Granzow, M. eds.: A practical approach to microarray data analysis. Kluwer Academic Publishers, Boston/Dordrecht/London (2003).
35. Eisen, M.B., Spellman, P.T., Brown, P.O. and Bosteon, D.: Cluster analysis and display of genome-wide expression patterns. Proc. Natl. Acad. Sci. USA, 95 (1998) 14863-14868.
36. Tamayo, P., Slonim, D., Mesirov, J., Zhu, Q., Kitareewan, S., Dmitrovsky, E. Lander, E.S., and Golub, T.R.: Interpreting patterns of gene expression with self-organizing maps: Methods and application to hematopoietic differentiation. Proc. Natl. Acad. Sci. USA, 96 (1999) 2907-2912.
37. Kohonen, T.: Self-organization and associative memory. Springer-Verlag, New York, Berlin, Heidelberg (1989).
38. Kohonen, T.: Self-organizazing map. Proc. of the IEEE, 78 (1990) 1464-1480.
39. Tavazoie, S., Hughes, J.D., Campbell, M.J., Cho, R.J., and Church, G.M.: Systematic determination of genetic network architecture. Nature Genet., 22 (1999) 281-285.
40. Akutsu, T., Miyano, S. and Kuhara, S.: Algorithms for identifying Boolean networks and related biological networks based on matrix multiplication and fingerprint function. J. Comput. Biol., 7 (2000) 331-343.
41. Liang, S., Fuhrman, S., and Somogyi, R.: Reveal, a general reverse engineering algorithm for inference of genetic network architectures. Pacific Symposium Biocomputing, 3 (1998) 18-29.
42. Friedman, N., Linial, M., Nachman, I., and Pe'er, D.: Using bayesian networks to analyze expression data. J. Comput. Biol., 7 (2000), 601-620.
43. Matsuno, H., Doi, A., Nagasaki, M., and Miyano, S.: Hybrid Petri net representation of gene regulatory network. Pacific Symposium Biocomputing, 5 (2000) 341-352.
44. Bishop, C.M.: Neural networks for pattern recognition. Oxford University Press, New York (1995).
45. Fukuoka, Y.: Artificial neural networks in medical diagnosis. 197-228. In Schmitt, M., Teodorescu, H.N., Jain, A., Jain, A., Jain, S., and Jain, L.C. eds.: Computational intelligence processing in medical diagnosis. Physica-Verlag, Heidelberg, New York (2002).
46. Ringner, M., Eden, P., and Johansson, P.: Classification of expression patterns using artificial neural networks. 201-215. In Berrar D.P., Dubitzky W., and Granzow M. eds.: A practical approach to microarray data analysis. Kluwer Academic Publishers, Boston/Dordrecht/London (2003).
47. Mateos, A., Herrero J., Tamames, J., and Dopazo, J.: Supervised neural networks for clustering conditions in DNA array data after reducing noise by clustering gene expression profiles. 91-103. In Lin, S.M., and Johnson, K.F. eds.: Methods of

microarray data analysis II. Kluwer Academic Publishers, Boston/Dordrecht/London (2002).

48. Brown, M.P.S., Grundy, W.N., Lin, D., Cristianini, N., Sugnet, C.W., Furey, T.S., Ares, M.Jr., and Haussler, D.: Knowledge-based analysis of microarray gene expression data by using support vector machines. Proc. Natl. Acad. Sci. USA, 97 (2000) 262-267.
49. Mukherjee, S.: Classifying microarray data using support vector machines. 166-185. In Berrar D.P., Dubitzky W., and Granzow M. eds.: A practical approach to microarray data analysis. Kluwer Academic Publishers, Boston/Dordrecht/London (2003).
50. Fukuoka, Y., Inaoka, H., and Kohane, I.S.: Inter-species differences of co-expression of neighbouring genes in eukaryotic genomes. BMC Genomics, 5 (2004) article no. 4.
51. Mohr, S., Leikauf, G.D., Keith, G., and Rihn, B.H.: Microarrays as cancer keys: an array of possibilities. J. Clin. Oncology, 20 (2002) 3165-3175.

8. Wearable Devices in Healthcare

Constantine Glaros and Dimitrios I. Fotiadis

Unit of Medical Tehcnology and Intelligent Information Systems, Dept. of Computer Science, University of Ioannina, GR 45110, Ioannina, Greece

8.1 Introduction

The miniaturization of electrical and electronic equipment is certainly not a new phenomenon, and its effects have long been evident in the healthcare sector. Nevertheless, reducing the size of medical devices is one thing, wearing them is quite another. This transition imposes a new set of design requirements, challenges and restrictions and has further implications on their use, as they are often intended for operation by non medical professionals in uncontrolled environments. The purpose of this chapter is to introduce the use of wearable devices in healthcare along with the key enabling technologies behind their design, with emphasis on information technologies. Furthermore, it aims to present the current state of development along with the potential public benefits in both technological and healthcare terms. The devices described are those involving some degree of digital information handling, thus excluding conventional wearable devices such as eyeglasses, hearing aids and prosthetic devices from the discussion.

A wearable medical device can be described as an autonomous, non-invasive system that performs a specific medical function such as monitoring or support. The term "wearable" implies that the device is either supported directly on the human body or a piece of clothing, and has an appropriate design enabling its prolonged use as a wearable accessory. In broad terms, this requires the device to have minimal size and weight, functional and power autonomy, to be easy to use and worn in comfort.

A typical device is built around a central processing unit and will normally provide a degree of physiological monitoring, data storage and processing, which may be combined with the use of microelectronics, an electrical or mechanical function, involve a degree of intelligence and telemedicine functions. Therefore, like any computer, a typical device will have a data input mechanism, a processing unit and an output mechanism. The input mechanisms deal with the collection of clinical and environmental information through physiological and other sensors, the direct data input by the users, and possibly other incoming information through wireless data transfer from a remote server. The role of the processing unit is to handle the incoming information, often in real time, in order to generate the appropriate feedback. This feedback is either accessed directly by the user in various forms providing monitoring, alerting, and decision support functions, or serves as a control mechanism for another component of the system providing supporting functions. Output mechanisms can therefore involve combinations of

C. Glaros and D.I. Fotiadis: *Wearable Devices in Healthcare*, StudFuzz **184**, 237–264 (2005)
www.springerlink.com

audio, visual, mechanical and electrical functions of a supporting device, or a telemetric service to a remote monitoring unit.

Wearable devices are of emerging interest due to their potential influence in certain aspects of modern healthcare practices, most notably in delivering point of care service, by providing remote monitoring, ambulatory monitoring within the healthcare environment, and support for rehabilitating patients, the chronically ill and the disabled. Other devices are designed as supporting tools for doctors within the healthcare environment, such as for monitoring patients during surgery or for keeping electronic patient records. Another distinct feature is their use by healthy individuals, either as health monitors or fitness assistants. The growing demand in such products can be attributed to a significant extent to an increase of the public's health awareness, and their increasing familiarity in using computer-based products on a daily basis. Apart from providing useful tools, the trend towards the widespread use of personal health assistants is also seen as a helpful step towards the transition of healthcare management into a more preventative model rather than the reactive, episodic model used today. Furthermore, wearable healthcare devices can help in changing the public's attitude towards personal healthcare in the sense that individuals are both asked and enabled to play a more active role in their care. This provides a striking resemblance to the way that the widespread use of wearable (wrist) watches changed people's awareness of the concepts of time and punctuality not so long ago. The incorporation of telemetric capabilities into wearable devices is also in line with the novel concept of pervasive healthcare, whereby wireless technologies allow citizens to transmit and access their health data, transmit and receive information about their current health condition anywhere and anytime.

Wearable healthcare devices have been around for quite some time. The most established medical device is the holter monitor, used to record the cardiac response of patients during normal activities, usually for a time period of 24 hours. Electrodes are placed on the patient's chest and are attached to a small, wearable, battery operated, recording monitor. Patients are required to keep a diary of their activities, which are later assessed by their therapists along with the recordings, by correlating any irregular heart activity with the patient's activity at the time. The next stage was to use wearables for real time applications, where physiological monitoring was supplemented with an alerting mechanism. Such an application is the sleep apnea monitor, which provides alerts when sleep patterns deviate from the expected breathing patterns beyond pre-set thresholds. More complex multi-signal monitoring and decision support devices were initially developed for high profile applications intended for astronauts and the military. NASA's LifeGuard system used multi-signal monitoring equipment for monitoring astronauts' vital signs and assessing their physiological responses in space. More demanding applications were pursued through the Land Warrior program of the US Army [1,2], seeking to develop wearable computers to assist soldiers with battlefield tasks. The primary medical task of these computers was to assess the health condition of the soldier on a continuous basis, to see if he is dead or alive, and if alive, to help the military commanders assess his ability to fight by using heart rate and breath rate as indicators of the soldiers general health, current level of fatigue, stress, anxiety, the severity of his wounds and the treatment requirements. To achieve the other military tasks of the system, the wearable prototypes integrated a range of functions and hardware, such as a video capture system for capturing still colour images, a helmet mounted display monitor with a speaker and a microphone, a navigation subsystem with GPS and a compass, soldier location and heading to a computer for map display, automatic position reporting and target location calculation, and wireless communications for communicating and exchanging digital information with his commanders.

This trend towards multifunctional devices could not escape the commercial health sector, as numerous wearable devices providing multi-signal monitoring, alerting mechanisms and telemetric functions have already reached the market, with many more promising and more complex ideas under research and development. Advancements in sensor technology and biosignal analysis allow not only the monitoring of vital signs such as heart response, respiration, skin temperature, pulse, blood pressure or blood oxygen saturation, but other important aspects of a person's condition such as body kinematics, sensorial, emotional and cognitive reactivity. Information technology is the key enabling factor, through the use of available miniaturized plug and play components, distributed computing, data security protocols, and communication standards. Other IT practices starting to find their way in wearable applications include the use of virtual reality, artificial intelligence techniques for automated diagnosis and decision support, and data fusion in multi-sensor systems. Data fusion is usually applied for control and assessment purposes in multi-sensor engineering systems with most applications being in robotics, military and transport [3-5]. However, it is starting to emerge in the medical field and is suitable for home-based and wearable multi-signal handling systems.

Wearable devices have the potential to become integral components of a modern healthcare system, as they can provide alternative options and solutions to numerous medical and social requirements. They do not only help to improve the provision of healthcare, the quality of life of the chronically ill and the disabled, but their use may also prove to be financially rewarding by saving the health service money through hospitalisation reductions, either through prevention or by helping provide the appropriate means for independent living. The financial considerations are considerable. In the United States alone, 90 million people suffer from chronic medical conditions like diabetes, asthma and heart disease, which account for approximately 75% of the total healthcare costs. However, up to now, a large proportion of commercial wearable medical products have been specifically developed for non-clinical applications such as for athletes, health aware individuals and as research tools for researchers seeking to increase the clinical understanding of certain health conditions. Those, along with the direct clinical applications have led to a dramatic increase in the market for medical devices in recent years but without a corresponding reduction in hospitalisations.

8.2 Wearable Technologies and Design

The ongoing development of wearable devices is closely linked with advances in a range of digital hardware technologies and is limited by certain ergonomic design restrictions and considerations. From the design point of view, their main distinguishing characteristic is that they are used in a very different manner than conventional medical equipment. The three main operational differences are: (a) they are usually worn by the patient, (b) they are usually operated by the patient, and (c) they normally function in an uncontrolled environment under various environmental conditions. This section provides a brief description of the key enabling technologies and the design requirements for wearable devices. This helps in clarifying the capabilities, limitations and the potential advancements of wearable medical products.

8.2.1 Wearable Hardware

The three main hardware components of a typical wearable medical device are: (a) the necessary physiological and peripheral sensors used to monitor a health condition and the surrounding environment, (b) the wearable computational hardware enabling the input, output and processing of information, and (c) the use of customised clothing acting as the supporting environment or even as a functional component of the device.

8.2.1.1 Sensors

Sensors are used to monitor the physical environment or an environmental process. Wearable devices make use of a wide range of sensors that can be broadly distinguished into medical and peripheral sensors. Medical sensors are those used for monitoring a clinical condition or a clinical process of an individual, and may involve the recording of physiological and kinesiological parameters. Peripheral sensors are those used to monitor the outer environment, enabling the provision of additional functional capabilities of a wearable system, or for enhancing the context awareness of the system assisting in the assessment of the measurements of the medical sensors.

For all kinds of sensors, wearability imposes a set of physical and functional restrictions affecting their selection, and thus limiting the range of available options. Apart from their physical attributes such as size and shape, wearable sensors should be non-invasive and easily attachable. Furthermore, they must have minimal power consumption and produce an electrical output so that measurements can be digitally processed. Operating conditions are also important, as the device must be durable and reliable in the intended conditions of use. For example, under certain conditions, the use of a piezoelectric sensor on a moving subject will produce overwhelming motion artefacts in the recorded signal, limiting the reliability of the measurements. In addition, physiological responses such as vibration and sweating may cause signal distortion or even sensor detachment with complete loss of the signal. The duration of use may also be important, as prolonged use may cause skin irritations or affect their reliability. For example, the contact resistance between the skin and an electrode may alter over time as gels in electrodes dry out.

Wearable devices can particularly benefit from the use of wireless sensors, which do not only minimise the hassle of setting up and using the device, but also help achieve freedom of movement and comfort during use. They are based on conventional sensing elements with an integrated wireless transmitter and an autonomous power supply. The use of wireless sensors removes the issue of cable management and facilitates the positioning of sensors on various anatomical locations and the development of more versatile system architectures. The increased electronic complexity of modern systems has also led to the development of intelligent sensors that perform functions beyond detecting a condition and that can provide a level of assessment. Such an application is the introduction of wireless intelligent sensors performing data acquisition and limited signal processing in personal and local area networks [6]. The use of intelligent sensors helps in reducing the processing workload of the wearable processor, and increases the speed of providing assessment. This processing assistance is particularly beneficial in real time applications, and in many cases eases the design processing requirements and specifications.

The medical sensors most commonly used for monitoring physiological responses in wearables include: skin surface electrodes for detecting surface potentials in bioelectric signal monitoring such as for electrocardiography (ECG), electromyography (EMG), electroencephalography (EEG), electrooculography (EOG); medical grade temperature thermistors for detecting skin surface temperature; galvanic skin response sensors for detecting skin conductance in relation to skin hydration; piezoelectric sensors used as pulse monitors for monitoring heart rate and in the form of belts placed in the chest an abdomen for monitoring respiratory effort; infrared emitter/receiver systems for photopletysmographic (PPG) measurements used for the detection of blood volume changes of a selected skin area providing indirect measures of blood pressure, and pulse oxymetry, which is a technique for detecting blood oxygen saturation and heart rate from a PPG signal. Some systems also incorporate kinesiological sensors for monitoring human motion and posture. For these applications the most commonly used sensors are: accelerometers for detecting motion; electrogoniometers for recording human joint angles in motion; proximity sensors for detecting distance from obstacles, and contact sensors. These sensors are based on a range of technologies such as electrical, mechanical, optical, ultrasonic, and piezoelectric. In medical wearables, they are usually used for monitoring human movement in relation to a clinical condition such as for gait abnormalities, tremor, Parkinson's disease, and for monitoring human movement with respect to the environment such as for obstacle detection for the visually impaired and for detecting physical contact.

Biosensors belong to another category of medical sensors used for monitoring biological properties and processes, but have found limited applications in wearable devices. Sensing strategies for biosensors include optical, mechanical, magnetic, calorimetric, and electrochemical detection methods. However, the requirements for small size and of providing an electrical output so that the measurements can be digitally processed mean that microelectronic biosensors are those with the greatest potential for use in wearables. Microelectronic biosensors are either calorimetric or electrochemical [7]. Calorimetric biosensors detect the heat of biological reactions with conventional thermistors or thermopile sensors in various arrangements. Electrochemical biosensors include potentiometric transducers such as the pH electrode and related ion-selective electrodes, and amperometric biosensors used for detecting and monitoring enzymes such as glucose, lactate and urea. There are ongoing research efforts aiming to produce multi-biosensor elements integrating amperometric and potentiometric sensors on one substrate forming an integrated lab on a chip.

Peripheral sensors are used for monitoring the physical environment, and in some cases for providing navigation assistance. Physical environment sensors monitor environmental conditions such as temperature, humidity, air quality, sound levels, and may also provide optical information. Therefore, environmental sensors can include thermometers and CO_2 monitors, microphones and even digital video cameras. Navigation aids make use of navigational sensors such as GPS and digital compasses for providing position and orientation. In a broader sense, any input mechanism providing information assisting in the assessment of the monitored conditions, medical or not, can be loosely described as a sensor. This may involve manual intervention by the user, such as the input of weight, height or other anthropometric measurements, or even the direct on-line accessibility of information from other devices such as electronic patient records, medical and other databases.

Apart from the above-mentioned sensors and technologies, there are emerging manufacturing and packaging approaches with the potential to be used either as components of or in conjunction with wearable devices. These include the use of micro electro-mechanical systems (MEMS), a very promising and rapidly expanding field with a wide range of applications, and Micro Total Analysis Systems (μTAS).

Devices based on micro electro-mechanical systems (MEMS) are manufactured with similar techniques to those used to create integrated circuits, and often have moving components that allow a physical or analytical function to be performed along with their electrical functions. Their distinguishing characteristic is that they have the capacity to transduce both physical and chemical stimuli to an electrical signal. MEMS have been used in the medical industry since 1980 for a variety of applications, and have the advantage of being small, reliable and inexpensive. The MEMS most commonly used in medical sensing applications are based on the Wheatstone bridge piezoresistive silicon pressure sensor that has been used in various forms to measure blood pressure, respiration and acceleration [8]. In addition, interest is growing for the use of MEMS in implantable devices. Implantable BioMEMS [9] combine sensing applications with their other capabilities of producing microreservoirs, micropumps, cantilevers, rotors, channels, valves and other structures. Current and emerging clinical applications based on BioMEMS include retinal implants to treat blindness, neural implants for stimulation, biosensors for the short term sensing of pH, analytes and pressure in blood, tissue and body fluids (but are not stable for long term implantation), and drug delivery with the use of a drug depot or supply within or on the device.

Another emerging research field deals with Micro Total Analysis systems (μTAS) [10], which are miniaturized systems for biochemical analysis operating completely automatic without the need of experienced operators. Such systems contain all the necessary components in one liquid handling board, like sample inlet facilities, micropumps, micromixers/reactors, sensors and the control electronics. They are used in clinical chemistry and although they are intended for bedside monitoring rather than for wearable applications, portable clinical analyzers can be used in conjunction or in association with wearable systems to provide continuous *in vivo* monitoring of many blood variables. These systems widen the scope of wearable monitoring devices.

8.2.1.2 Computing Hardware

The miniaturization of computational hardware has led to the development of processing and supporting accessories enabling wearability. Wearable computing is a broader field used in many applications such as manufacturing, medicine, the military, in maintenance, and entertainment. In these applications the user wears a computer and a visual display, and may be wirelessly connected to a broader network enabling exchange of information. A feature that is often found in these applications is the provision of augmented reality, where a user wears a see through display that allows graphics or text to be projected in the real world [11]. The adaptation of computing hardware for wearable computing as well as for other portable and mobile applications has made available a range of components that can be used in the design of medical devices. These include the necessary input and output mechanisms, the processing units, the data storage devices, power supply and the means for wireless telemetry. Furthermore, they are mostly plug and play components that are easy to use and facilitate the development of modular systems allowing usage flexibility. This is particularly important for medical wearables as they also make use of sensors as well as other hardware [12]

The main objective of wearable input/output devices is to facilitate human-computer interaction with minimal hindering of other activities. Data entry or text input devices have included body mounted keyboards, hand held keyboards, trackballs, data gloves and touch screens. For complete hands free operation, many applications have made use of speech recognition software, and even posture, EMG, and EEG based devices. Output devices have included small sized liquid crystal displays, head mounted displays such as clip-on monitors and monitors embedded in glass frames, and speakers. An emerging technology for enhancing the realism of wearable augmented and virtual reality environments for certain applications involves the use of haptic/tactile interfaces [13]. These devices allow the users to receive haptic feedback output from a variety of sources, allowing them to actually feel virtual objects and manipulate them by touch.

Processing units are identical or downgraded versions of current desktop and notebook personal computers placed on compact motherboards. Handheld computers and personal digital assistants (PDA's) are two well-known commercial examples having compact processing power. Many research prototypes have been based on the PC 104 motherboard, and user programmable integrated circuits such as field programmable gate arrays (FPGA's), electronically programmable logic devices (EPLD's) and complex programmable logic devices (CPLD's). The functions of these circuits are user programmable and not set by the manufacturer. Generally speaking, the integration of hardware with software components maximizes the overall processing speed of the system and minimizes the processing unit's requirements. Wearable medical devices particularly benefit from the use of digital signal processing microchips. Memory chips and more recently Compact Flash® memory cards are used for data storage. They are light and small and not vulnerable to failure with movement, making them ideal for use in mobile and wearable applications. In addition, the memory cards do not require a battery to retain data indefinitely. Power autonomy is achieved through the use of high capacity rechargeable batteries, in conjunction with an optimisation of the processing, storing and transmission requirements for lower power consumption, according to the intended capabilities and scope of the wearable. Effort has been made to investigate alternative means to supplement wearable's power supply. These include the use of solar cells woven on clothing, piezoelectric inserts in shoes, and alternative means for generating power by using body heat, breath or human motion [14].

Wireless communications are required to transfer data between sensors and the device, the device and the telemedicine server, and for providing internet access. Most wireless applications have been based on radio transmission and IrDA serial data links. The recent trend is to create wireless personal area networks (wPAN's) for communication between the device and sensors, or generally between the wearable components of a device, usually based on the Bluetooth™ protocol operating in the 2.4 GHz ISM band (incorporated in IEEE Std 802.15). Communication between the wearable device and the telemedicine server is achieved through a wireless local area network (wLAN) based on the IEEE 802.11 standard, also operating in the 2.4GHz ISM band. It is essentially a wireless extension of the Ethernet and is often referred to as wireless fidelity (Wi-Fi). Cellular mobile phone technologies such as GSM, GPRS, and the 3rd generation UMTS protocols provide the means for mobile communication and internet access, and are also described as wireless mobile area networks (wMAN).

8.2.1.3 Clothing

Clothing is the necessary supporting element for devices that are not directly attached to the human body. Custom designed clothing is used to minimize the hassle of wearing the device, make it more comfortable while in use, practical to use, and provides the necessary supporting mechanism for placing the hardware components and sensors. Clothing also provides a certain level of protection from environmental conditions such as temperature changes, humidity, rain, and direct sun exposure. It can also help moderate physiological responses through the use of sweat absorbent fabrics and act as a vibration damper during motion.

Nevertheless, clothing becomes more interesting when it is designed to form an integral part of the device and not just a means of fixation. The term computational clothing refers to pieces of clothing having the ability to process, store, send and retrieve information [15]. This can be achieved in two ways, either by attaching or embedding electronic systems into conventional clothing and clothing accessories, or by merging textile and electronic technologies during fabric production (e-broidery) to produce electronic textiles (e-textiles) [16].

Multi-sensor clothing has been used in applications of context awareness and medical monitoring, allowing for multiple sensor data fusion of distributed or centralized sensors [17]. Prototype applications include the development of internet connected shoes allowing one to run with a jogging partner located elsewhere, and the use of physiological sensors attached on a bathing suit for monitoring individuals during sleep, assessing their discomfort for adjusting room heating [18]. Computing hardware components and sensors have also been embedded and integrated into fashion accessories, such as jewellery, gloves, belts, eyeglasses and wristwatches in a number of applications. Eyeglass based head mounted displays and multimedia systems that include cameras, microphones and earphones are already commercially available.

One of the first prototype applications of e-broidery was the wearable motherboard [19], which was formed by a mesh of electronically and optically conductive fibres integrated into the normal structure of the fibres and yarns used to create the garment. The shirt consisted of sensing devices containing a processor and a transmitter. A strategic objective of the e-textile approach is to create fabrics that can be crushed, washed and retain their properties unaffected. This requires the use of textile materials with electric properties, such as piezoelectric materials, lycra textiles treated with polypyrrole and carbon filled rubber materials for creating strain sensing fabrics, and conductive fibres of metallic silk organza which is a finely woven silk fabric with a thin gold, silver or copper foil wrapped around each thread. E-textile applications have included the production of complete clothing accessories to detect motion and posture, and local embroidery on a normal garment to create keypads for performing a function such as for generating text or music.

8.2.2 Wearable Ergonomics

Wearable ergonomics deal with issues such as the physical shape of wearables, their active relationship with the human anatomy in motion, their acceptability as a function of comfort, fashion, and purpose, the relationship between the wearable device and the work environment, the physical factors affecting their use, and the human – device interaction [20]. A list of general guidelines for wearable product design is presented below [21]:

1. Placement: The selection of the location for placing the wearable on the body to be unobtrusive.
2. Form Language: The shape of the wearable must ensure a comfortable and stable fit, while protecting it from accidental bumps.
3. Human Movement: The wearable should allow for joint freedom of movement, shifting of flesh, flexion and extension of muscles.

4. Proxemics: It refers to the aura around the body that the brain perceives as part of the body (0-13cm, 0-5 inches off the body). The rule of thumb is to minimize the thickness as much as possible.
5. Sizing: The wearable must be designed to fit as many types of users as possible.
6. Attachment: Refers to the form of the wearable and the means for its attachment to the body.
7. Containment: The degree to which containment of the required components can be achieved often dictates the overall shape and nature of the device.
8. Weight: The total weight of the wearable should be kept to a minimum. Weight distribution is also important as heavier loads can be carried closer to the centre of gravity. Loads should also be balanced to avoid altering the body's natural movement and balance.
9. Accessibility: Refers to the location of the wearable on the body to make it usable. This depends on the need for visual, tactile, auditory or kinaesthetic access on the human body.
10. Sensory Interaction: The way the user interacts with the wearable, whether passively or actively, should be kept simple and intuitive.
11. Thermal Aspects: There are functional, biological and perceptual thermal aspects of designing objects for the body, as it needs to breathe and is very sensitive to products that create, focus or trap heat.
12. Aesthetics: The culture and context of use dictates the shapes, materials, textures and colours of the wearable.
13. Long-term effects: The long-term effects of using wearable devices on the human body are currently unknown, and if any, they depend on their nature and the use conditions.

Naturally, not all of the above guidelines can be met and the design will always involve tradeoffs between them depending on the nature and the prospective use of the wearable. For instance, physiological sensors can only be placed in specific anatomical locations of the human body, dictating to a great extent the containment of the wearable.

8.3 Information Handling

Digital information handling is the main function of a wearable computer and involves all aspects of information flow from the acquisition and storage of data, the processing of the data for the extraction of useful information, and the means for providing feedback. The main purpose of wearable devices in healthcare is to provide clinical feedback for monitoring purposes through visual representations, alerts and decision support, often in real time.

This section focuses on the handling of sensor-derived physiological information and introduces the processing techniques that provide an add-on value to wearable devices. Furthermore, it introduces the potential of virtual and augmented reality applications as information feedback methodologies for medical wearables.

8.3.1 Signal Acquisition and Processing

Biomedical signal processing is a vast research area of which most wearable medical devices deal only with one-dimensional signals. The collection of multiple biosignals will normally require the use of multi-channel input hardware, upon which they are rooted and connected. This is therefore a necessary add-on to the hardware requirements of a wearable. Once recording has started the signals are then processed to provide the required feedback. The main signal processing stages for monitoring and interpreting a biological process can be seen in Figure 1.

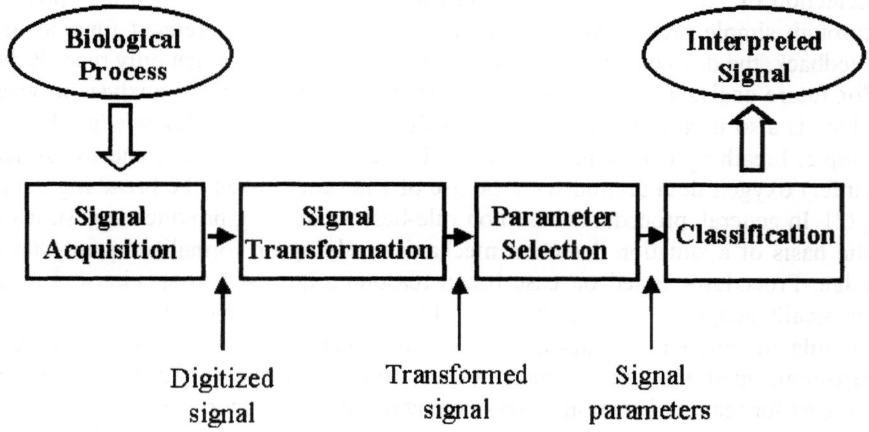

Figure 1. Signal processing stages

The first stage of signal processing involves the digitisation of the analogue signals. The Shannon-Nyquist theorem specifies that the sampling rate should be twice the maximum frequency of the signal. Furthermore, real time measurements require the use of time stamps and the synchronisation of the measurements, due to possible use of different sampling rates in the analogue/digital converter. The second stage is the signal transformation or pre-processing stage in which the signal is transformed to remove excess information, while keeping the useful information. It involves the application of algorithms for noise filtering and signal distortion correction. The third stage is the parameter selection or feature extraction stage, in which the signal characteristics that can provide discriminatory power to detect, predict or infer a medical state are evaluated. Feature extraction methodologies can range from being very simple, such as for the detection of a signal value or through the application of a pre-determined threshold, to being more complicated through the use of rule based, statistical, or machine learning techniques. Feature extraction may involve signal examination in both time and frequency domains, for providing a vital sign (e.g. heart rate, breath rate) or even for detecting a medical condition and for assessing its progress (e.g. arrhythmia, myopathy, gait abnormalities). The final stage is the classification stage, in which the derived signal parameters are used to assign the signal to a class (e.g. type of arrhythmia, myopathy, degree of rehabilitation). This is normally a component of more advanced decision support systems.

Wearable devices can potentially perform all the processing stages described above. However, the incorporation of complex processing algorithms is limited by memory availability, processing capabilities and power autonomy considerations that are all restricted in wearable systems. Even though advances are continuously made, wearables will always be less versatile in these terms than desktop computers. Therefore, most commercial devices tend to keep the processing requirements to a minimum, as the computational requirements particularly for real time processing and feedback can be very demanding. They limit their analysis to the detection of vital signs and only reach a classification stage when it is possible through simple processing applications. If there is no requirement for real time feedback, the device is then designed as a monitoring device that only records data for future analysis. Apart from estimating vital signs, biosignal analysis in wearables is also used to infer a clinical condition based on prior knowledge. For example, breathing curves have been used to estimate breath rate, and to estimate (infer) oxygen desaturation with the use of Cheyene-Stokes-like breathing curves [22]. In general, procedures based on rule-based reasoning provide suggestions on the basis of a situation detection mechanism relying on formalized prior knowledge. Procedures based on case based reasoning are used to specialise and dynamically adapt the rules on the basis of the patient's characteristics and of the accumulated experience. Multi modal reasoning methodologies use combinations of reasoning methodologies to reach a more reliable assessment [23]. The methodologies for feature detection, assessment and decision support can also involve the use of intelligent information processing, such as fuzzy logic, neural networks, and genetic algorithms (e.g. automated breath detection on long duration signals using feed forward back propagation artificial neural networks for monitoring sleep apnea [24]). The most demanding algorithms are those incorporating intelligent functions for real time multi-sensor assessments. These are prone to the *curse of dimensionality*, whereby increases in the number of sensors used will slow down the learning process exponentially [25]. Other characteristic signal processing issues in wearable systems include the presence of noise due to motion and body fat movements, possible power line interference from subcomponents of the device, and the uncontrolled conditions of the measuring environment [26].

A typical example of a complex multi-monitoring and assessment system is the MIThrill platform [27], which provides a modular framework for the real time understanding of wearable sensor data. The system makes use of pattern recognition techniques for modelling and interpreting the output of the sensors. The four modules involve: (a) Sensing: A digital sensing device measures something in the real world, resulting in a digital signal of sampled values. For example, a microphone sensor converts continuous fluctuations in air pressure (sound) into discrete sampled values with a specified resolution, encoding, and sampling rate. (b) Feature extraction: The raw sensor signal is transformed into a feature signal more suitable for a particular modelling task. For example, the feature extraction stage for a speaker-identification-classification task might involve converting a sound signal into a power-spectrum feature signal. (c) Modelling: A generative or discriminative statistical model such as a Gaussian mixture model, support vector machine hyperplane classifier, or hidden Markov model classifies a feature signal in real time. For example, a Gaussian mixture model could be used to classify accelerometer spectral features as walking, running, sitting, and so on. (c) Inference: The results of the modelling stage, possibly combined with other information, are fed into a Bayesian inference system for complex interpretation and decision-making.

8.3.2 Multi-Sensor Management and Information Fusion

Multi-sensor management [28] is a system or process that seeks to manage or coordinate the usage of a suite of sensors or measurement devices in a dynamic, uncertain environment, to improve the performance of data fusion and ultimately, that of perception [3]. The sensor manager can have a centralized, decentralized or hierarchical architecture and is responsible for answering questions like: which observation tasks are to be performed and what are their priorities; how many sensors are required to meet an information request; when are extra sensors to be deployed and in which locations; which sensor sets are to be applied to which tasks; what is the action or mode sequence for a particular sensor; what parameter values should be selected for the operation of sensors.

Information fusion is the broad term used to describe the integration of information from multiple sources. The process is often referred to as data fusion or sensor fusion, depending on the source of the data. It is essentially a method, or a range of methods for integrating signals from multiple sources, aiming to achieve improved accuracies and better inference about the environment than could be achieved by a single source alone [29]. The concept of sensor fusion has a direct biological analogy, in the same way as humans use all their senses to evaluate their surrounding environment. One of its main advantages is that it increases the robustness and reliability of a monitoring system. The use of sensor fusion algorithms is mostly found in target tracking, robotic and military applications, for providing guidance, navigation and control. Medical applications are emerging, but limited.

Multi sensor fusion for wearable medical applications implies the use of physiological and in some cases kinesiological and environmental sensors. Furthermore, input variables can also be extracted from databases such as electronic patient records, or other datasets. Sensor fusion algorithms can be classified into three different groups, as seen in Table 1 [4]:

Table 1. Sensor fusion algorithms

Probabilistic Models	Least-Square Techniques	Intelligent Fusion
Bayesian Reasoning	Kalman Filtering	Fuzzy Logic
Evidence Theory	Optimal Theory	Neural Networks
Robust Statistics	Regularization	Genetic Algorithms
Recursive Operators	Uncertainty Ellipsoids	

It is beyond the scope of this chapter to present the merits and limitations of each algorithm. Their selection depends on the problem in question and the approach the investigator is most comfortable with, as the same problem can often be handled by diverse approaches. For demonstration purposes the Kalman filter [30] is presented, which is the most commonly used method in engineering sensor fusion applications, and has been used with various adaptations depending on the nature of the problem in hand, such as the fuzzy Kalman filter [4] for non Gaussian noise and the extended Kalman Filter used to estimate system states that can only be observed indirectly or inaccurately by the system itself. The filter is often used to combine data from many sensors and produce the optimal estimate in a statistical sense. If a system can be described with a linear model and both the system error and the sensor error can be modelled as Gaussian noise, then the Kalman filter provides a unique statistically optimal estimate of the fused data. It is therefore able to find the best estimate based on the correctness of each individual measurement.

Consider a linear system described by the following two equations [31]:

State equation:

$$x_{k+1} = Ax_k + Bu_k + w_k$$

Output equation:

$$y_k = Cx_k + z_k,$$

where A, B and C are matrices, k the time index, x the state of the system, u a known input to the system, y the measured output, w the process noise and z the measurement noise. X cannot be measured directly, so we measure y, which is a function of x corrupted with noise z.

Two criteria are set. For the first criterion, we want the average value of the state estimate to be equal to the average value of the true state so that the expected value of the estimate should be equal to the expected value of the state. The second criterion is that we want a state estimate that varies from the true state as little as possible, so we want to find the estimator with the smallest possible error variance. The Kalman filter is the estimator satisfying the above criteria.

We further make the assumptions that the averages of w and z are zero, and that no correlation exists between w and z. The noise covariance matrices are then defined as:

Process noise covariance:

$$S_w = E\left(w_k w_k^T\right),$$

Measurement noise covariance:

$$S_z = E\left(z_k z_k^T\right).$$

The Kalman filter then consists of three equations, each involving matrix manipulation given below:

$$K_k = AP_k C^T \left(CP_k C^T + S_z\right)^{-1},$$

$$\hat{x}_{k+1} = \left(A\hat{x}_k + Bu_k\right) + K_k\left(y_{k+1} - C\hat{x}_k\right),$$

$$P_{k+1} = AP_k A^T + S_w - AP_k C^T S_z^{-1} CP_k A^T,$$

where K is the Kalman gain matrix, and P the estimation error covariance matrix. The first component of the state estimate equation ($\hat{x}$) derives the estimate as if we didn't have a measurement, while the second term called the correction term represents the amount by which to correct the propagated state estimate due to our measurement. By examining the first equation it can be seen that when the measurement noise is large, S_z is large and K will be small won't give much credibility to the measurement y when computing the next state estimate. Inversely, when the measurement noise is small, so will S_z, and K will be large giving a lot of credibility to the measurement when computing the next state estimate.

Sensor fusion applications in medicine involve two approaches. The first approach involves using redundant sensors to achieve more reliable results. The second approach is to fuse information from different sensors to obtain assessments that are not obtainable by any single sensor alone. In some medical applications, information fusion methodologies have been used to combine clinical images obtained from different diagnostic modalities on the same location to improve diagnostic efficiency. Nevertheless, image fusion is not relevant for wearable devices, which deal with one-dimensional signals.

A sensor fusion method for heart rate estimation was presented by Ebrahim et al [32] and evaluated by Feldman et al [33]. The sensors used were independent, in the sense that each signal origin and the causes for artefacts were different in each case. They used electrocardiography (ECG), pulse oxymetry (SpO_2) and an invasive arterial pressure (IAP) sensor to obtain heart rate information. Sensor fusion was based upon the consensus between sensors, consistency with past estimates and physiologic consistency. The fusion algorithm applied consisted of four steps, which can be seen in Figure 2.

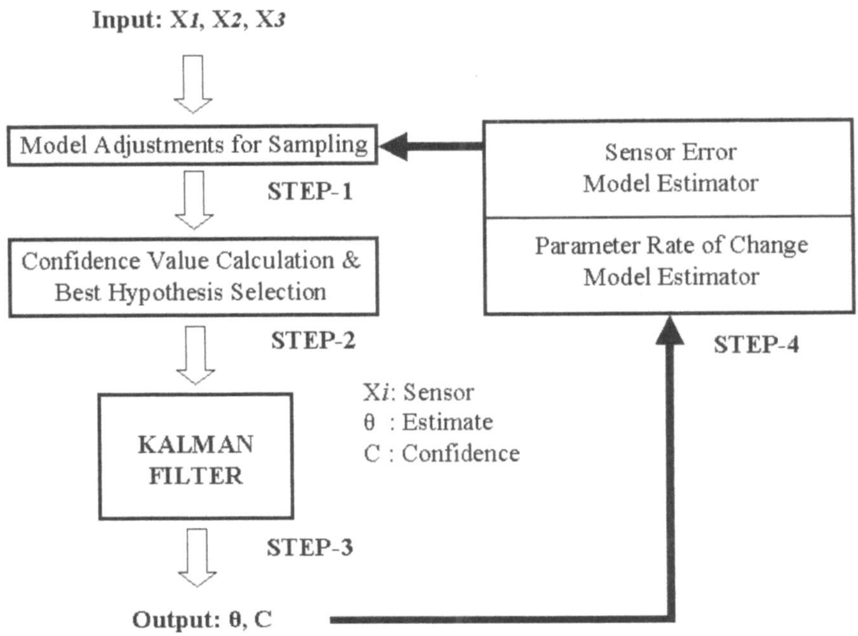

Figure 2. Sensor fusion flowchart for HR estimation [32]

In Step 1, adjustments are made to the models to account for differences in the time stamps of the most recent estimates. In Step 2 individual sensor measurements and the heart rate prediction are identified as good or bad, and the confidence value of the decision is computed. In Step 3, a Kalman filter derives the optimal fused estimate based on the good estimates identified in Step 2. Finally, in Step 4 the fused estimate is used to refine sensor error models and the prediction error model using assessed data. They found that the fused heart rate estimate was consistently either as good as or better than the estimate obtained by any individual sensor. It also reduced the incidence of false alarms without missing any true alarms.

8.3.3 Data Handling and Feedback Mechanisms

Apart from the processes of data acquisition and processing previously described, a wearable device has to store and transmit information while keeping in mind privacy and security issues, and provide the necessary feedback mechanisms for its users. Data handling deals with the means and decisions on the amount and nature of data to be retrieved, recorded, stored and transmitted, and depends on the clinical and functional requirements of the system. It may involve the use of data mining techniques, encryption and encoding for security and the protection of sensitive medical data, and compatibility and compliance issues with hospital medical informatics systems and medical databases such as electronic patient records (COAS, CIAS, HRAO, CDSA, HL7).

Feedback mechanisms are selected according to the nature of the device and their selection affects the nature, frequency and quality of the feedback provided to the users. Feedback can involve combinations of audio, visual, and tactile forms, which often need to be provided in real time in monitoring and other applications. User interface design is very important for the effectiveness, safety and proper use of the device, and must be provided in a way that is comprehensible, relevant and friendly to the person using it. Since most wearables are intended for use by the patients, an element of fashion and fun is also important. All wearable devices use conventional user-feedback mechanisms through monitors or speakers for visualising information and for providing warnings, which can even involve virtual and augmented reality environments and speech synthesis.

In virtual reality applications, the user wears a head mounted display to experience an immersive representation of a computer-generated simulation of a virtual world. With augmented reality, the display allows graphics or text to be projected in the real world [11]. Both approaches have very promising prospects in applications of medical wearables. Virtual reality systems have already been used for the user-friendly visualisation of monitoring activities and the stimulation of patients in rehabilitation programs. Rehabilitation applications aim to improve the patient's experience during physiotherapy, to assist and complement in the physiotherapy process, in the form of games and tasks, and have been used as components of greater telemonitoring and teletherapy systems. They have been used primarily for patients rehabilitating from traumatic injuries, pathological causes, strokes, and traumatic brain injuries. Although most of these are designed for home use, they often incorporate wearable components due to the size and transportation requirements. Virtual reality therapy (VRT) systems provide exposure therapy for the treatment of psychological conditions such as acrophobia [34] and fear of flying [35], and aim to provide the virtual environment simulating the real conditions that are to be treated.

A range of applications has also been designed for medical personnel in the forms of wearable training tools for doctors, for simulating a surgery, for surgery planning, and for providing augmented reality during surgery. In the case of augmented reality, the generated images are overlaid onto patient, which requires accurate registration of the computer-generated imagery with the patient's anatomy. The application of computational algorithms and virtual reality visualizations to diagnostic imaging, preoperative surgical planning, and intraoperative surgical navigation is referred to as computer-aided surgery (CAS). Applications include minimally invasive surgical procedures, neurosurgery, orthopaedic surgery, plastic surgery, and coronary artery bypass surgery [36].

8.4 Wearable Applications

Wearable devices can be broadly categorised according to their primary function into monitoring systems, rehabilitation assistance devices and long-term medical aids. The primary function of monitoring devices is to provide dedicated monitoring of specific medical conditions. Rehabilitation devices are those that can actively assist in the rehabilitation process while retaining a monitoring element. Long-term medical aids are the devices used to improve the user's quality of life, and have been described as assistive technology devices (ATD's). They allow their users to experience higher levels of independence and social and vocational participation.

Most commercial applications tend to focus around monitoring, and often have built in telemetry functions. Some are designed for use within the healthcare environment under medical supervision, others for occasional use at home by patients, and others for continuous use in all environments. Polysomnographs are typical examples of devices designed for use under supervision by researchers and medical personnel, within a medical laboratory or a healthcare unit. Polysomnographs are wearable, modular, multi-data recorders, measuring ECG, EMG, EOG, EEG, thoracic and abdominal effort, body position, and pulse oximetry, and provide real time monitoring with wireless telemetry. Numerous companies have developed wrist-wearable blood pressure monitoring devices, intended for the occasional and hassle free monitoring of blood pressure at home. The measurements are automatic at the push of a button, providing pulse and pressure readings that can also be stored for future reference. Continuous use devices include the sport wristwatch heart monitors aiming to help habitual and professional athletes in their training sessions. Many of these allow the setting of training limits within user-specified target zones, and provide audio and visual alarms when these limits are exceeded. Most versions of the sports monitors allow the storing of multiple readings and their subsequent uploading on a personal computer for comparison with previous training session profiles and with suggested training programs through the internet. Another example is the GlucoWatch® biographer, which is a wearable non-invasive glucose monitor for patients with diabetes [37]. The device extracts glucose through intact skin via reverse iontophoresis where it is detected by and amperometric biosensor, and can provide glucose readings every 20 min for 12 hours. It is a wrist-watch device with all the necessary functions to perform the iontophoresis and biosensor functions. It has a liquid-crystal display, PC communication capabilities, temperature and skin conductivity sensors to detect skin temperature fluctuations and perspiration, and a disposable component which comprises of the biosensor and iontophoresis electrodes and hydrogel disks.

Other devices provide both monitoring and alerting functions for the prevention of possible or even impending life threatening situations. Sleep apnea monitors are monitoring and warning devices used at home or hospital for patients in periods of high risk [38], such as infants susceptible to the sudden infant death syndrome (SIDS). The infant wears a respiratory effort belt while sleeping, and an alert is provided to the parents or doctors when the breathing patterns cause reasons for concern. Other systems designed specifically for prevention use continuous monitoring of vital signs and ECG for individuals with a known family history of heart disease, or for those recovering from a heart attack or heart surgery. Such systems would look for early signs of heart problems before the person becomes symptomatic [39].

The LifeVest™ wearable defibrillator (www.lifecor.com) is one of the few wearable commercial prototypes designed to perform a function beyond monitoring and alerting. It was designed as an intermediate-treatment option for people in high risk for sudden cardiac arrest, for patients that do not require to be hospitalised and do not necessarily have long-term risks where they are often candidates for an implantable cardioverter defibrillator. It continuously monitors the patient's heart with dry, non-adhesive sensing electrodes to detect life threatening abnormal heart rhythms, and provides prompt defibrillation when needed.

A number of emerging applications are aiming to integrate and take full advantage of wireless communication and GPS combinations. Medical Intelligence (www.medicalintelligence.ca) has developed a wireless wearable cardiac alert system linked to a GPS integrated in a mobile phone or a pocket PC. The Vital Positioning System™ consists of a belt incorporating ECG and heart activity sensors, GPS and Bluetooth, and alerts designated emergency services that a person is having a heart attack and provides positioning. It makes use of self-learning artificial intelligence to predict signs of an upcoming incident, calling for an ambulance before the condition develops, giving a bit more valuable time for the emergency services to react. It is also an autonomous monitoring system storing measurements for use by physicians. There have also been considerable efforts to develop GPS-based navigation and guidance aids for the visually impaired [40]. Prototype systems make use of a GPS receiver to position the patients within their surrounding environment and who are represented in a spatial database forming part of the geographic information system (GIS) within the computer. A compass is used to determine orientation and a mobile phone for communicating with a central server to retrieve information. A synthetic speech display provides information about locations of nearby streets, points of interest and instructions for travelling to desired destinations.

Future applications are likely to have increased complexity, through the merging of a wider range of technologies. As previously stated, augmented reality involves the use of a head mounted display used as a means for projecting computer derived information in the physical environment for augmenting real objects. Wearable medical applications of augmented reality include the use of virtual reality and feedback assistance to doctors during surgery and to function as memory aids for the elderly suffering from memory loss and Alzheimer's disease. Memory glasses function like a reliable human assistant, storing reminder requests and delivering them under appropriate circumstances. Such systems differ qualitatively from a passive reminder system such as a paper organizer, or a context-blind reminder system such as a modern PDA, which records and structures reminder requests but which cannot know the user's context [27]. In another research prototype using augmented reality functions, this time for patients with Parkinson's disease (www.parreha.com), the patients wear a head-mounted display on one eye superimposing computer generated geometric shapes, giving visual cues with sensory data to help navigation. It was found that the system greatly enhanced patient awareness, motor skills and coordination specifically related to walking.

The Dromeas system was designed to monitor athletes recovering from leg injuries and to assess their physical condition during rehabilitation [41]. It performs real time monitoring in normal training conditions at the early stages of rehabilitation. It combines both physiological and kinesiological sensors, such as ECG, a respiratory effort belt for monitoring breath rate, local skin temperature in the site of the injury and the equivalent position on the other leg, and a pain level button for the user supplied pain condition at the site of injury according to pre-defined levels. Leg motion is monitored with six electrogoniometers placed in each hip, knee and ankle. The recovering athlete has no control on the system, apart from the pain button. The signals are fed into a wearable computer producing alerts and visual feedback to the patient and at the same time are wirelessly transferred to a nearby computer where they are used to provide decision support on the condition of the injury and the overall physical condition of the athlete to the monitoring personnel. The monitoring interface (Figure 3) provides real time presentation of the recorded signals, the alerts and warnings of the device. A virtual reality module displays a virtual athlete whose movement is synchronized with the recordings taken by the goniometers [42]. This virtual reality representation is also used to provide feedback to the athlete through a clip-on monitor. The system keeps full backups of the monitoring sessions and stores them into an internet portal for access by researchers and health professionals.

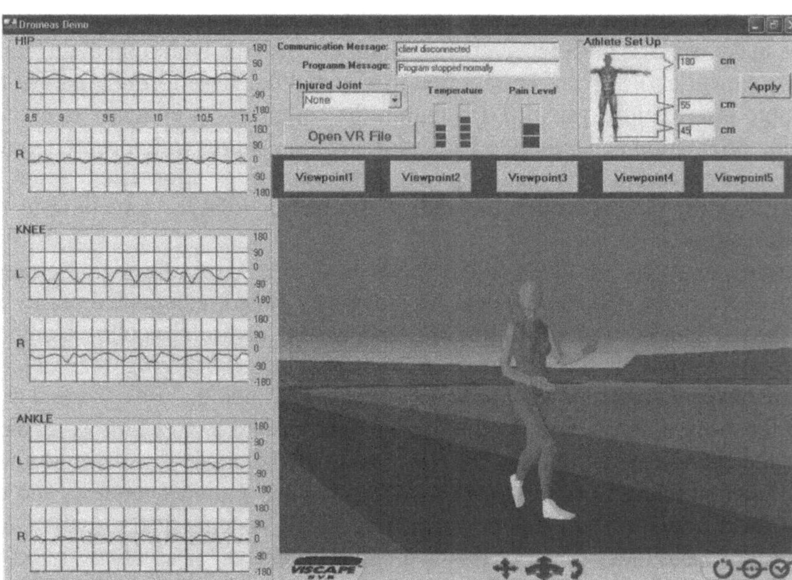

Figure 3. Monitoring interface with virtual reality module

There is also much interest in devices that actively assist in the rehabilitation process. A technology with great prospects involves the use of external electrical nerve stimulation. Small electrical impulses applied by transcutaneous electrical nerve stimulation and functional electrical stimulation (FES) motivates weak or paralysed muscles, assisting in the restoration of gait and movement in persons with paraplegia, celebral palsy, or when recovering from heart strokes. Devices based on the FES principle have been commercially available in wearable as sporting equipment for exercising several muscle groups. Another example is the wearable accelerometric motion analysis system (WAMAS) [43], which monitors people with balance disorders, acts as a diagnostic tool, a biofeedback device during therapy and a fall prevention aid for institutionalised and community living fall-prone elderly. It consists of two triaxial accelerometers attached of eyeglass frames for measuring head motion, and two more accelerometers attached on a belth at the waist. The system interacts wirelessly with the accelerometers and provides real-time visual, speech and/or non-verbal auditory feedback to the user, communicating the patient status to a remote clinician and recognizes if the system is unused or used incorrectly.

Prospective uses of wearables are even greater when combined with other systems to provide a different service, such as wearable/implantable systems or wearable/fixed systems. A glucose-monitoring device can be potentially used to control an implantable insulin infusion pump as part of the same system. USBONE is a prototype wearable ultrasound platform for the remote monitoring and acceleration of the healing process of long bones [44]. The system is designed for patients with open fractures treated with external fixation devices. It consists of pair of miniature ultrasound transducers implanted into the affected region in either side of the fracture, an ultrasound wearable device, and a centralised monitoring unit located in a clinical environment. The wearable device is mounted onto the frame of the external fixator and is responsible for the initiation of LiUS therapy session, for carrying out ultrasound measurements and for wirelessly communicating the data with the centralised unit.

Combined wearable and fixed component systems have been used to develop health-safe environments, such as for complete home monitoring platforms for the elderly, the critically ill and the disabled. Health smart homes may involve the use of a wearable medical monitoring device with a range of cameras positioned in all rooms, continuously monitoring the whereabouts and movement patterns of the subjects. They aim to provide medical security by detecting sudden abnormal events like a fall or a chronic pathologic activity, and raising the appropriate alarms [45]. Systems based on the same principles have also been used for research purposes, such as for recognising physiological patterns related to stress in various environments. One application has aimed to quantify driver stress [46], by examining driver behaviour features in conjunction with physiological information, video and other information about the driver's behaviour and context. The physiological recordings included an electrocardiogram, skin conductivity, respiration, blood volume pressure, and electromyogram signals.

8.5 Discussion

The use of wearable devices in healthcare is currently limited, but the increasing interest has been greatly assisted by the general trend to move into a more preventative healthcare model, in which the public plays a more energetic role in personal health management. The development of novel portable and wearable devices both follows and assists this trend, and provides the means for shifting healthcare from the hospital at home, and subsequently to personal care. The extent to which this transition will eventually take place is currently unknown, and certainly has its limits. It will depend on their acceptance by all the prospective users, such as patients, medical personnel, researchers, and the general public, and their ability to provide the safe and reliable means for a more effective and versatile health service, for the better quality of living for the chronically ill and the disabled, and their usefulness as research tools. Equally important are the financial considerations that often dictate the means and procedures for healthcare provision, the continuous optimisation of the related costs and benefits, along with the assessment of their impact on the quality of service provided.

The increasing interest in wearable devices has gone hand in hand with continuing technological achievements in the fields of sensor development, wearable computing and information technology, broadening their scope and capabilities. Sensors and sensor systems are becoming cheaper, smaller, more reliable and more versatile in use than ever before. The miniaturization of computing hardware and its adaptation to wearable applications, along with advancements in a range of information technology practices, has reached a level where wearable products can now provide powerful and effective tools to their users. These IT advancements encompass the ongoing research efforts in scientific fields like biomedical signal processing, artificial intelligence in medicine for pattern recognition and for medical decision support, and novel human-computer interaction technologies such as speech recognition and virtual reality. Continuing progress on all of these aspects along with the use of wireless telemetry and the ability to provide telemedicine functions can only help in their further establishment in daily healthcare practices. Their use is also in line with the emerging concept of ambient intelligence.

Ambient intelligence describes a potential future in which we will be surrounded by intelligent objects and in which the environment will recognize the presence of persons and will respond to it in an undetectable manner [47]. Ambient intelligence is based on three key technologies [48]:

- Ubiquitous Computing, describing the fact that microprocessors are embedded into everyday objects and are therefore available throughout the physical environment while being invisible to the user.
- Ubiquitous Communication, enabling these objects to communicate by means of wireless technologies with other devices, hosts and users.
- Intelligent User Interfaces, enabling citizens to interact with such an intelligent environment in a natural and personalised way.

Modern mobile phones are good examples of devices that combine all three of the ambient intelligence key technologies. A number of wearable healthcare device prototypes also have the same potential. Nevertheless, it is almost certain that a range of wearable medical devices will be integrated with or will be supplied as add-ons of mobile phones, making use of their capabilities and their communication networks. This has the added advantage of easier user acceptance, as mobile phones are already part of daily life, while simplifying the medical wearables' design and reducing its production costs. To an extent, this is already starting to materialize, as some mobile phone manufacturers have already tapped into the fitness market by incorporating fitness monitors in selected products, along with other potentially exploitable functions for medical devices such as GPS, GIS, digital compasses, environmental sensors etc.

Most commercial products currently evolve around personal health monitoring either within or out of the immediate health service environment, or as fitness assistants for health aware individuals. Wearable devices in healthcare provide remote monitoring of vital signs for patients in periods of need or of high risk, such as during rehabilitation after surgery, or a heart attack. Some applications further provide the means for pervasive healthcare and telemedicine functions. They are also useful tools for the management of chronic diseases such as asthma, diabetes and heart conditions. Other applications aim to provide effective supporting devices for patients with permanent or temporary disabilities, such as memory deficiency, the deaf, the visually impaired, and the paraplegic. Furthermore, they are extensively used as research tools for understanding the physiological responses of a range of clinical conditions in a laboratory, clinical or natural environment. Some applications are also intended for use by health professionals, providing clinical and management assistance tools for facilitating and assisting their daily clinical practices. Nevertheless, most commercial devices primarily involve the monitoring of vital signs for various purposes, usually in real time, and often provide a degree of telemedicine capabilities. Even though these are important services, the challenge for further applications lies in the potential ability of wearable devices to provide an add on value such as decision support and even functional assistance, either as stand alone devices or in conjunction with other devices within the immediate health service, at home, or during normal daily activities.

One of the emerging trends is therefore to include the element of medical decision support to provide immediate assessment of the progress of the monitored clinical condition for the benefit of both the doctors and patients. This assessment would be even more significant if it could be used to control the patient's treatment. The possibility of using wearable devices not just for assessment and prevention but also as integral components of a treatment system is of great interest. This could entail the use of a combination of wearable and implantable technologies for dealing with chronic conditions such as diabetes and paralysis. It can involve the use of implantable infusion pumps or BioMEMS for drug delivery of insulin or antibiotics, the management of a heart condition in conjunction with pacemakers, or even a wearable computer-controlled functional electrical stimulation system with real time motion feedback for controlling paralysed muscles. Wearable devices may also be used as integral components of larger medical systems such as for home monitoring systems for the elderly and the disabled [45], in which the medical systems will exhibit collective intelligence built upon the intelligence of their individual components.

Progress depends also on the handling of more basic issues such as user acceptability, safety, reliability, compatibility, security, and even clinical knowledge. Any wearable device aiming to be acceptable must necessarily provide a distinct sense of purpose that is evident to the user, must be comfortable to wear and easy to use without overwhelming and confusing features. In some cases fashion will also dictate the acceptance of such devices, particularly those intended for the general public for non-critical medical situations. This has been achieved in fitness applications where hi-tech health gadgets are seen to be trendy. Nevertheless, a device provided through the healthcare system will be used regardless of its fashion characteristics as long as it serves its medical purpose. Ease of use is also an important safety aspect as possible misuse may at best make it ineffective or even give rise to use-related hazards. Prompted by the increase in home-based and wearable medical devices, the US Food and Drug Administration's centre for devices and radiological health has issued industrial guidelines for the use-safety of medical devices, incorporating human factor engineering into risk management [49]. In addition, as any medical device, a wearable device must comply with the relevant standards, codes and regulations minimising the device failure hazards and receive regulatory approval by the appropriate legal body. Reliability concerns may involve a number of issues not unique to wearables, such as power autonomy and wireless data transfer. A particular problem in wearables is the handling of noise from biometric signals, particularly in uncontrolled environments, as well as possible sensor detachment or failure. In both respects, the use of sensor fusion techniques can improve the reliability and robustness of systems, as well as to provide the means for clinical assessment. Compatibility with conventional medical devices is also an important issue, both in terms of software (e.g. for access and exchange of information with hospital EPR's) and hardware, such as the standardization of wireless transmission protocols for the interoperability of devices, and their communication with existing hospital information systems. In doing this, issues of data transfer security for ensuring patient confidentiality and protection of personal medical data, must also be addressed.

Continuing research in all of the related technological and medical fields can only help in the advancement and broadening of the use of wearables. One of the arising issues is to make appropriate medical assessments with available sensors, taking into account the sensor design limitations placed on wearables. In a sense, this is an inverse way of thinking, as a doctor handling a clinical problem would try and use all the appropriate monitoring facilities, whereas in a wearable the monitoring facilities are limited and we want to examine what clinical conditions can be assessed with the available sensors. Further research is therefore required on the use of available sensor combinations for assessing specific medical conditions as well as for the use of information fusion and other techniques for providing decision support. Naturally, in many cases information that cannot be obtained through a wearable would be required to reach a reliable assessment of the patient's condition. For some situations, a possible solution would be to examine the possibility of inferring one medical condition by examining another, along with the reliability of doing this for the particular monitoring conditions. For example, this could involve the examination of the coupling patterns between different signals in various conditions such as heart rate variability, blood pressure variability and respiration [50]. This is not a simple task, and can only serve as a useful indicator and not as an accurate and conclusive assessment. However, it can improve the decision support characteristics of the wearable prior to proper examination.

Finally, any healthcare system will need to take into account the financial and logistical issues that arise through the use of wearable devices. These do not only deal with the cost of purchasing, supplying and maintaining the devices but may involve other management and financial issues. For some wearable applications, such as the use of polysomnographs within the hospital environment, the associated costs and benefits can be more easily evaluated with the main parameters being the cost of purchasing and maintaining the devices, the degree to which they can free up more expensive monitoring equipment or intensive care units, and the degree to which they help provide a better quality of care to the patients. However, this becomes much more complicated once the patient leaves the hospital, particularly as the degree of possible hospitalisation reductions associated with the increasing use of wearables is yet unknown. Furthermore, other associated costs may become significant, such as the cost of maintaining a telemedicine service targeted for a much wider and ever growing audience, requiring the availability of further dedicated personnel and hardware within the health service. Systems targeted for use by healthy individuals, medical professionals and those aiming to improve the quality of life of the chronically ill and the disabled are mostly financed by their prospective users. Other logistical issues that need to be resolved involve when, by what means and how often a communication is performed between the wearable/user and the health service, in what circumstances this should be in real time, what kind of response is required by the health service in emergency and non-critical situations, what is the cost/benefit of each approach, and so on.

References

1. Zieniewicz, M.J., Johnson, D.C., Wong, D.C., and Flatt, J.D.: The evolution of army wearable computers. Pervasive Computing (2002) 30-40.
2. Tappert, C.C., Ruocco, A.S., Langdorf, K.A., Mabry, D.M., Heineman, K.J., Brick, T.A., Cross, D.M., and Pellissier, S.V.: Military applications of wearable computers and augmented reality. In Fundamentals of Wearable Computers and Augmented Reality, Barfield, W., and Caudell, T. (eds) Laurence Erlbaum Associates (2001) 625-647.
3. Xiong, N., and Svensson, P.: Multi-sensor management for information fusion: issues and approaches. Information fusion 3 (2002) 163-186.
4. Sasiadek, J.Z.: Sensor fusion. Annual Reviews in Control 26 (2002) 203-228.

5. Dailey, D.J., Harn, P., and Lin, P.: ITS Data Fusion. Final research report - Research project T9903, Washington State Transportation Commission and US Department of Transportation (1996).
6. Jovanov, E., Raskovic, D., Price, J., Chapman, J., Moore, A., and Krishnamurthy, A.: Patient monitoring using personal area networks of wireless intelligent sensors. Biomed Sci Instrum 37 (2001) 373-378.
7. Urban, G.: Microelectronic biosensors for clinical applications. Handbook of biosensors and electronic noses: medicine, food and the environment, Kress-Rogers, E. (ed), CRC Press (1997).
8. Joseph, H., Swafford, B., and Terry, S.: MEMS in the medical world. Sensors online (www.sensorsmag.com) Apr. (2003).
9. Richards Grayson, A.C., Shawgo, R.S., Johnson, A.M., Flynn, N.T., Li, Y., Cima, M.J., and Langer, R.: A BioMEMS review: MEMS technology for physiologically integrated devices. Proc. IEEE 92:1 (2004) 6-21.
10. Bergveld, P.: Bedside clinical chemistry: From catheter tip sensor chips towards micro total analysis systems. Biomedical Microdevices 2:3 (2000) 185-195.
11. Barfield, W., and Caudell, T.: Basic concepts in wearable computers and augmented reality. In Fundamentals of wearable computers and augmented reality, Barfield, W. and Caudell, T. (eds) Laurence Erlbaum Associates (2001) 3-26.
12. Crowe, J., Hayes-Gill, B., Sumner, M., Barratt, C., Palethorpe, B., Greenhalgh, C., Storz, O., Friday, A., Humble, J., Setchell, C., Randell, C., and Muller, H.L.: Modular sensor architecture for unobtrusive routine clinical diagnosis. In Proc. Int. Workshop on Smart Appliances and Wearable Computing (2004).
13. Tan, H.J, and Pentland, S.: Tactual displays for wearable computing. In. Proc 1st Int. Symp. Wear. Comp. IEEE Comp. Soc. Press (1997) 84-89.
14. Starner, T.: Human-powered wearable computing. IBM Systems Journal 35:3&4 (1996) 618-629.
15. Barfield, W., Mann, S., Baird, K., Gemperle, F., Kasabach, C., Stirovic, J., Bauer, M., Martin, R., and Cho, G.: Computational Clothing and Accessories. In Fundamentals of wearable computers and augmented reality, Barfield, W. and Caudell, T. (eds) Laurence Erlbaum Associates (2001) 471-509.
16. Post, E.R., Orth, M., Russo, P.R., and Gershenfeld, N.: E-broidery: Design and fabrication of textile-based computing. IBM Systems Journal 39:3-4 (2000) 840-860.
17. Van Laerhoven, K., Schmidt, A., and Gellersen, H.W.: Multi-sensor context aware clothing. In. Proc 6th Int. Symp. Wear. Comp. IEEE Comp. Soc. Press (2002) 49-56.
18. Mann, S.: Smart clothing: The "wearable computer" and WearCam. Personal Technologies 1:1 (1997).
19. Park, S., and Jayaraman, S.: Enhancing the quality of life through wearable technology. IEEE Eng. Med. Biol. 22:3 (2003) 41-48.
20. Baber, C., Knight, J., Haniff D., and Cooper, L.: Ergonomics of wearable computers. Mobile Networks and Applications 4 (1999) 15-21.
21. Gemperle, F., Kasabach, C., Stivoric, J., Bauer, M., and Martin, R.: Design for wearability. Proc. 2nd Int. Symp. Wear. Comp., IEEE Comp. Soc. Press (1998) 116-122.
22. Nishida, Y. Suehiro, T., and Hirai, S.: Estimation of oxygen desaturation by analysing breath curve. J. Robotics and Mechatronics 11:6 (1999) 483-489.
23. Montani, S., Bellazzi, R., Portinale, L., and Stefanelli, M.: A multi-modal reasoning methodology for managing IDDM patients. Int. J. Medical Informatics 58-59 (2000) 243-256.

24. Sá, C.R., and Verbandt, Y.: Automated breath detection on long-duration signals using feedforward backpropagation artificial neural networks. IEEE Trans. Biomed. Eng. 49:10 (2002) 1130-1141.
25. Van Laerhoven, K., Aidoo, K.A., and Lowette, S.: Real-time analysis of data from many sensors with neural networks, In. Proc 5th Int. Symp. Wear. Comp. IEEE Comp. Soc. Press (2001).
26. Martin, T., Jovanov, E., and Raskovic, D.: Issues in wearable computing for medical monitoring applications: A case study of a wearable ECG monitoring device. In. Proc 4th Int. Symp. Wear. Comp. IEEE Comp. Soc. Press (2000) 43-49.
27. Pentland A.: Healthwear – Medical technology becomes wearable. IEEE Computer May (2004) 34-41.
28. Ng, G.W., and Ng, K.H.: Sensor management – what, why and how. Information Fusion 1 (2000) 67-75.
29. Boss, T., Diekmann, V., Jürgens, R., and Becker, W.: Sensor fusion by neural networks using spatially represented information. Biological Cybernetics 85 (2001) 371-385.
30. Kalman, R.E.: A new approach to linear filtering and prediction problems. Trans. ASME – Journal of Basic Engineering 82:D (1960) 35-45.
31. Simon, D.: Kalman filtering. Embedded Systems Programming (2001) 72-79.
32. Ebrahim, M.H., Feldman, J.M., and Bar-Kana, I.: A robust sensor fusion method for heart rate estimation. J. Clinical Monitoring 13 (1997) 385-393.
33. Feldman, J.M., Ebrahim, M.H., and Bar-Kana, I.: Robust sensor fusion improves heart rate estimation: clinical evaluation. J. Clinical Monitoring 13 (1997) 379-384.
34. Jang, D.P., Ku, J.H., Choi, Y.H., Wiederhold, B.K., Nam, S.W., Kim, I.Y., and Kim, S.I.: The development of virtual reality therapy (VRT) system for the treatment of acrophobia and therapeutic case. IEEE Trans. Inf. Tech. Appl. in Biomedicine 6:3 (2002) 213-217.
35. Banos, R.M., Botella, C., Perpina, C., Alcaniz, M., Lozano, J.A., Osma, J., and Gallardo, M.: Virtual reality treatment of flying phobia. IEEE Trans. Inf. Tech. Appl. in Biomedicine 6:3 (2002) 206-212.
36. Kania, K.: Virtual reality moves into the medical mainstream. MDDI Magazine (2000).
37. Tierney, M.J., Tamada, J.A., Potts, R.O., Jovanovic, L., and Garg, S.: Clinical evaluation of the GlucoWatch biographer: a continual, non-invasive glucose monitor for patients with diabetes. Biosensors & Bioelectronics 16 (2001) 621-629.
38. Bowman, B.R., and Schuck, E.: Medical instruments and devices used in the home. The Biomedical Engineering Handbook, Bronzino, J.D. (ed), CRD&IEEE Press (1995).
39. Satava, R.M., and Jones, S.B.: Medical applications for wearable computing. In Fundamentals of wearable computers and augmented reality, Barfield, W. and Caudell, T. (eds) Laurence Erlbaum Associates (2001) 649-662.
40. Loomis, J.M., Golledge, R.G., and Klatzky, R.L.: GPS-based navigation systems for the visually impaired. In Fundamentals of wearable computers and augmented reality, Barfield, W. and Caudell, T. (eds) Laurence Erlbaum Associates (2001) 429-446.
41. Glaros, C., Fotiadis, D.I., Likas, A., and Stafylopatis, A.: A wearable intelligent system for monitoring health condition and rehabilitation of running athletes. Proc 4th IEEE Conf. on Information Technology Applications in Biomedicine (2003) 276-279.

42. Trastogiannos, C., Glaros, C., Fotiadis, D.I., Likas, A., and Stafylopatis, A.: Wearable virtual reality feedback for the real time health monitoring of running athletes. Proc. VIIth IOC Olympic World Congress on Sport Sciences, Athens, Greece 7-11 Oct. (2003) 26C.
43. Sabelman, E.E., Schwandt, D.F., and Jaffe, D.L.: The wearable accelerometric motion analysis system (WAMAS): combining technology development and research in human mobility. Proc. Conf. Intellectual Property in the VA – Changes, Challenges and Collaborations (2001).
44. Protopappas, V., Baga, D., Fotiadis, D.I., Likas, A., Papachristos, A., and Malizos, K.N.: An intelligent wearable system for the monitoring of fracture healing of long bones. Proc. IFMBE (EMBEC'02) (2002) 978-979.
45. Demongeot, J., Virone, G., Duchene, F., Benchetrin, G., Herve, T., Noury, N., and Rialle, V.: Multi-sensors acquisition, data fusion, knowledge mining and alarm triggering in health smart homes for elderly people. C R Biol. 325:6 (2002) 673-682.
46. Healey, J., Seger, J., and Picard, R.: Quantifying driver stress: developing a system for collecting and processing biometric signals in natural situations. Biomed. Sci. Instrum. 35 (2001) 193-198.
47. European Community Information Society Technologies Advisory Group: Scenarios for ambient intelligence in 2010, Final Report. European Community (2001).
48. Gouaux, F., Simon-Chautemps, L., Adami, S., Arzi, M., Assanelli, D., Fayn, J., Forlini, M.C., Malossi, C., Martinez, A., Placide, J., Ziliani, G.L., and Rubel, P.: Smart devices for the early detection and interpretation of cardiological syndromes. Proc. 4th IEEE Conf on Information Technology Applications in Biomedicine (2003) 291-294.
49. Kaye, R., and Crowley, J.: Medical device use-safety: Incorporating human factors engineering into risk management – Identifying, understanding and addressing use-related hazards. Guidance for industry and FDA premarket and design control reviewers. U.S. Food and Drug Administration – Center for Devices and Radiological Health (2000) www.fda.gov/cdrh/HumanFactors.html.
50. Censi, F., Calcagnini, G., and Cerutti, S.: Coupling patterns between spontaneous rhythms and respiration in cardiovascular variability signals. Computer Methods and Programs in Biomedicine 68 (2002) 37-47.

Index

MIX
Papier aus verantwortungsvollen Quellen
Paper from responsible sources
FSC® C105338

If you have any concerns about our products,
you can contact us on
ProductSafety@springernature.com

In case Publisher is established outside the EU,
the EU authorized representative is:
Springer Nature Customer Service Center GmbH
Europaplatz 3, 69115 Heidelberg, Germany

Printed by Libri Plureos GmbH
in Hamburg, Germany